T0259605

Advances in Colorectal Neoplasia

Editor

SEAN J. LANGENFELD

SURGICAL CLINICS
OF NORTH AMERICA

www.surgical.theclinics.com

Consulting Editor
RONALD F. MARTIN

June 2017 • Volume 97 • Number 3

ELSEVIER

1600 John F. Kennedy Boulevard • Suite 1800 • Philadelphia, Pennsylvania, 19103-2899

http://www.surgical.theclinics.com

SURGICAL CLINICS OF NORTH AMERICA Volume 97, Number 3
June 2017 ISSN 0039–6109, ISBN-13: 978-0-323-53033-0

Editor: John Vassallo, j.vassallo@elsevier.com
Developmental Editor: Colleen Dietzler

Surgical Clinics of North America (ISSN 0039–6109) is published bimonthly by Elsevier Inc., 360 Park Avenue South, New York, NY 10010-1710. Months of publication are February, April, June, August, October, and December. Business and Editorial Offices: 1600 John F. Kennedy Blvd., Suite 1800, Philadelphia, PA 19103-2899. Periodicals postage paid at New York, NY and additional mailing offices. Subscription prices are $386.00 per year for US individuals, $756.00 per year for US institutions, $100.00 per year for US students and residents, $469.00 per year for Canadian individuals, $958.00 per year for Canadian institutions, $525.00 for international individuals, $958.00 per year for international institutions and $250.00 per year for Canadian and foreign students/residents. To receive student/resident rate, orders must be accompanied by name of affiliated institution, date of term, and the *signature* of program/residency coordinator on institution letterhead. Orders will be billed at individual rate until proof of status is received. Foreign air speed delivery is included in all *Clinics* subscription prices. All prices are subject to change without notice. POSTMASTER: Send address changes to *Surgical Clinics*, Elsevier Health Sciences Division, Subscription Customer Service, 3251 Riverport Lane, Maryland Heights, MO 63043. **Customer Service (orders, claims, online, change of address): Telephone: 1-800-654-2452 (U.S. and Canada); 314-447-8871 (outside U.S. and Canada). Fax: 314-447-8029. E-mail: journalscustomerservice-usa@elsevier.com (for print support); journalsonline support-usa@elsevier.com (for online support).**

Reprints. For copies of 100 or more, of articles in this publication, please contact the Commercial Reprints Department, Elsevier Inc., 360 Park Avenue South, New York, New York 10010-1710. Tel. 212-633-3874, Fax: 212-633-3820, E-mail: reprints@elsevier.com.

The Surgical Clinics of North America is also published in Spanish by McGraw-Hill Interamericana Editores S.A., P.O. Box 5-237 06500 Mexico D.F. Mexico; and in Portuguese by Interlivros Edicoes Ltda., Rua Comandante Coelho 1085, CEP 21250, Rio de Janeiro, Brazil; and in Greek by Paschalidis Medical Publications, Athens Greece.

The Surgical Clinics of North America is covered in *MEDLINE/PubMed (Index Medicus), EMBASE/Excerpta Medica, Current Contents/Clinical Medicine, Current Contents/Life Sciences, Science Citation Index,* and *ISI/BIOMED.*

Contributors

CONSULTING EDITOR

RONALD F. MARTIN, MD, FACS
Colonel (ret.), United States Army Reserve, York Hospital, York, Maine

EDITOR

SEAN J. LANGENFELD, MD, FACS, FASCRS
Assistant Professor of Surgery, Associate Program Director, General Surgery Residency, Department of Surgery, University of Nebraska Medical Center, Omaha, Nebraska

AUTHORS

SERGIO EDUARDO ALONSO ARAUJO, MD, PhD
Assistant Professor of Surgery, Hospital Israelita Albert Einstein, São Paulo, Brazil

TESS HANNAH AULET, MD
General Surgery Resident, Department of Surgery, University of Vermont Medical Center, Burlington, Vermont

CANAAN BAER, MD
Colon and Rectal Clinic, Swedish Medical Center, Seattle, Washington

AMIR BASTAWROUS, MD, MBA
Colon and Rectal Clinic, Swedish Medical Center, Seattle, Washington

SARAH BASTAWROUS, DO
Department of Radiology, Puget Sound Veteran's Affairs Administration Hospital, University of Washington, Seattle, Washington

JENIFER S. BEATY, MD, FACS, FASCRS
Assistant Clinical Professor of Surgery, Creighton University Medical Center, Associate Clinical Professor of Surgery, University of Nebraska College of Medicine, Omaha, Nebraska

KYLE G. COLOGNE, MD
Assistant Professor of Clinical Surgery, Division of Colorectal Surgery, University of Southern California Keck School of Medicine, Los Angeles, California

MARIANNE V. CUSICK, MD
Assistant Professor of Surgery, Colon & Rectal Surgery, University of Texas/McGovern Medical School, Houston, Texas

TIMOTHY F. FELDMANN, MD
Department of Surgery, Capital Medical Center, Olympia, Washington

LEANDRO FEO, MD, FACS, FASCRS
Colorectal Service, Department of Surgery, Catholic Medical Center, Manchester, New Hampshire

LAURA MELINA FERNANDEZ, MD
Angelita & Joaquim Gama Institute, São Paulo, Brazil

JASON M. FOSTER, MD, FACS
Associate Professor of Surgery, Division of Surgical Oncology, University of Nebraska Medical Center, Omaha, Nebraska

ANGELITA HABR-GAMA, MD, PhD
Professor of Surgery, Angelita & Joaquim Gama Institute, São Paulo, Brazil

BRADLEY HALL, MD
Department of General Surgery, University of Nebraska Medical Center, Omaha, Nebraska

LYEN C. HUANG, MD
Fellow, Division of Colon & Rectal Surgery, Mayo Clinic, Rochester, Minnesota

ANJALI S. KUMAR, MD, MPH, FACS, FASCRS
Director, Colorectal Surgery Program, Section of General, Thoracic, and Vascular Surgery, Virginia Mason Medical Center, Seattle, Washington

SEAN J. LANGENFELD, MD, FACS, FASCRS
Assistant Professor of Surgery, Associate Program Director, General Surgery Residency, Department of Surgery, University of Nebraska Medical Center, Omaha, Nebraska

SLAWOMIR MARECIK, MD
Advocate Lutheran General Hospital, Associate Professor of Clinical Surgery, University of Illinois at Chicago College of Medicine, Park Ridge, Illinois

RAMAN MENON, MD
Colon and Rectal Clinic, Swedish Medical Center, Seattle, Washington

AMIT MERCHEA, MD, FACS, FASCRS
Consultant, Division of Colon & Rectal Surgery, Assistant Professor of Surgery, Mayo Clinic, Jacksonville, Florida

JESSE SAMUEL MOORE, MD, FACS, FASCRS
Assistant Professor, Department of Surgery, University of Vermont Medical Center, Burlington, Vermont

GARRETT M. NASH, MD, MPH, FACS, FASCRS
Colorectal Service, Department of Surgery, Memorial Sloan Kettering Cancer Center, New York, New York

YOSEF NASSERI, MD, FACS, FASCRS
Surgery Group of Los Angeles, Los Angeles, California

JAMES PADUSSIS, MD
Assistant Professor of Surgery, Division of Surgical Oncology, University of Nebraska Medical Center, Omaha, Nebraska

AJIT PAI, MD
Consultant Surgical Oncologist, Apollo Hospitals, Apollo Cancer Institute, Chennai, India

JOHN PARK, MD
Advocate Lutheran General Hospital, Associate Professor of Surgery, Chicago Medical School, Park Ridge, Illinois

JAMES MICHAEL PARKER, MD
Department of Surgery, Middlesex Hospital Surgical Alliance, Middletown, Connecticut

RODRIGO OLIVA PEREZ, MD, PhD
Angelita & Joaquim Gama Institute, Colorectal Surgery Division, University of São Paulo School of Medicine, A Beneficência Portuguesa de São Paulo - Digestive Surgical Oncology Division, São Paulo, Brazil

MARK J. PIDALA, MD
Assistant Professor of Surgery, Colon & Rectal Surgery, University of Texas/McGovern Medical School, Houston, Texas

MICHAEL POLCINO, MD, FACS
Division of Colorectal Surgery, St. Barnabas Hospital, Bronx, New York

MICHAEL G. PORTER, MD, FACS, FASCRS
Associate Professor, Program Director, Department of Surgery, University of Kansas School of Medicine–Wichita, Wichita, Kansas

LEELA PRASAD, MD
Advocate Lutheran General Hospital, Professor of Surgery, University of Illinois at Chicago College of Medicine, Park Ridge, Illinois

GUILHERME PAGIN SÃO JULIÃO, MD
Angelita & Joaquim Gama Institute, São Paulo, Brazil

SCOTT M. STOEGER, MD, PhD
General Surgery Resident, Department of Surgery, University of Kansas School of Medicine–Wichita, Wichita, Kansas

CHARLES A. TERNENT, MD, FACS, FASCRS
Associate Clinical Professor of Surgery, Creighton University Medical Center, Clinical Professor of Surgery, University of Nebraska College of Medicine, Omaha, Nebraska

BRUNA BORBA VAILATI, MD
Angelita & Joaquim Gama Institute, São Paulo, Brazil

KATERINA WELLS, MD, MPH
Department of Surgery, Director of Colorectal Research, Baylor University Medical Center, Dallas, Texas

PAUL E. WISE, MD
Professor of Surgery, Director, Washington University Inherited Colorectal Cancer and Polyposis Registry, Program Director, Washington University General Surgery Residency, Washington University in St Louis School of Medicine, St Louis, Missouri

MORIAH WRIGHT, MD
Research Fellow, Colon and Rectal Surgery, Inc, Omaha, Nebraska

DANIEL OWEN YOUNG, MD
Colorectal Surgery Program, Section of General, Thoracic, and Vascular Surgery, Virginia Mason Medical Center, Seattle, Washington

Contents

with poor short- and long-term outcomes. For abnormality localizing to the colon proximal to the splenic flexure, surgical management with hemicolectomy is often a safe and appropriate approach. Obstructions are more common in the distal colon, however, where there is an evolving spectrum of surgical and nonsurgical options, most notably by the development of endoluminal stents. Perforation and bleeding are managed similarly to benign causes, as malignancy may be only part of a differential diagnosis at the time of an operation.

Laparoscopic colorectal surgery has now become widely adopted for the treatment of colorectal neoplasia, with steady increases in utilization over the past 15 years. Common minimally invasive techniques include multiport laparoscopy, single-incision laparoscopy, and hand-assisted laparoscopy, with the choice of technique depending on several patient and surgeon factors. Laparoscopic colorectal surgery involves a robust learning curve, and fellowship training often lays the foundation for a high-volume laparoscopic practice. This article provides a summary of the various techniques for laparoscopic colorectal surgery, including operative steps, the approach to difficult patients, and the learning curve for proficiency.

Robotic colorectal surgery has become increasingly prevalent, with several reported benefits for surgeons and patients alike. Although its use is well-supported for pelvic surgery, there is less evidence that it is beneficial for abdominal surgery. There are several technical limitations of robotic surgery, and newer generations of robot platforms have addressed these, which may lead to increased use in the near future. In general, robotic surgery is more beneficial for surgeons than it is for patients.

Local excision (LE) of early-stage rectal cancer avoids the morbidity associated with radical surgery but has historically been associated with inferior oncologic outcomes. Newer techniques, including transanal endoscopic microsurgery (TEM) and transanal minimally invasive surgery (TAMIS), have been developed to improve the quality of LE and extend the benefits of LE to tumors in the more proximal rectum. This article provides an overview of conventional LE, TEM, and TAMIS techniques, including indications for their use and pertinent literature on their associated outcomes for rectal cancer.

In recent years, our understanding of rectal cancer has improved, including how locally advanced disease responds to chemotherapy and radiation. This has led to new innovations and advances in the treatment of rectal cancer, which includes organ-preserving strategies for responsive disease, and minimally invasive approaches for the performance of total mesorectal excision/protectomy for persistently advanced disease. This article discusses new strategies for rectal cancer therapy, including Watch and Wait, local excision, minimally invasive proctectomy, and transanal total mesorectal excision particularly in the setting of preoperative multimodality treatment.

Awareness of hereditary colorectal cancer syndromes is important to facilitate their identification because affected patients are at increased risk for early onset, synchronous, and metachronous colorectal malignancies, and certain extracolonic malignancies depending on the syndrome. Identification of an affected individual allows for screening and early interventions for patients and their at-risk kindred. Genetic counseling and testing is important to the care of these patients. As knowledge of the genetic basis of these syndromes grows, unique genotype-phenotype profiles allow clinicians to tailor surveillance and treatment strategies based on individual risk.

Inflammatory bowel disease is associated with an increased risk of dysplasia and cancer. Improvements in medical management and endoscopic surveillance have reduced these risks. Patients can develop cancer even in the absence of dysplasia or with indefinite or low-grade dysplasia. Most guidelines recommend starting surveillance colonoscopy 6 to 10 years after initial diagnosis with interval surveillance afterward every 1 to 5 years depending on risk and/or individual characteristics. Most patients should undergo total proctocolectomy with end ileostomy or reconstruction with ileal pouch anal anastomosis because segmental and subtotal resections carry a higher risk of metachronous cancers.

Primary colorectal lymphoma, carcinoids (neuroendocrine tumors), and gastrointestinal stromal tumors comprise a small subset of all colorectal cancers. Their features are unique, and their treatment varies from that of colorectal adenocarcinoma. Appropriate identification is key in the management of these tumors.

Management of metastatic colorectal cancer requires accurate staging and multidisciplinary evaluation, leading to a consensus treatment plan with the ultimate goal of increasing survival and improving the quality of life, while taking into consideration the patient's performance status, disease burden, and goals of care. Since the introduction of multidrug chemotherapeutic regimens, survival of patients with metastatic colorectal cancer has improved. Many patients with unresectable disease are undergoing surgery for asymptomatic primary tumors despite evidence that it is usually a futile intervention. Palliative measures for local control of the primary tumor include colonic stents, laser therapy, and fulguration.

Historically, patients with peritoneal carcinomatosis secondary to colorectal cancer have a poor overall prognosis. Recent data support the use of cytoreductive surgery and heated intraperitoneal chemotherapy (CRS + HIPEC) to specifically address the peritoneal disease. Retrospective studies on CRS + HIPEC have been promising, showing significant improvements in OS compared with systemic chemotherapy alone. However, CRS + HIPEC carries morbidity similar to other advance oncology procedures such as liver resection and pancreatoduonectomy. It is hoped that ongoing clinical trials will clarify its role in the treatment of patients with peritoneal metastatic colorectal cancer.

Colorectal cancers develop through at least 3 major pathways, including chromosomal instability, mismatch repair, and methylator phenotype. These pathways can coexist in a single individual and occur in both sporadic and inherited colorectal cancers. In spite of the unique molecular and genetic signatures of colorectal cancers, nonspecific chemotherapy based on the antineoplastic effects of 5-fluorouracil is the cornerstone of therapy for stage III and some stage II disease. Techniques to recognize colorectal cancer at the molecular level have facilitated development of new signature drugs designed to inhibit the unique pathways of colorectal cancer growth and immunity.

SURGICAL CLINICS
OF NORTH AMERICA

Foreword

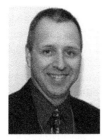

Ronald F. Martin, MD, FACS
Consulting Editor

In this issue of the *Surgical Clinics of North America*, we explore in some depth the neoplastic disorders of the colon. This is again another topic that brings us to the question of which topics belong to the world of the generalist and which topics belong to the world of the subspecialist.

In the field of medicine, there is a great deal of language to be learned and used. Much of it is technical and requires great precision to use it well. However, there is a whole separate unofficial language that governs medical day-to-day life as well. The slang and jargon we use among ourselves is as much a part of everyday life as with any other profession or craft. We are ruled by acronyms and euphemisms as much as we are by facts and analysis. Some of the terminology is effective shorthand, but some of the language we use may actually hinder our better efforts. One concept that has always intrigued me—in a negative way—is the concept of the "turf battle." I never really understood how a turf battle was in the interest of the patients. It always seemed to be about putting the interest of the provider, service, or discipline ahead of the better interest of the patient. It also seems to be more often motivated by greed or ego than by some sort of zealous belief that the afflicted citizens would be better served.

For patients with colon problems, there are several disciplines that are brought to bear to help them: general surgery, colorectal surgery, minimally invasive surgery, acute care surgery, gastroenterology, diagnostic imaging, medical genetics, medical oncology, and radiation oncology, to name just some and not to mention all the other disciplines and persons who support all of those efforts. Everybody in that list has something that she or he could potentially do to help patients with colonic problems. In theory, it is an enormous support system with lots of backup potential. In reality, it is a great support system in many places, but upon very close inspection, the seams and cracks are highly visible. For well-reimbursed services for some patients in some places, there is usually great support; however, for those patients who live in places with less access to services or are less capable of providing reimbursement, the access to parts or all of the care may be more limited.

It seems to me that turf battles are usually less about a jealous desire to "own" the responsibility to address a set of patient problems than it is to optimize our own access

http://dx.doi.org/10.1016/j.suc.2017.04.002
0039-6109/17/© 2017 Published by Elsevier Inc.
surgical.theclinics.com

as providers to desirable or lucrative work. On an individual level, I get it—who doesn't? On a system level, it is perhaps not the best way to provide for the whole. Whether it is the differential access for those with resources, the differential access for those who show up electively during the weekdays versus those who present more urgently on nights or weekends, or those who live nearer to broader services or live farther away, we end up with a variable—sometimes highly variable—ability to respond to the needs of patients. Some of those differences might be mitigated by changes on our system of compensation and risk sharing; others perhaps not.

Regardless of whether we could create a better system someday or not, we have what we have today. Care will be divided and overlapping for better or for worse for the foreseeable future. Resources will be heterogeneously distributed both geographically and economically for some time to come. All of the providers listed above will be regularly involved in the care of these patients or perhaps sporadically involved in the care of such patients. It would therefore stand to reason that no matter which group one falls into—the specialist, the generalist, the everyday provider, or the occasional provider—it would be of benefit to have the best comprehensive knowledge set to address the problems one may encounter. To that end, Dr Langenfeld and his colleagues have assembled an outstanding collection of reviews to help us all be as educated and prepared as we can be.

To answer the question of which topics belong to the generalist and which to the specialists, the answer will almost always be all belong to both, if for no other reason than we all need to effectively communicate with one another as best we can. Any real division of knowledge would be predicated on the idea that we can truly eliminate overlap in our collective responsibility to care for patients. If we believe that we should care for the person rather than limit our efforts to addressing a patient's specific isolated problem, then we should not fractionate our care or knowledge. Perhaps if we all worried less about who owns the turf and focus a bit more on the fact that there is only one turf and we all live on it, then we might actually develop a better system.

Ronald F. Martin, MD, FACS
Colonel (ret.), United States Army Reserve
York Hospital
16 Hospital Drive, Suite A
York, ME 03909, USA

E-mail address:
rmartin@yorkhospital.com

Preface

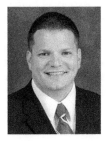

Sean J. Langenfeld, MD, FACS, FASCRS
Editor

Colorectal cancer remains one of the deadliest and most common malignancies that patients encounter. Thankfully, it is also a cancer that responds very well to surgical therapy. When I was making career decisions as a surgical resident, I knew that I wanted to take out cancer as a major part of my practice. However, I was discouraged by the poor long-term survival, even after resection with curative intent, for malignancies such as pancreatic, liver, and lung cancer, where aggressive tumor biology often trumped the quality of the surgical resection. Conversely, other less-aggressive tumors tended to follow indolent courses regardless of the surgeon's talents.

What I enjoyed most about colorectal cancer was that in the absence of metastatic disease, the quality of the surgical resection often dictated whether the patient ultimately lived or died. That is a responsibility that I've taken very seriously in my practice. However, the colorectal cancer surgeon is much more than a simple technician. He or she is the captain of the ship and must lead the multidisciplinary team from diagnosis to definitive treatment, ensuring the best possible outcome for the patient.

Despite the increasing subspecialization of the surgical workforce, most colectomies are still performed by general surgeons, with only 11.5% of colectomies and 22% of proctectomies performed by board-certified colorectal surgeons.[1] A query of the American Board of Surgery looking at 1995-1997 showed that, on average, general surgeons performed 11 partial colectomies per year (14 colectomies = 70th percentile and 23 colectomies = 90th percentile).[2,3] One can only assume that these numbers have continued to decline, and a 2016 study found the median number of open colectomies among surgeons in "large rural" communities (population 10,000-50,000) to be 7 per year, and the median number of laparoscopic colectomies to be 1 per year, with 76% performing less than 10 colectomies per year.[4] The number is more difficult to predict in the urban setting, where there is competition for cases with subspecialty surgeons.

Given that most colectomies are performed by general surgeons, and most of these surgeons are considered "low volume," it is essential that evidence-based, up-to-date resources be available to the general surgery workforce. The goal of this issue is to provide a concise yet comprehensive review of the management of colon and rectal

Surg Clin N Am 97 (2017) xv–xvi
http://dx.doi.org/10.1016/j.suc.2017.04.001
0039-6109/17/© 2017 Published by Elsevier Inc.

surgical.theclinics.com

cancer. It is hoped that this can be used to guide the practicing surgeon through the decision-making process and definitive surgery, while also helping them identify cases that are complex enough to require referral to a subspecialty center.

I want to thank the authors, who dedicated their time and expertise to this issue. I believe you will find that their work was of the highest quality, and I am privileged to call them colleagues and friends. I would also like to thank the publishing team from Elsevier, who demonstrated an unparalleled level of organization and support. Last, I would like to thank Dr Ronald Martin for giving me the opportunity to be Guest Editor for this issue. He is an outstanding Consulting Editor and a model surgeon, and I am grateful for the opportunity to participate in such an incredible publication.

Sean J. Langenfeld, MD, FACS, FASCRS
Department of Surgery
University of Nebraska Medical Center
983280 Nebraska Medical Center
Omaha, NE 68198-3280, USA

E-mail address:
sean.langenfeld@unmc.edu

REFERENCES

1. Etzioni DA, Cannom RR, Madoff RD. Colorectal procedures: what proportion is performed by American Board of Colon and Rectal Surgery-certified surgeons? Dis Colon Rectum 2010;53:713–20.
2. Hyman N. How much colorectal surgery do general surgeons do? J Am Coll Surg 2002;194:37–9.
3. Langenfeld SJ, Thompson JS, Oleynikov D. Laparoscopic colon resection: is it being utilized? Adv Surg 2013;47:29–43.
4. Moore J, Pellet A, Hyman N. Laparoscopic colectomy and the general surgeon. J Gastrointest Surg 2016;20(3):640–3.

Colorectal Cancer Screening

Jesse Samuel Moore, MD[a],*, Tess Hannah Aulet, MD[b]

KEYWORDS

- Colorectal cancer • Screening • Prevention • Colonoscopy • CT colonography

KEY POINTS

- Guaiac fecal occult blood testing is the only screening modality with high-quality evidence shown in randomized trials to decrease both the incidence and mortality in colorectal cancer.
- Endoscopic testing has the benefit of diagnostic and therapeutic tools, which allows for removal of premalignant adenomas in a 1-step procedure as well as being able to biopsy existing cancers.
- The best screening test is the one that individual patients complete and repeat as necessary.

INTRODUCTION

Colorectal cancer (CRC) is common in the United States. Based on data from 2010 to 2012, the lifetime incidence for average-risk individuals is 4.5%. Although it accounts for only 8% of all new cancers, it is the third leading cause of cancer death in men and women. Approximately 50,000 deaths in the United States are attributed to CRC each year.[1,2] Nearly all CRCs begin as small adenomatous polyps, so it is a disease in which screening, particularly with colonoscopy, is likely to be effective. The rates of screening for patients 50 to 75 years old from 2002 to 2010 increased from 52% to 65%,[3] and the annual incidence of new colon cancers in the same time period declined by 2% to 4%.[1]

It is important for surgeons to understand the rationale for screening, cancer risk stratification, available screening procedures, current guidelines, and the outcomes of screening. This understanding allows careful counseling of patients and their families. Cancers found during screening are typically earlier stage and more likely to be curable.

Disclosures: The authors have nothing to disclose.
[a] Department of Surgery, University of Vermont Medical Center, 111 Colchester Avenue, Mailstop 320FL4, Burlington, VT 05401, USA; [b] Department of Surgery, University of Vermont Medical Center, 111 Colchester Avenue, Mail-stop 341BA1, Burlington, VT 05401, USA
* Corresponding author.
E-mail address: Jesse.Moore@uvmhealth.org

Surg Clin N Am 97 (2017) 487–502
http://dx.doi.org/10.1016/j.suc.2017.01.001
0039-6109/17/© 2017 Elsevier Inc. All rights reserved.

CAUSE AND PATHOPHYSIOLOGY
Risk Factors

For most individuals, age is the most significant risk factor in developing CRC.[4,5] The average age of diagnosis is 68 years.[4] Between 2009 to 2013, 94.3% of new CRC cases were diagnosed in individuals more than the age of 45 years, with the highest percentage of cases, 24%, diagnosed in patients aged 65 to 74 years.[2] In the United States, male sex is associated with a higher incidence of CRC, with 47.1 per 100,000 men diagnosed per year compared with 36 per 100,000 in women.[2]

Race and ethnicity affect individuals' risk for CRC in the United States. There is a higher incidence of CRC in both male and female African Americans compared with white individuals.[2,5] Hispanic and Asian/Pacific Islander groups have a lower overall incidence compared with white Americans.[2]

There are several hereditary factors that contribute to risk of developing CRC. CRC caused by genetic factors is estimated to occur in approximately 30% of cases.[6] Not all of these genetic influences are well defined and understood.[7] Hereditary nonpolyposis CRC (HNPCC), also known as Lynch syndrome, and familial adenomatous polyposis (FAP) are the most common familial syndromes associated with the development of CRC. Despite being the most common, these two syndromes account for approximately 5% of CRC cases.[6,8] HNPCC is the result of mismatch repair gene mutations.[7] A mutation in the adenomatous polyposis gene (APC) is responsible for the development of FAP.[8]

Patients with a personal history of CRC or adenomas are at higher risk for the development of CRC. Individuals with a family history of CRC have also been well shown in the literature to have a higher incidence of CRC.[9] Population-based cohort studies have identified an increased risk of developing CRC in patients with first-degree relatives found to have adenomas on colonoscopy.[9–11]

Inflammatory bowel disease has been shown to increase the risk of developing CRC. This relationship has been best shown in ulcerative colitis (UC). Based on pooled estimates from a meta-analysis of 116 studies, the overall prevalence of CRC in patients with UC was 3.7%.[12] Risk of CRC in patients with UC is influenced by the duration, extent, and severity of the disease. Crohn colitis is associated with an increased risk of CRC, but the extent of the relationship is not as well understood.[5]

Diets high in processed and red meats have been shown in epidemiologic studies to be associated with an increased risk for CRC.[13,14] Alcohol use (2 or more drinks per day) and tobacco use are associated with an increased risk of CRC. Smoking has been associated with an almost 2-fold increase in diagnosis of an adenoma and a higher CRC mortality in active smokers.[13,14] Multiple prospective and case-control studies have supported an association between obesity and risk of CRC. The exact mechanism behind this is not known, but could be related to a proinflammatory states or insulin metabolism.[13]

Protective Factors

Physical activity has been well studied as showing a protective effect in risk of CRC development. In a meta-analysis of 52 studies, individuals who were physically active had a 20% to 30% lower risk of CRC compared with individuals who were less active. Maintaining a healthy body weight and routine physical activity has been supported as being associated with lower risks for CRC.[13]

Aspirin (acetylsalicylic acid [ASA]) and nonsteroidal antiinflammatory drugs (NSAIDs) have been studied for use in the prevention of CRC and several studies have shown their potential benefit. A Cochrane Review identified 9 randomized trials for inclusion and examined change in polyp burden and adverse events with NSAID and ASA use. This review noted that ASA reduced the recurrence of sporadic adenomas in 3 of the studies and there was some evidence to support adenoma regression with NSAIDs, but further study was needed.[15] The use of ASA and NSAIDs is not being recommended for chemoprevention of CRC in the general population because of concern that the risks outweigh the benefits.[13] However, the US Preventive Services Task Force (USPSTF) has recommended daily low-dose aspirin supplementation for prevention of cardiovascular disease (CVD) and CRC in adults aged 50 to 59 years with a 10% or greater risk 10-year CVD risk.[16]

Dietary supplementation with vitamins A, C, E, and D; folate; and fiber has been hypothesized as having preventive effects on the development of CRC. Despite extensive studies, there is no consistent or high-quality evidence that these decrease the risk of colorectal adenoma or cancer.[5,13,17–19] Calcium supplementation has been supported in the literature from both observational and randomized experimental studies as having an impact in preventing CRC.[5,13]

Adenoma-Carcinoma Sequence

Adenomatous polyps are precursors for most CRCs.[9] The adenoma-carcinoma sequence in CRC has been well studied and accepted as an explanation for the pathogenesis of CRC.[10] The adenoma-carcinoma sequence describes the evolution of histologic changes that occur from adenoma to carcinoma as various mutations are acquired.[5] It is estimated that it takes approximately 10 years for an adenoma to transform into a carcinoma, which is why screening intervals are generally 10 years for the average-risk population.[20,21]

Prevalence of adenomas in the population is largely based on age, sex, and family history, whereas smoking and obesity are also risk factors.[22] Cross-sectional imaging studies have suggested that 25% to 40% of asymptomatic patients older than 50 years in the United States have 1 or more adenomas.[23] Size and histology of adenomas are important because not every adenomatous polyp transforms into a cancer.[24] Adenomatous polyps are associated with a higher risk of CRC. These polyps are the most common type and make up approximately 50% to 66% of polyps.[24]

SCREENING RATIONALE

Symptoms for CRC often develop late in the natural course of the disease. Precursor or early lesions rarely cause symptoms, which is why early detection with screening is important. The detection of adenomas and removal with screening disrupts the adenoma-carcinoma sequence.[25] Once a patient is diagnosed with adenomas or CRC, they are no longer in the screening category and are placed in a surveillance program.[4]

Defining Patients' Risk

Understanding how to define the risk of CRC for each patient is critical in being able to provide the optimal screening recommendations. Patients are categorized into average-risk, increased-risk, and high-risk populations, as summarized in **Table 1**.[24,26] Professional organizations differ in their classification systems and how they define risk. Ensuring a detailed and accurate family history is crucial in determining an individual's risk.

Average risk is defined as having no personal history of CRC or adenomas, no history of inflammatory bowel disease (IBD), and no family history of CRC or genetic syndromes.[4,5] Personal history of adenomatous polyp or CRC and family history places

Table 1
Defining risk of colorectal cancer by clinical history

	Risk Category		
	Average Risk	**Increased Risk**	**High Risk**
Family history	No history	Adenomatous polyps or CRC in an FDR	Yes, history of hereditary syndrome
Personal history of adenoma or CRC	No history or history of hyperplastic polyps[a]	Yes	No history
History of IBD	No history	Crohn and UC[b]	Crohn and UC[b]
Hereditary syndromes	No history	No history	HNPCC, FAP

Abbreviations: FDR, first-degree relative; IBD, inflammatory bowel disease.
[a] Except with hyperplastic polyposis syndrome, these individuals are at increased risk.
[b] Depends on source; National Comprehensive Cancer Network guidelines list IBD as increased risk, whereas the US Multi-Society Task Force lists this as high risk.
Data from Refs.[5,24,26]

individuals at an increased risk for CRC.[26] According to most sources, family history can be defined as patients with a first-degree relative (parent, sibling, child) with adenomatous polyps or CRC. The age of diagnosis of the affected relative may influence the age to initiate screening and the screening interval.[5,24]

IBD is classified as both increased and high risk depending on which guidelines are reviewed.[24,26] Individuals with a history of genetic syndromes, such as Lynch syndrome and FAP, are classified as high risk and follow specific screening recommendations.[24]

Decisions regarding surveillance and screening intervals are largely based on pathology results from colonoscopy specimens.[23] Polyps are typically classified into 2 broad categories, adenoma or hyperplastic polyps, with the latter having little risk of malignant transformation (aside from hyperplastic polyposis syndrome).[25] Patients with hyperplastic polyps are considered average risk.[25] Diagnosis of an advanced adenoma, defined as an adenoma larger than 10 mm, containing high-grade dysplasia, or containing significant villous histology, generally decreases the interval to the next surveillance colonoscopy.[9,23,24]

SCREENING PROCEDURES

There are several options for CRC screening. Stool-based tests are better at detecting early cancers and some advanced adenomas. They are safe and can be done by patients at home. Radiographic testing provides structural images of the colon with low risk of perforation. However, they often require bowel preparation and do not allow for removal of polyps or biopsy of larger lesions. Endoscopic testing has the benefit of being able to remove premalignant adenomas in a 1-step procedure and biopsy existing cancers, albeit with higher risk of perforation. Ultimately, the best screening test is the one that individual patients complete and repeat as necessary. Therefore, it is imperative that physicians are aware of all available screening modalities.

Stool-Based Tests

Hemoglobin in the gut is broken down into heme and globin moieties. Guaiac fecal occult blood testing (gFOBT) detects heme via a peroxidase reaction. In the past, patients were instructed to follow a restrictive diet in the days leading up to testing, including avoidance of red meats and certain fruits and vegetables, which are foods that can hypothetically lead to a false-positive test. This practice has been shown to decrease compliance with testing without difference in test results, and avoidance of these foods is no longer recommended.[27] High doses of vitamin C, typically higher than those in a multivitamin, can cause a false-positive and should be avoided before testing. Patients apply stool to a guaiac card from 3 consecutive bowel movements. Cards are sent back to the physician's office where they are tested with a reagent. There are several older reagents (Hemoccult, Hemoccult-II, and Hemoccult-R) that are no longer considered sensitive enough for screening. The Hemoccult-SENSA (Beckman Coulter) reagent has an acceptable sensitivity of 64% to 80% for detection of CRC, but a much lower sensitivity for detection of precancerous polyps.[28,29] A positive gFOBT requires follow-up colonoscopy.

Fecal immunochemical tests (FITs) use antibodies that are specific to the globin moiety of hemoglobin. They are not reliant on peroxidase activity and therefore no pretesting dietary changes are needed. They are performed the same way as gFOBT, except only a single stool card is needed. The combination of only requiring a single stool sample and no dietary restrictions may increase patients' compliance with testing.[30] FIT tests are specific to blood that is colonic in origin, decreasing the chance of a false-positive test as a result of upper intestinal bleeding.[28] Sensitivity for detection of CRC is similar to the sensitivity of gFOBT.[31]

The most recent advance in stool-based testing combines FIT testing for hemoglobin with DNA (Cologuard; Exact Sciences) testing for cells that have been shed into the stool by a colorectal neoplasm. The combination of FIT-DNA has higher single-test sensitivity than FIT alone. The specificity is lower than that of FIT alone, which may lead to a higher rate of false-positives and subsequent colonoscopy, with its inherent risks.[32]

Stool-based tests have some advantages compared with radiographic or endoscopic techniques. They are done easily at home and without significant disruption of daily routine or assumption of risk to the patient. In the case of gFOBT, a nonphysician can test the completed stool cards in the office. It is important to realize that studies showing the efficacy of stool-based testing have been done on stool samples collected at home. Testing stool obtained in the office during a digital rectal examination has a sensitivity of 5% and is not considered appropriate for screening.[33] Stool-based testing is unable to detect most polyps because most polyps do not bleed. Any patient with an abnormal stool-based test requires subsequent colonoscopy and a small number of these are false-positives. The annual (gFOBT, FIT) or every-3-year (fecal DNA) interval may be more frequent than some patients wish to endure.

Radiographic Tests

Computed tomography colonography (CTC) appears in guidelines of the American College of Gastroenterology, the American College of Radiology (ACR), the US Multi-Society Task Force (USMSTF), and National Comprehensive Cancer Network (NCCN).[24,26,34,35] Protocols for CTC remain variable across studies. Most studies and guidelines include a full mechanical bowel prep before CTC, but other studies have been performed on unprepped colons. In addition, the number of scanner detectors, the reconstruction techniques, and the slice thickness have not been standardized. Studies have been designed to assess diagnostic accuracy by having all subjects undergo colonoscopy after CTC. Because of a low incidence of cancers in the study populations, the ability of CTC to detect cancer has not been assessed. In studies that used bowel preparation, the sensitivity for adenomas larger than

10 mm was 66% to 94% and specificity was 86% to 98%.[36] Note that CTC interpretation requires special expertise, and not all radiologists are adequately trained to read CTC scans.

The recommendations on what to do with the findings of CTC colonoscopy are still evolving. There is agreement that lesions larger than 10 mm need to be referred for colonoscopy. For lesions between 6 and 9 mm there is less consensus. Some guidelines recommend follow-up CTC in 3 years, whereas the ACR recommends colonoscopy.[35,37] The ideal interval for repeat CTC after a negative study has yet to be defined.

The risks of CTC are not typically related to perforation. In more than 22,000 screening CTC examinations there was 1 (0.005%) perforation.[38] Whether there is a real increase in lifetime cancer risk as a result of episodic radiation exposure from radiographic studies is debated. The estimated dose of radiation with a CTC is 7 to 13 mSv.[24] The Health Physics Society has stated that the health effects of radiation exposure less than 50 to 100 mSv are "too small to be observed or are non-existent. Calculation of collective dose...over large populations carries uncertainties too high to make it useful for estimating health effects."[39] One study used linear, no-threshold radiation risk estimates and calculated an additional 0.044% lifetime risk of colon cancer for a 50-year-old patient undergoing a CTC.[40]

CTC provides images of the entire abdomen and pelvis, not just the colon. Incidental extracolonic findings are reported in 15% to 69% of CTC with 4.5% to 11% being deemed clinically significant.[41–44] Clinically irrelevant incidental findings can lead to unnecessary imaging studies, additional radiation exposure, risk and pain from biopsy procedures, as well as time away from work and mental distress for patients.

Double-contrast barium enema (DCBE) is included in the guidelines of the USMSTF, ACR, and American College of Physicians.[24,37,45] This test requires a full cathartic bowel preparation. It is performed without sedation and involves instillation of air and rectal contrast, which can be uncomfortable for the patient. The quality of the study relies on the technician or radiologist performing the examination and the radiologist interpreting it. In patients with a history of prior polypectomy who received DCBE as surveillance, the sensitivity for adenomas greater than 10 mm was 48% and 73% for adenomas greater than 7 mm.[24] The use of DCBE has been declining in recent years.[46] This decline is likely to lead to fewer training opportunities for radiology residents. Combined with low interest from radiologists in practice to perform DCBE, there may be insufficient radiologists to perform DCBE in the future.[24]

Endoscopic

Endoscopic screening can be performed with either sigmoidoscopy or colonoscopy. With this technique, direct visualization of the large intestinal mucosa is possible with the goal of identifying early or precancerous lesions. Removal of adenomas has served as the primary prevention of CRC.[47] Although direct visualization techniques have been widely adopted, and offer the advantage of both diagnostic and therapeutic capabilities, they are invasive procedures and involve risk.

Sigmoidoscopy

Flexible sigmoidoscopy (FSIG) allows endoscopic examination of the rectum, sigmoid, and descending colon. It is performed with a flexible scope inserted through the anus and into the lower colon to allow direct visualization of the mucosa. Sigmoidoscopes are 60 cm in length.[5,24] With this procedure, if a lesion is identified, it may be removed or biopsied.[21] Data on the sensitivity of this procedure are limited, with most estimates coming from colonoscopy studies.[36] It has been stated that FSIG is 60% to 70% as sensitive for detecting CRC and advanced adenomas as colonoscopy.[24] The sensitivity of this screening modality may vary with age, gender, and race because some studies have shown variability in the prevalence of proximal adenomas based on these factors.[24,48]

FSIG can be performed in the office and often with little or no need for sedation.[24] Patients are typically in a lateral recumbent or prone jack-knife position.[5] In preparation for an FSIG, enemas are typically used either before arrival or in the office, with no oral prep required.[49] This procedure typically takes less time than a colonoscopy. Because the proximal colon is not examined, there is a potential to miss as many as one-third of adenomas and CRCs.[21] Effectiveness of FSIG for detection of lesions depends on the endoscopist's ability to perform a complete, high-quality examination. One of the quality indicators for FSIG is insertion of the scope to at least 40 cm.[24]

If a sigmoidoscopy is abnormal, patients may be referred for a full endoscopic examination with colonoscopy. The rate of referral to a colonoscopy after a screening FSIG is variable because of the lack of standard referral criteria, and ranges from 5% to 33%.[50]

The most common risks associated with sigmoidoscopy include bleeding and perforation.[4] Based on pooled data, the risk of perforation is 1 in every 10,000 procedures. Risk for major bleeding events is estimated to be 2 in 10,000 procedures.[50] However, screening sigmoidoscopy may lead to referral for colonoscopy and additional risk for perforation and bleeding may occur. There is variability in the screening interval recommendations for FSIG. In general, FSIG should be performed every 5 years after a normal examination,[4,24,26] and may be combined with fecal-based studies to increase sensitivity.[4,24]

Colonoscopy

Colonoscopy is widely used as a screening method for early detection of polyps and colorectal neoplasm.[51] It possesses the highest sensitivity for both cancer and precancerous polyps. It is not only diagnostic, with the ability to identify and biopsy lesions, it is also therapeutic, with the ability to remove polyps and early cancers, treat symptoms such as bleeding and obstruction, and tattoo lesions to assist with surgical planning.[52]

The sensitivity of colonoscopy for CRC has been estimated in several small studies and ranges from 85% to 96%.[53] Sensitivity of colonoscopy to detect adenomas 10 mm or larger ranges from 89% to 98%, but it is less sensitive (74.6%–92.8%) for adenomas 6 to 10 mm.[50] After completion of a full cathartic bowel preparation, colonoscopy is performed in specialized endoscopy suites or in the operating room using conscious sedation.

Ideally, bowel preparation is cathartic, without causing dehydration, electrolyte disturbances, or mucosal alterations.[54] There have been a multitude of studies comparing the type, volume, timing, and safety of administration of various bowel preparations. Bowel preparation formulas have continued to evolve with the goal of increasing patient tolerance and compliance.[55] Because some bowel preparations on the market have been associated with complications in children, the elderly, patients with renal insufficiency, and patients on angiotensin-converting enzyme inhibitors or angiotensin receptor blockers, it is important to consider the patient's comorbid conditions, age, and medications when selecting a bowel preparation.[55] Studies have suggested that the timing of administration is the most important factor, and there is evidence to support superiority of split-dose regimens.[55,56] Preparation quality has been shown to decline as the time interval between completion of bowel prep to time of procedure increases.[22]

In order to ensure adequate visualization, insufflation and distension of the colon is required. Air, carbon dioxide, and water have all been used as techniques for insufflation. Although room air is readily available, it is not absorbed well by the gastrointestinal (GI) tract and, despite suctioning before endoscope removal, it has been associated with increased abdominal pain, cramping, and distension.[57] Carbon dioxide is readily absorbed by the GI mucosa. Randomized control trials have shown that carbon dioxide is associated with less abdominal distension and postprocedural pain, but have found no difference in cecal intubation rate compared with air.[57] Water insufflation during colonoscopy has also been studied with regard to patient tolerance and screening effectiveness. A recent Cochrane Review found no difference between water and air insufflation with regard to cecal intubation, but did find a slightly higher adenoma detection rate (ADR) with water insufflation. Patients also had significantly less abdominal pain with water insufflation techniques compared with air.[51]

Quality parameters of a high-quality examination have been identified and are important to track and document in practice.[22] ADR is a quality measure defined as the percentage of patients in whom 1 or more adenomas were identified on screening colonoscopy.[22] Based on prevalence studies, it has been recommended that individual colonoscopists should identify at least 1 adenoma in 25% of men and 15% of women undergoing screening colonoscopy.[22,23]

Another quality metric that has been examined is colonoscopy withdrawal time, which is defined as the time of colonoscopy withdrawal from the cecum to the anus. The withdrawal phase of colonoscopy is when meticulous examination of the mucosa occurs and most adenomas are detected.[58] Longer withdrawal times have been shown to correlate with an increased ADR.[22,50,58–60] The minimum withdrawal time in average-risk patients has been consistently recommended to be 6 minutes or greater.[22,23,53,58,59]

Reaching the ileocecal valve and the appendiceal orifice is known as cecal intubation.[22,23] Visualizing the entire colon, including the cecum, is important for detection of neoplasms, because low cecal intubation rates have been associated with higher rates of interval CRCs.[22] Cecal intubation rates have been reported as high as 97% to 99% in the literature among screening populations.[22,23] Visualization of the terminal ileum is not required but adds additional certainty to having achieved cecal intubation. Another sign that is referred to in verifying cecal intubation is called the crow's foot. This sign is caused by the impression of the taenia coli in the cecal wall. Although this sign is good to recognize, it is not reliable in confirming cecal intubation. Similarly transillumination through the abdominal wall to confirm location and cecal intubation is not reliable.[23] Documentation of cecal intubation should be done in 100% of cases both for quality improvement and medical-legal purposes.[23] Retroflexed view of the rectum as a technique is widely described and practiced, but there are no randomized studies on the efficacy of this technique.[53,61,62]

An inadequate bowel preparation for colonoscopy can result in cancellation, incomplete examination, increased costs, longer procedure time, complications, and missed lesions.[22,24,55,56] Poor bowel prep may occur in as many as 20% to 25% of colonoscopies, but there is little in the literature about what to do after a poor preparation.[54,56,63] It is recommended that patients undergo repeat examination, but the interval is not well studied.[55,63] Adenoma miss rates have been reported from 20% to 49% when there is not adequate bowel prep.[63,64] There is variability in the documentation of bowel prep because of the use of several scales and subjectivity in assigning scores.[54] The US Multisociety Task Force on CRC stated that adequate bowel prep was defined as one in which polyps larger than 5 mm could reliably be seen.[23]

Complications can result from the preparation (dehydration or electrolyte abnormalities), the procedure as a result of technical errors (bleeding or perforation), or also from the sedation (respiratory distress or cardiovascular event). It is important for these complications, in addition to the possibility of a missed lesion or incomplete examination, to be included in an informed consent.[22] The incidence of perforations is 4 per 10,000 colonoscopies and the incidence of major bleeding events is 8 per 10,000 colonoscopies performed.[4,50] Approximately 36% of perforations and 96% of major bleeding events occur with polypectomy.[4,50] Few randomized trials have studied major cardiopulmonary adverse events associated with colonoscopy, but they occur with increased frequency in the elderly, patients with higher ASA scores, and with comorbidities.[50,65]

In a Cochrane Review of the use of propofol during colonoscopy, most of the literature is based on healthy outpatient populations and there is limited literature concerning propofol administration by anesthesiologists versus nonanesthesiologists. In generally healthy patients, propofol for sedation can lead to faster recovery and discharge times and increased patient satisfaction, without significant adverse events compared with traditional benzodiazepines or narcotics used for conscious sedation.[66]

SCREENING RECOMMENDATIONS

There are several professional organizations that put forth screening guidelines for CRC. The USPSTF provides recommendations based on both the risks and benefits of the procedure to the patient, and do not factor in cost. The USPSTF focuses its recommendations on average-risk populations and makes recommendations with the goal of maximizing screening. Thus, their recommended screening tests are not ranked or placed in preferential order.[4] Most US guideline organizations recommend several options for screening techniques. Among organizations there is variability and no complete consensus with recommendations.[36] The NCCN stratifies risk into 3 groups and makes its recommendations for screening based on risk.[26] Screening recommendations are fluid and may change based on findings with initial screening test and health status of the patient.

Recommendations for Average Risk

For average-risk individuals, screening is recommended to begin at 50 years old.[4,24,26,36] A summary of screening recommendations for average-risk patients by professional organization and screening modality is presented in **Table 2**. There is agreement among most organizations that colonoscopy should be performed every 10 years and gFOBT and FIT performed annually.[4,5,24,26] Studies have supported a 10-year screening interval being safe in an average-risk population after a negative colonoscopy.[20] Recommendations for screening FSIG by the USPSTF are every 5 years alone or every 10 years with yearly FIT.[4] The NCCN has stated that FSIG should be performed every 5 years with or without a stool-based test at year 3.[26]

Recommendations for Personal History of Colorectal Cancer or Adenoma

The NCCN has stated that individuals with a history of adenomatous polyps should be placed in a surveillance program.[26] In patients with prior adenoma removal, screening interval recommendation depends on size, histology, degree of removal, and quantity.[24] Individuals with advanced adenomas (>10 mm, villous features, or high-grade dysplasia) should undergo colonoscopy every 3 years.[5,25] Patients who undergo resection for CRC should have colonoscopy at 1 year for surveillance.[5,24,26]

Table 2
Screening modality recommendations for average-risk patients by professional organization

Society or Professional Organization	Colonoscopy	FSIG	gFOBT	FIT	CTC	DCBE
USPSTF (2016)	Every 10 y	Every 5 y Or Every 10 y + annual FIT	Annually	Annually	Every 5 y	NA
NCCN (2016)	Every 10 y	Every 5 y ± FOBT or FIT at year 3	Annually	Annually	Every 5 y	NA
ACS, USMSTF, and ACR (2008)	Every 10 y	Every 5 y	Annually	Annually	Every 5 y	Every 5 y

Abbreviations: ACS, American Cancer Society; FOBT, fecal occult blood testing; NA, not addressed.
Data from Refs.[4,24,26,36]

Recommendations for Family History

Among organizations, definitions of family history and CRC risk are variable and thus screening recommendations based on family history may vary by professional organization. The USMSTF along with the American Cancer Society (ACS) and ACR published joint guidelines in 2008, which stated that individuals with a family history of either CRC or adenomatous polyp in a first-degree relative should initiate screening with colonoscopy at 40 years of age or 10 years before first diagnosis.[24] If adenoma or CRC is diagnosed in a first-degree relative before the age of 60 years, the screening interval should be 5 years; otherwise they follow the interval of average-risk individuals.[24] NCCN guidelines differ in that, if a first-degree relative with CRC is more than 60 years of age, they recommend initiating screening at age 50 years. Both the USMSTF and NCCN state that an individual with 2 first-degree relatives with CRC at any age should initiate screening at age 40 years or 10 years before earliest diagnosis of CRC and undergo 5-year interval screening.[24,26]

Recommendations for Lynch Syndrome and Familial Adenomatous Polyposis

The USMSTF/ACS/ACR guidelines from 2008 recommended initiating screening in patients diagnosed or at increased risk for hereditary nonpolyposis colorectal cancer (HNPCC) with colonoscopy. Screening was recommended to be every 1 to 2 years starting at age 20 to 25 years or 10 years before the earliest diagnosis of CRC in a first-degree relative.[24] For patients with diagnosed or suspected FAP, initiating screening with FSIG annually starting at age 10 to 12 years is recommended. This approach allows for assessment of gene expression.[24] Colonoscopy can also be performed as a screening method. For both HNPCC and FAP, counseling on genetic testing is recommended.[24]

Recommendations for Inflammatory Bowel Disease

Patients with IBD have a high risk of CRC and thus are screened for CRC based on the duration of disease, which is defined as the time from onset of symptoms.[22] The USMSTF/ACS/ACR guidelines from 2008 recommend initiating screening colonoscopy with biopsies for dysplasia every 1 to 2 years, 8 years after a diagnosis of pancolitis or 12 to 15 years after diagnosis of left-sided colitis.[24] The NCCN recommends initiation of surveillance with colonoscopy 8 to 10 years after the onset of symptoms for both patients with UC and patients with Crohn's disease.[26]

Recommendations for the Elderly

In considering when to stop screening individuals for CRC, it becomes more important to balance the risks and benefits of each screening modality. After the age of 75 years, the benefit of early detection and intervention from screening declines.[4] The decision to screen patients for CRC in patients aged 76 to 85 years should be individualized and should include a conversation between the patient and physician.[26] Factors such as presence of comorbidities that may limit life expectancy or preclude treatment if cancer is detected, as well as prior screening history, are important to include when counseling these patients. Patients in this age group who have never been screened are more likely to benefit from screening.[4] The USPSTF does not recommend screening in individuals more than 86 years old.[4]

CLINICAL OUTCOMES OF SCREENING TECHNIQUES

There have been 5 randomized controlled trials (RCTs) examining the effectiveness of gFOBT on colon cancer incidence and mortality.[67–71] These trials include 404,396 patients screened biennially with Hemoccult-II for 11 to 30 years. Screened patients, compared with those who received no screening, experienced a reduction in colon cancer–specific mortality of 9% to 22%. After 20 years of screening, the relative risk for colon cancer–specific mortality was 0.91 (95% confidence interval [CI], 0.84–0.98) and at 30 years the relative risk was 0.78 (95% CI, 0.56–0.82).[36] Most US guidelines recommending gFOBT suggest annual testing. Annual gFOBT testing was compared with biennial testing in the Minnesota Colon Cancer Control Study. With more than 60,000 patients and 30 years of follow-up there was lower incidence of CRC (relative risk [RR], 0.81; 95% CI, 0.71–0.93) and risk of CRC-related mortality (RR, 0.68; 95% CI, 0.56–0.82) in patients screened annually.[72–74]

The impact of screening with FSIG has been evaluated in 4 recently published RCTs.[47,75–77] All trials used minimal bowel prep and 1 combined FIT testing with FSIG.[47] Criteria for referral for colonoscopy varied but it was generally indicated when adenomas greater than 10 mm, multiple polyps, or CRC were discovered. A total of 458,002 patients with a median follow-up of 11 years were included. Compared with no screening, FSIG reliably decreased CRC incidence (pooled incidence rate ratio [IRR], 0.79; 95% CI, 0.75–0.85) and CRC-related mortality (pooled IRR, 0.73; 95% CI, 0.66–0.82).[36]

There are no RCTs that evaluate colonoscopy's impact on CRC incidence or mortality. The National Polyp Study followed 1418 patients who underwent colonoscopy and had removal of adenomatous polyps. The incidence of new CRC in this group was compared with 3 reference groups of patients who had not undergone polypectomy. Depending on the reference group, the incidence of CRC was decreased by 76% to 90%.[78] A subsequent report with 23 years of follow-up reported CRC mortality to be decreased by 53%.[79] The largest prospective cohort study followed 57,166 women from the Nurses' Health Study and 31,736 men from the Health Professionals Follow-up Study. Study participants self-reported receiving colonoscopy or sigmoidoscopy and the reason for it. Compared with study members who did not undergo endoscopy, CRC incidence over 22 years was 47% lower after self-reported screening endoscopy with polypectomy, 53% lower with self-reported negative screening colonoscopy, and 44% lower with self-reported negative screening sigmoidoscopy. CRC-related mortality over 24 years was 68% lower with self-reported screening colonoscopy and 41% lower with self-reported screening sigmoidoscopy.[80]

The impact of CTC and DCBE on cancer incidence and mortality has not been studied.[24,36] Studies that attempt to compare the effectiveness of one screening technique with another are limited. Studies usually only evaluate a single round of screening during which the numbers of cancers detected are too low to make meaningful comparisons regarding reductions in CRC incidence or mortality and are unreliable.[36]

SUMMARY

Screening and early intervention of CRC reduces mortality.[4] It is important for physicians to understand basic screening rationale and how to risk stratify patients, and to have a familiarity with the recommendations in order to make the appropriate recommendations based on the individual's risk of CRC. Although there are several screening techniques and screening recommendations, it is essential to take a patient-centered approach to screening in order to ensure compliance. Colonoscopy remains the screening tool with the highest sensitivity for cancer and precancerous polyps, and it is also the only modality to allow therapeutic interventions for the entire colon.

REFERENCES

1. Siegel RL, Miller KD, Jemal A. Cancer statistics, 2015. CA Cancer J Clin 2015; 65(1):5–29.
2. SEER stat fact sheets: colon and rectum cancer. Available at: http://seer.cancer. gov/statfacts/html/colorect.html. Accessed September 16, 2016.
3. Centers for Disease Control and Prevention (CDC). Vital signs: colorectal cancer screening, incidence, and mortality–United States, 2002-2010. MMWR Morb Mortal Wkly Rep 2011;60(26):884–9.
4. US Preventive Services Task Force, Bibbins-Domingo K, Grossman DC, et al. Screening for colorectal cancer: US Preventive Services Task Force Recommendation Statement. JAMA 2016;315(23):2564–75.
5. Beck D, Roberts P, Saclarides T, et al, editors. The ASCRS textbook of colon and rectal surgery. 2nd edition. New York: Springer Science+Business Media; 2011.
6. Da Silva FC, Wernhoff P, Dominguez-Barrera C, et al. Update on hereditary colorectal cancer. Anticancer Res 2016;36(9):4399–406.
7. Laken SJ, Petersen GM, Gruber SB, et al. Familial colorectal cancer in Ashkenazim due to a hypermutable tract in APC. Nat Genet 1997;17(1):79–83.
8. Burt RW, DiSario JA, Cannon-Albright L. Genetics of colon cancer: impact of inheritance on colon cancer risk. Annu Rev Med 1995;46:371–9.
9. Tuohy TM, Rowe KG, Mineau GP, et al. Risk of colorectal cancer and adenomas in the families of patients with adenomas: a population-based study in Utah. Cancer 2014;120(1):35–42.
10. Winawer SJ, Zauber AG, Gerdes H, et al. Risk of colorectal cancer in the families of patients with adenomatous polyps. National Polyp Study Workgroup. N Engl J Med 1996;334(2):82–7.
11. Ahsan H, Neugut AI, Garbowski GC, et al. Family history of colorectal adenomatous polyps and increased risk for colorectal cancer. Ann Intern Med 1998; 128(11):900–5.
12. Eaden JA, Abrams KR, Mayberry JF. The risk of colorectal cancer in ulcerative colitis: a meta-analysis. Gut 2001;48(4):526–35.
13. Chan AT, Giovannucci EL. Primary prevention of colorectal cancer. Gastroenterology 2010;138(6):2029–43.e10.
14. Larsson SC, Wolk A. Meat consumption and risk of colorectal cancer: a meta-analysis of prospective studies. Int J Cancer 2006;119(11):2657–64.

15. Asano TK, McLeod RS. Non steroidal anti-inflammatory drugs (NSAID) and aspirin for preventing colorectal adenomas and carcinomas. Cochrane Database Syst Rev 2004;(2):CD004079.

16. Final Recommendation Statement: Aspirin use to prevent cardiovascular disease and colorectal cancer: preventive medication. Available at: https://www.us preventiveservicestaskforce.org/Page/Document/RecommendationStatementFinal/ aspirin-to-prevent-cardiovascular-disease-and-cancer. Accessed September 28, 2016.

17. Ibrahim EM, Zekri JM. Folic acid supplementation for the prevention of recurrence of colorectal adenomas: metaanalysis of interventional trials. Med Oncol 2010;27(3):915–8.

18. Negri E, Franceschi S, Parpinel M, et al. Fiber intake and risk of colorectal cancer. Cancer Epidemiol Biomarkers Prev 1998;7(8):667–71.

19. Kunzmann AT, Coleman HG, Huang WY, et al. Dietary fiber intake and risk of colorectal cancer and incident and recurrent adenoma in the Prostate, Lung, Colorectal, and Ovarian Cancer Screening Trial. Am J Clin Nutr 2015;102(4):881–90.

20. Singh H, Turner D, Xue L, et al. Risk of developing colorectal cancer following a negative colonoscopy examination: evidence for a 10-year interval between colonoscopies. JAMA 2006;295(20):2366–73.

21. Holme O, Bretthauer M, Fretheim A, et al. Flexible sigmoidoscopy versus faecal occult blood testing for colorectal cancer screening in asymptomatic individuals. Cochrane Database Syst Rev 2013;(9):CD009259.

22. Rex DK, Schoenfeld PS, Cohen J, et al. Quality indicators for colonoscopy. Gastrointest Endosc 2015;81(1):31–53.

23. Rex DK, Bond JH, Winawer S, et al. Quality in the technical performance of colonoscopy and the continuous quality improvement process for colonoscopy: recommendations of the U.S. Multi-Society Task Force on Colorectal Cancer. Am J Gastroenterol 2002;97(6):1296–308.

24. Levin B, Lieberman DA, McFarland B, et al. Screening and surveillance for the early detection of colorectal cancer and adenomatous polyps, 2008: a joint guideline from the American Cancer Society, the US Multi-Society Task Force on Colorectal Cancer, and the American College of Radiology. Gastroenterology 2008;134(5):1570–95.

25. Brooks DD, Winawer SJ, Rex DK, et al. Colonoscopy surveillance after polypectomy and colorectal cancer resection. Am Fam Physician 2008;77(7):995–1002.

26. National Comprehensive Cancer Network. NCCN clinical practice guidelines in oncology (NCCN guidelines): colorectal cancer screening. 2016. Available at: https://www.nccn.org/professionals/physician_gls/pdf/colorectal_screening. pdf. Accessed September 10, 2016.

27. Pignone M, Campbell MK, Carr C, et al. Meta-analysis of dietary restriction during fecal occult blood testing. Eff Clin Pract 2001;4(4):150–6.

28. Allison JE, Sakoda LC, Levin TR, et al. Screening for colorectal neoplasms with new fecal occult blood tests: update on performance characteristics. J Natl Cancer Inst 2007;99(19):1462–70.

29. Allison JE, Tekawa IS, Ransom LJ, et al. A comparison of fecal occult-blood tests for colorectal-cancer screening. N Engl J Med 1996;334(3):155–9.

30. Hol L, van Leerdam ME, van Ballegooijen M, et al. Screening for colorectal cancer: randomised trial comparing guaiac-based and immunochemical faecal occult blood testing and flexible sigmoidoscopy. Gut 2010;59(1):62–8.

31. Lee JK, Liles EG, Bent S, et al. Accuracy of fecal immunochemical tests for colorectal cancer: systematic review and meta-analysis. Ann Intern Med 2014;160(3): 171.

32. Imperiale TF, Ransohoff DF, Itzkowitz SH, et al. Multitarget stool DNA testing for colorectal-cancer screening. N Engl J Med 2014;370(14):1287–97.

33. Collins JF, Lieberman DA, Durbin TE, et al, Veterans Affairs Cooperative Study #380 Group. Accuracy of screening for fecal occult blood on a single stool sample obtained by digital rectal examination: a comparison with recommended sampling practice. Ann Intern Med 2005;142(2):81–5.

34. Rex DK, Johnson DA, Anderson JC, et al. American College of Gastroenterology guidelines for colorectal cancer screening 2009 [corrected]. Am J Gastroenterol 2009;104(3):739–50.

35. Yee J, Rosen MP, Blake MA, et al. ACR appropriateness criteria on colorectal cancer screening. J Am Coll Radiol 2010;7(9):670–8.

36. Lin JS, Piper MA, Perdue LA, et al. Screening for colorectal cancer: a systematic review for the U.S. Preventive Services Task Force. Rockville (MD): Agency for Healthcare Research and Quality; 2016.

37. McFarland EG, Fletcher JG, Pickhardt P, et al. ACR Colon Cancer Committee white paper: status of CT colonography 2009. J Am Coll Radiol 2009;6(11): 756–72.e4.

38. Pickhardt PJ. Incidence of colonic perforation at CT colonography: review of existing data and implications for screening of asymptomatic adults. Radiology 2006;239(2):313–6.

39. Health Physics Society. Radiation risk in perspective. 2016. Available at: hps.org/documents/risk_ps010–3.pdf. Accessed September 14, 2016.

40. Brenner DJ, Georgsson MA. Mass screening with CT colonography: should the radiation exposure be of concern? Gastroenterology 2005;129(1):328–37.

41. Pickhardt PJ, Taylor AJ. Extracolonic findings identified in asymptomatic adults at screening CT colonography. AJR Am J Roentgenol 2006;186(3):718–28.

42. Yee J, Kumar NN, Godara S, et al. Extracolonic abnormalities discovered incidentally at CT colonography in a male population. Radiology 2005;236(2):519–26.

43. Gluecker TM, Johnson CD, Wilson LA, et al. Extracolonic findings at CT colonography: evaluation of prevalence and cost in a screening population. Gastroenterology 2003;124(4):911–6.

44. Hara AK, Johnson CD, MacCarty RL, et al. Incidental extracolonic findings at CT colonography. Radiology 2000;215(2):353–7.

45. Qaseem A, Denberg TD, Hopkins RH Jr, et al. Screening for colorectal cancer: a guidance statement from the American College of Physicians. Ann Intern Med 2012;156(5):378–86.

46. Robertson RH, Burkhardt JH, Powell MP, et al. Trends in colon cancer screening procedures in the US Medicare and Tricare populations: 1999-2001. Prev Med 2006;42(6):460–2.

47. Holme O, Loberg M, Kalager M, et al. Effect of flexible sigmoidoscopy screening on colorectal cancer incidence and mortality: a randomized clinical trial. JAMA 2014;312(6):606–15.

48. Castiglione G, Ciatto S, Mazzotta A, et al. Sensitivity of screening sigmoidoscopy for proximal colorectal tumours. Lancet 1995;345(8951):726–7.

49. Phillips J, Ridd C, Thomas K, et al. Screening sigmoidoscopy and colonoscopy for reducing colorectal cancer mortality in asymptomatic persons. Cochrane Database Syst Rev 2013;9:CD005201.

50. Lin JS, Piper MA, Perdue LA, et al. Screening for colorectal cancer: updated evidence report and systematic review for the US Preventive Services Task Force. JAMA 2016;315(23):2576–94.
51. Hafner S, Zolk K, Radaelli F, et al. Water infusion versus air insufflation for colonoscopy. Cochrane Database Syst Rev 2015;(5):CD009863.
52. Luo H, Zhang L, Liu X, et al. Water exchange enhanced cecal intubation in potentially difficult colonoscopy. Unsedated patients with prior abdominal or pelvic surgery: a prospective, randomized, controlled trial. Gastrointest Endosc 2013; 77(5):767–73.
53. Rex DK. Maximizing detection of adenomas and cancers during colonoscopy. Am J Gastroenterol 2006;101(12):2866–77.
54. Landreneau SW, Di Palma JA. Update on preparation for colonoscopy. Curr Gastroenterol Rep 2010;12(5):366–73.
55. Wexner SD, Beck DE, Baron TH, et al. A consensus document on bowel preparation before colonoscopy: prepared by a task force from the American Society of Colon and Rectal Surgeons (ASCRS), the American Society for Gastrointestinal Endoscopy (ASGE), and the Society of American Gastrointestinal and Endoscopic Surgeons (SAGES). Gastrointest Endosc 2006;63(7):894–909.
56. Johnson DA, Barkun AN, Cohen LB, et al. Optimizing adequacy of bowel cleansing for colonoscopy: recommendations from the US multi-society task force on colorectal cancer. Gastroenterology 2014;147(4):903–24.
57. Committee AT, Lo SK, Fujii-Lau LL, et al. The use of carbon dioxide in gastrointestinal endoscopy. Gastrointest Endosc 2016;83(5):857–65.
58. Lee TJ, Blanks RG, Rees CJ, et al. Longer mean colonoscopy withdrawal time is associated with increased adenoma detection: evidence from the Bowel Cancer Screening Programme in England. Endoscopy 2013;45(1):20–6.
59. Barclay RL, Vicari JJ, Doughty AS, et al. Colonoscopic withdrawal times and adenoma detection during screening colonoscopy. N Engl J Med 2006;355(24): 2533–41.
60. Gellad ZF, Weiss DG, Ahnen DJ, et al. Colonoscopy withdrawal time and risk of neoplasia at 5 years: results from VA Cooperative Studies Program 380. Am J Gastroenterol 2010;105(8):1746–52.
61. Tellez-Avila F, Barahona-Garrido J, Garcia-Osogobio S, et al. Diagnostic yield and therapeutic impact of rectal retroflexion: a prospective, single-blind study conducted in three centers. Clin Endosc 2014;47(1):79–83.
62. Aranda-Hernandez J, Hwang J, Kandel G. Seeing better–Evidence based recommendations on optimizing colonoscopy adenoma detection rate. World J Gastroenterol 2016;22(5):1767–78.
63. Chokshi RV, Hovis CE, Hollander T, et al. Prevalence of missed adenomas in patients with inadequate bowel preparation on screening colonoscopy. Gastrointest Endosc 2012;75(6):1197–203.
64. Rex DK, Katz PO, Bertiger G, et al. Split-dose administration of a dual-action, low-volume bowel cleanser for colonoscopy: the SEE CLEAR I study. Gastrointest Endosc 2013;78(1):132–41.
65. ASGE Standards of Practice Committee, Fisher DA, Maple JT, et al. Complications of colonoscopy. Gastrointest Endosc 2011;74(4):745–52.
66. Singh H, Poluha W, Cheung M, et al. Propofol for sedation during colonoscopy. Cochrane Database Syst Rev 2008;(4):CD006268.
67. Scholefield JH, Moss SM, Mangham CM, et al. Nottingham trial of faecal occult blood testing for colorectal cancer: a 20-year follow-up. Gut 2012;61(7):1036–40.

68. Lindholm E, Brevinge H, Haglind E. Survival benefit in a randomized clinical trial of faecal occult blood screening for colorectal cancer. Br J Surg 2008;95(8): 1029–36.
69. Kronborg O, Jorgensen OD, Fenger C, et al. Randomized study of biennial screening with a faecal occult blood test: results after nine screening rounds. Scand J Gastroenterol 2004;39(9):846–51.
70. Faivre J, Dancourt V, Lejeune C, et al. Reduction in colorectal cancer mortality by fecal occult blood screening in a French controlled study. Gastroenterology 2004; 126(7):1674–80.
71. Hardcastle JD, Chamberlain JO, Robinson MH, et al. Randomised controlled trial of faecal-occult-blood screening for colorectal cancer. Lancet 1996;348(9040): 1472–7.
72. Shaukat A, Mongin SJ, Geisser MS, et al. Long-term mortality after screening for colorectal cancer. N Engl J Med 2013;369(12):1106–14.
73. Mandel JS, Church TR, Bond JH, et al. The effect of fecal occult-blood screening on the incidence of colorectal cancer. N Engl J Med 2000;343(22):1603–7.
74. Mandel JS, Bond JH, Church TR, et al. Reducing mortality from colorectal cancer by screening for fecal occult blood. Minnesota Colon Cancer Control Study. N Engl J Med 1993;328(19):1365–71.
75. Schoen RE, Pinsky PF, Weissfeld JL, et al. Colorectal-cancer incidence and mortality with screening flexible sigmoidoscopy. N Engl J Med 2012;366(25): 2345–57.
76. Segnan N, Armaroli P, Bonelli L, et al. Once-only sigmoidoscopy in colorectal cancer screening: follow-up findings of the Italian Randomized Controlled Trial–SCORE. J Natl Cancer Inst 2011;103(17):1310–22.
77. Atkin WS, Edwards R, Kralj-Hans I, et al. Once-only flexible sigmoidoscopy screening in prevention of colorectal cancer: a multicentre randomised controlled trial. Lancet 2010;375(9726):1624–33.
78. Winawer SJ, Zauber AG, Ho MN, et al. Prevention of colorectal cancer by colonoscopic polypectomy. The National Polyp Study Workgroup. N Engl J Med 1993; 329(27):1977–81.
79. Zauber AG, Winawer SJ, O'Brien MJ, et al. Colonoscopic polypectomy and long-term prevention of colorectal-cancer deaths. N Engl J Med 2012;366(8):687–96.
80. Nishihara R, Wu K, Lochhead P, et al. Long-term colorectal-cancer incidence and mortality after lower endoscopy. N Engl J Med 2013;369(12):1095–105.

Imaging for Colorectal Cancer

Yosef Nasseri, MD[a],*, Sean J. Langenfeld, MD[b]

KEYWORDS

• Imaging • Colorectal cancer • MRI • Endorectal ultrasonography • CT

KEY POINTS

• Plain films and abdominal ultrasonography have limited roles in modern staging of colorectal cancer.
• Patients are often referred for surgery with inadequate imaging, and it is the surgeon's responsibility to ensure proper preoperative staging.
• Rectal cancer requires additional local staging with endorectal ultrasonography or pelvic MRI to determine whether neoadjuvant chemoradiation will be beneficial.
• After curative resection, yearly computed tomography scans of the chest, abdomen, and pelvis are recommended for most patients.

INTRODUCTION

A comprehensive approach to colorectal cancer includes thorough radiologic imaging, which allows appropriate initial staging of the disease, as well as subsequent surveillance for disease recurrence. Several imaging modalities are used with different associated advantages and disadvantages. This article provides an overview of appropriate modern imaging in the evaluation of colon and rectal cancer. Recommendations mirror those of the American Society of Colon and Rectal Surgeons (ASCRS)[1–3] as well as the National Comprehensive Cancer Network (NCCN).[4,5]

DIFFERENT IMAGING MODALITIES
Plain Films

Before the widespread adoption of more capable imaging modalities, plain films were the mainstay of diagnosis and staging for colorectal cancer. However, its role in

Disclosures: The authors have nothing to disclose.
[a] Surgery Group of Los Angeles, 8635 West 3rd Street, Suite 880W, Los Angeles, CA 90048, USA;
[b] General Surgery Residency, Department of Surgery, University of Nebraska Medical Center, 983280 Nebraska Medical Center, Omaha, NE 68198-3280, USA
* Corresponding author.
E-mail address: yosefnasseri@gmail.com

modern medicine has diminished. In general, plain films do not possess adequate sensitivity for the identification of primary and metastatic lesions, so they are only useful when the findings are advanced and dramatic.

Chest radiographs (CXRs) can be used to detect pulmonary lesions, which may represent primary or malignant tumors. However, the sensitivity for detection of colorectal metastases is poor.[2] One retrospective review found that CXR detected only 36.7% of pulmonary metastases.[6] Abdominal radiographs may be useful for identification of the large bowel obstructions that can occur from a locally advanced primary tumor (**Fig. 1**). Abdominal films can be aided by the administration of Gastrografin to better identify the offending tumor (**Fig. 2**).

Ultrasonography

Ultrasonography of the abdomen has a low sensitivity for primary tumors. Its main historical significance was for the detection of liver metastases. Several important studies on staging and surveillance of colorectal cancer, including the GILDA (Gruppo Italiano di Lavaro per la Diagnosi Anticipata) trial,[7] used ultrasonography as the primary method for detecting liver lesions. However, current guidelines have abandoned abdominal ultrasonography in favor of computed tomography (CT) because of its increased sensitivity and reproducibility. Endorectal ultrasonography remains an important element in the local staging of rectal cancer, and it is discussed in greater detail later in this article.

Computed Tomography

CT has become a mainstay in the diagnosis and staging of colorectal cancer. It can be used to assess the location and extent of the primary tumor (**Fig. 3**), involvement of adjacent organs, enlargement of regional and distant lymph nodes, and the presence or absence of metastatic disease. CT is the most common modality used to stage colorectal hepatic metastases.[8] With the advent of helical CT (also called spiral CT),

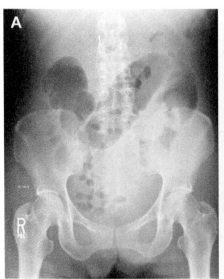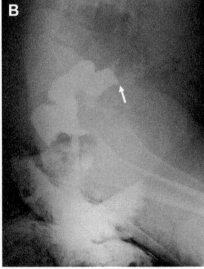

Fig. 1. Large bowel obstruction on plain film. (*A*) Proximal colon dilatation caused by sigmoid mass. (*B*) Gastrografin enema revealing obstructing sigmoid colon cancer (*arrow*).

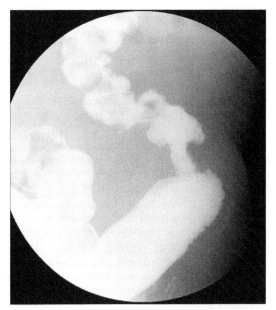

Fig. 2. Radiograph of apple core lesion. Gastrografin enema showing a rectal apple core sign caused by partially obstructing mass.

which images many slices at once (as opposed to original CT scans, which captured images slice by slice), CT's reliability in correctly detecting hepatic metastases preoperatively has improved, with an estimated sensitivity of 85%, positive predictive value of 96%, and false-positive rate of 4%.[9] At present, most tertiary and quaternary

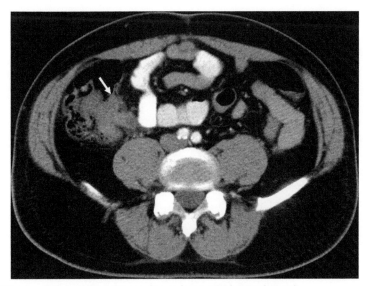

Fig. 3. CT scan of the abdomen, revealing a large cecal mass (*arrow*).

centers have 32-slice and 64-slice CT scanners with remarkable resolution and speed compared with prior generations.

Chest CT plays an important role in the pulmonary metastatic work-up of a primary colorectal cancer (**Fig. 4**). Its overall accuracy in detecting lung metastases preoperatively is 83.9%, with a sensitivity and specificity of up to 73% and 74%, respectively.[10,11] However, CT detects many indeterminate lesions, most of which are benign, which in turn necessitates further evaluation. Great disagreement therefore exists about the need for preoperative CT scans of the chest.

MRI

MRI is used extensively to evaluate hepatic metastases, because it provides increased detail that may affect resectability (**Fig. 5**). It is also used to evaluate primary tumors that encroach on or invade adjacent structures, once again to determine resectability and/or the need for neoadjuvant therapy. The role of pelvic MRI in the local staging of rectal cancer is discussed later in this article.

Like CT, MRI technology has also improved dramatically in recent years, improving both the speed and resolution of images. There have been increases in the strength of the magnetic field, with current machines using 3-T and even 7-T technology.[12] For pelvic MRI, high-resolution MRI scans via endorectal or phased-array coil methods provide a clear view of rectal wall anatomy, thereby allowing the accurate assessment of the depth of rectal tumor invasion (**Fig. 6**).

PET and PET/Computed Tomography

PET scans, by themselves or in conjunction with a CT scan (PET/CT) (**Fig. 7**), have a less-defined role in the evaluation of colorectal cancer. Although it does not have a role in the routine staging of colorectal cancer, it does have utility in the detection of occult disease as well as further evaluation of indeterminate lesions, and may be helpful in identifying metastatic disease when uncertainty exists regarding the benefit of surgical resection. It can also be used to assess changes in tumor metabolism, because cancers often show a decrease in glucose avidity after systemic treatment.

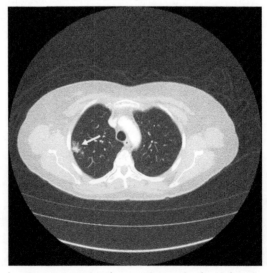

Fig. 4. CT of lung showing metastatic adenocarcinoma in the right upper lobe (*arrow*).

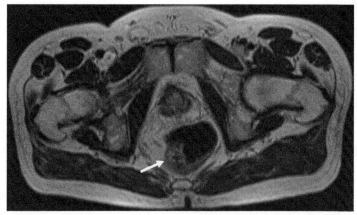

Fig. 5. Sagittal and axial MRI of the abdomen revealing colorectal liver metastases (*arrow*).

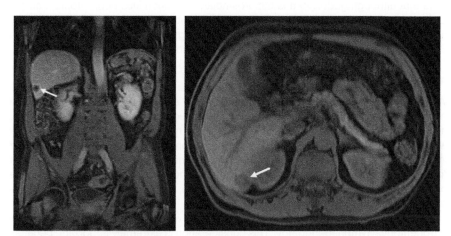

Fig. 6. MRI of abdomen and pelvis revealing colorectal liver metastases (*arrows*).

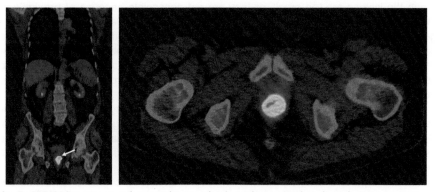

Fig. 7. PET/CT images reveal a rectal tumor both in the sagittal and axial views (*arrow*).

INITIAL STAGING OF COLORECTAL CANCER

When a patient has a new diagnosis of colon or rectal cancer, the next step is to determine the cancer's stage, because this has a large impact on prognosis and treatment options. Therefore, one of the first bifurcations in the decision tree is based on the presence or absence of metastatic disease.

For colon and rectal cancer, both the ASCRS practice parameters and the NCCN guidelines recommend routine preoperative radiographic staging with a CT scan of the chest, abdomen, and pelvis.[2–5] Based on these recommendations, chest radiograph is no longer adequate for preoperative pulmonary evaluation. The CT scan should be done with both oral and intravenous (IV) contrast, and rectal contrast is generally unnecessary.

Patients often arrive to the surgeon's clinic with preexisting laboratory tests and imaging of varying extent and quality. It is the surgeon's responsibility to ensure proper preoperative imaging. A noncontrasted CT scan should be considered inadequate for staging purposes, and should be repeated with contrast when necessary. When patients have allergy to IV contrast, an acceptable alternative is to obtain a gadolinium-enhanced MRI scan of the abdomen along with a noncontrasted CT of the chest. Note that although gadolinium is hyperosmolar, it is much less nephrotoxic than the iodine-based contrasts used for CT scans,[13] and it is also associated with a lower risk of allergic reaction. If neither of these imaging modalities are possible, then a PET/CT scan may be ordered knowing that it may not detect smaller lesions.

Approach to Positive Radiologic Findings

When abnormalities are detected on staging CT scan, more information is often necessary. CT scans cannot always accurately categorize liver lesions, and so cysts, hemangiomas, and metastatic tumors may appear radiologically similar. When available, a gadolinium-enhanced MRI scan of the abdomen may better characterize liver lesions. If found to be cysts or hemangiomas, then no further work-up is necessary. If found to be indeterminate or worrisome for malignancy, core-needle biopsy should be performed by the interventional radiology (IR) team, either using CT or ultrasonography to assist with the biopsy.

Another common finding on CT scan that may be worrisome for systemic disease is retroperitoneal lymphadenopathy. This consideration is extremely important, because retroperitoneal spread of colorectal cancer is associated with a very poor prognosis,[14] and resection of the primary tumor may be unnecessary and even counterproductive. When these nodules are large enough, they can often be safely biopsied by IR as well. When the lesions are too small, or they are not accessible because of proximity to other retroperitoneal structures such as the aorta and inferior vena cava, then the surgeon may want to proceed with surgery with curative intent, with plans to monitor the nodules with serial imaging. However, if adequate suspicion exists for metastatic disease, then it is often appropriate to initiate a trial of primary systemic chemotherapy to see whether (1) the nodules shrink with therapy, and/or (2) the patient manifests more conventional evidence of systemic disease.

When there are abnormal findings on CT of the chest, the surgeon must balance the risk of pulmonary metastasis with the likelihood of nonpathologic pulmonary nodules. Once again, IR-guided biopsy is often feasible. The surgeon may also want to use the assistance of a thoracic surgeon for further work-up, and possibly therapeutic intervention.

Another important consideration is for locally advanced colon cancers that are found to encroach or invade adjacent structures. This situation may be as simple as a cecal cancer abutting the anterior abdominal wall, or it may include more distal cancers that invade the liver, duodenum, pancreas, and major vessels. However, this occurrence is uncommon, but it can typically be detected through preoperative imaging, allowing the surgeon to plan accordingly to ensure a safe R0 resection.

LOCAL STAGING FOR RECTAL CANCER

Colon cancer is generally more straightforward than rectal cancer to diagnose and treat. Once it has been established that there is no metastatic disease, the next step is to surgically remove the offending colonic segment. In contrast, rectal cancer involves a more complex decision tree, in which the next step is to locally stage the tumor to determine whether it is early (stage 1 [T1–2N0]) or locally advanced (stage II [T3–4N0]) or stage III (TxN1–2)]. Early tumors are treated with immediate surgery. Locally advanced tumors require neoadjuvant chemotherapy and radiation before surgical intervention.

When the surgeon receives a referral for sigmoid, rectosigmoid, or rectal cancer, an important component of the initial office examination is rigid proctosigmoidoscopy to determine the distance from the anal verge. Often, tumors that seem colonic on flexible endoscopy actually lie within the extraperitoneal rectum. Therefore, surgeons should never rely on endoscopic pictures or the endoscopist's estimation, and a digital examination is not adequate to exclude extraperitoneal disease. There is no hard cutoff for labeling rectal cancers based on distance from the anal verge, and gender and body habitus affect this determination. However, most experts agree that tumors less than or equal to 12 cm from the anal verge should be considered for neoadjuvant therapy when locally advanced.

The ASCRS practice parameters and the NCCN guidelines both recommend routine preoperative staging with either endorectal ultrasonography (ERUS) or high-resolution pelvic MRI. If the lesion is determined to be locally advanced (stage II or III), patients should undergo neoadjuvant chemotherapy and radiation. For the NCCN, MRI is preferred to ERUS,[5] but neither technique has proved to be universally superior. Both are described later, along with their relative strengths and weaknesses.

Endorectal Ultrasonography

ERUS is a reliable approach to the local staging of rectal cancer, and is typically performed by a specialty-trained surgeon rather than a radiologist. ERUS involves a transducer covered with a water-filled balloon that is passed through a proctoscope, which is inserted into the patient's rectum,[15] allowing a 360° view of the rectal lumen. There are normally 5 rings seen in the images (**Fig. 8**). Radially outward, these layers correspond with (1) the area between the balloon and rectal mucosa, (2) mucosa and muscularis mucosa, (3) submucosa, (4) muscularis propria, and (5) the area between the muscularis propria and perirectal fat. Occasionally, 7 layers are observed, when the muscularis propria appears as 2 darker rings surrounding a lighter, white ring.[15]

T stage is determined by invasion of the layers of the rectal wall that were mentioned earlier, prefixed by a *u;* for example, uT1 and uT2. ERUS is better than MRI and CT for determining T stage, with an overall accuracy of 84%, sensitivity of 81% to 96%, and specificity of 91% to 98%, depending on stage.[16,17] Mesorectal lymph nodes (LNs) can also be assessed (**Fig. 9**), with a sensitivity of 67% and specificity of 78%.[2] Nodes are deemed to be positive when larger than 5 to 10 mm. However, reliance on LN size may understage a significant number of patients, because nodal metastasis occurs in up to 50% of nodes smaller than 5 mm.[17,18]

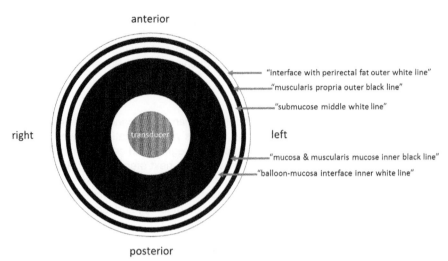

Fig. 8. Cartoon rendering of an ERUS image. The various dark and light rings correlate with anatomic structures.

ERUS is a more dynamic and less expensive study than MRI, but it is operator dependent and requires special training to perform. ERUS is also sometimes hindered by stenotic lesions, bulky lesions, and patient discomfort.

Pelvic MRI

Pelvic MRI is an acceptable alternative to ERUS for the local staging of rectal cancer. Although earlier studies showed sensitivity and specificity to be similar to ERUS, advances in technology and image resolution have led many experts to switch to routine staging with MRI. Specifically, high-resolution imaging with phased-array coils have

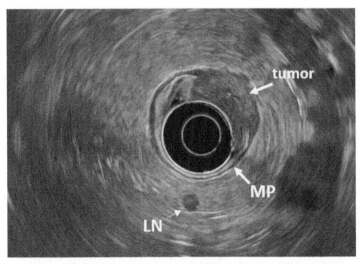

Fig. 9. ERUS image with clinically positive mesorectal lymph node. Midrectal tumor invading the muscularis propria (MP) and an involved LN (T3N1 lesion).

improved accuracy and eliminated the need for an endorectal coil, which is often found by patients to be uncomfortable.[17]

A 2012 meta-analysis of T and N staging with MRI showed significant heterogeneity among studies, many of which used older technology.[18,19] The investigators reported a pooled sensitivity and specificity of 87% and 75%, respectively, for T stage, and 77% and 71% for N stage. In general, MRI is better than ERUS for detecting morphologic abnormalities among LNs smaller than 10 mm, including mixed signal intensity and/or irregular borders, perhaps allowing the detection of subcentimeter metastatic nodes.[2] Importantly, MRI has a 94% specificity for involvement of the circumferential radial margin, which is an important factor that cannot be accurately assessed with ERUS. MRI can also assess other threatened margins, along with involvement of adjacent pelvic organs such as the prostate or vagina, which may also assist in preoperative planning.

Compared with ERUS, MRI is more expensive and more time consuming. It is more likely to overstage T2 tumors than ERUS, and it has difficulty differentiating active tumor from treatment-related scarring and fibrosis.[20] However, MRI does have the advantage of improved patient comfort; improved reproducibility; better understanding of related pelvic anatomy, including the levators and the mesorectal envelope; and better characterization of subcentimeter mesorectal LNs. At present, experts still disagree on which test is the most appropriate for tumor staging, and unbiased clinicians are likely to find uses for both techniques in their practices depending on patient and tumor characteristics.

SURVEILLANCE AFTER CURATIVE RESECTION OF COLORECTAL CANCER

After patients have received surgery with curative intent, serial imaging plays an important role in the subsequent cancer surveillance. There is great disagreement among major organizations regarding the intensity of surveillance, as well as the need for surveillance in patients with stage 1 cancer. Discussions regarding these topics are outside the scope of this article.

When an intense surveillance program has been chosen for patients with colon and rectal cancer, serial laboratory tests, office examinations, and endoscopic evaluations are warranted. In addition, both the ASCRS and the NCCN recommend annual CT scans of the chest, abdomen, and pelvis for the first 5 years after resection.[1,4,5] At present, there is no role for routine PET/CT, MRI, or ultrasonography for patients after curative resection. However, these tests are used selectively when necessary, as previously outlined.

When abnormalities are found on surveillance imaging, it is important to reference the initial preoperative scans. Indeterminate nodules that are unchanged in size can be closely monitored, typically with reduced imaging intervals. However, new nodules or enlarging nodules require biopsy to exclude metastatic disease. In addition, restaging CT scans should be obtained whenever a patient has shown other signs or symptoms concerning for recurrent malignancy, including weight loss and failure to thrive, new-onset abdominal complaints, shortness of breath, and increases in serum carcinoembryonic antigen level.

SUMMARY

Radiologic imaging plays a crucial role in the diagnosis and treatment of colon and rectal cancer. It is often the responsibility of the surgeon to ensure that proper staging has been completed. A strong understanding of the different available tests, their strengths and weaknesses, and their relative indications can allow for outstanding patient care, and avoid costly and time-consuming tests that are not ultimately beneficial.

ACKNOWLEDGMENTS

Meka Uffenheimer, BS, worked closely with Dr Y. Nasseri on drafting this article and conducting the research.

REFERENCES

1. Steele SR, Chang GJ, Handren S, et al. Practice guidelines for the surveillance of patients after curative treatment of colon and rectal cancer. Dis Colon Rectum 2015;58:713–25.
2. Monson JRT, Weiser MR, Buie WD, et al. Practice parameters for the management of rectal cancer (revised). Dis Colon Rectum 2013;56:535–50.
3. Chang GJ, Kaiser AM, Mills S, et al. Practice parameters for the management of colon cancer. Dis Colon Rectum 2012;55:831–43.
4. Available at: https://www.nccn.org/professionals/physician_gls/pdf/colon.pdf. Accessed October 1, 2016.
5. Available at: https://www.nccn.org/professionals/physician_gls/pdf/rectal.pdf. Accessed October 1, 2016.
6. Lazzaron AR, Vieira MV, Damin DC. Should preoperative chest computed tomography be performed in all patients with colorectal cancer? Colorectal Dis 2015;17(10):O184–90.
7. Rosati G, Ambrosini G, Barni S, et al. A randomized trial of intensive versus minimal surveillance of patients with resected Dukes B2-C colorectal carcinoma. Ann Oncol 2016;27:274–80.
8. Biasco G, Derenzini E, Grazi G, et al. Treatment of hepatic metastases from colorectal cancer: many doubts, some certainties. Cancer Treat Rev 2006;32(3):214–28.
9. Valls C, Andía E, Sánchez A, et al. Hepatic metastases from colorectal cancer: preoperative detection and assessment of resectability with helical CT. Radiology 2001;218(1):55–60.
10. Cho YK, Lee WY, Yi LJ, et al. Routine chest computed tomography as a preoperative work-up for primary colorectal cancer: is there any benefit in short-term outcome? J Korean Surg Soc 2011;80(5):327–33.
11. Oh BY, Noh GT, Hong KS, et al. The availability of computed tomography for pulmonary staging in colorectal cancer. Ann Surg Treat Res 2014;86(4):212–6.
12. Wood R, Bassett K, Foerster V, et al. 1.5 tesla magnetic resonance imaging scanners compared with 3.0 tesla magnetic resonance imaging scanners: systematic review of clinical effectiveness. CADTH Technol Overv 2012;2(2):e2201.
13. Perazella MA. Gadolinium-contrast toxicity in patients with kidney disease: nephrotoxicity and nephrogenic systemic fibrosis. Curr Drug Saf 2008;3(1):67–75.
14. Gagniere J, Dupre A, Chabaud S, et al. Retroperitoneal nodal metastases from colorectal cancer: curable metastases with radical retroperitoneal lymphadenectomy in selected patients. Eur J Surg Oncol 2015;41(6):731–7.
15. Blomqvist L, Machado M, Rubio C, et al. Rectal tumour staging: MR imaging using pelvic phased-array and endorectal coils vs endoscopic ultrasonography. Eur Radiol 2000;10(4):653–60.
16. Puli SR, Bechtold ML, Reddy JBK, et al. How good is endoscopic ultrasound in differentiating various T stages of rectal cancer? Meta-analysis and systematic review. Ann Surg Oncol 2009;16:254–65.

17. Marcet J. Rectal cancer: preoperative evaluation and staging. In: Steele SR, Hull TL, Read ThE, et al, editors. The ASCRS textbook of colon and rectal surgery. 3rd edition. New York: Springer; 2016. p. 471–9.
18. Akasu T, Sugihara K, Moriya Y, et al. Limitations and pitfalls of transrectal ultrasonography for staging of rectal cancer. Dis Colon Rectum 1997;40:S10–5.
19. Al-Sukhni E, Milot L, Fruitman M, et al. Diagnostic accuracy of MRI for assessment of T category, lymph node metastases, and circumferential resection margin involvement in patients with rectal cancer: a systematic review and meta-analysis. Ann Surg Oncol 2012;19(7):2212–23.
20. Kekelidze M, D'Errico L, Pansini M, et al. Colorectal cancer: current imaging methods and future perspectives for the diagnosis, staging and therapeutic response evaluation. World J Gastroenterol 2013;19(46):8502–14.

The Difficult Colorectal Polyp

Mark J. Pidala, MD[a],*, Marianne V. Cusick, MD[b]

KEYWORDS

- Colorectal polyps • Colonoscopy • Polypectomy • Endoscopic mucosal resection
- Endoscopic submucosal dissection • Laparoscopic colon surgery

KEY POINTS

- The definition of a "difficult" polyp is a moving target, but traditionally refers to polyps not amenable to endoscopic removal by the average endoscopist.
- Many patient-specific and polyp-specific factors impact the approach to difficult polyps.
- Conventional and advanced endoscopic techniques are usually successful in removing precancerous polyps with low complication rates.
- Almost 20% of polyps that are premalignant on initial biopsy will harbor an invasive malignancy that is discovered after complete resection.

INTRODUCTION

The direct relationship between neoplastic colorectal polyps and colorectal cancer has been well established.[1] Known as the adenoma to carcinoma sequence, this relationship has become the cornerstone of colorectal cancer prevention.[2,3] Screening colonoscopy with polypectomy has been linked to a decrease in the incidence of colorectal cancer and its associated mortality.[4–6]

Of the various screening modalities available for early detection of colorectal cancer, only endoscopic polypectomy offers the ability to remove premalignant lesions before they develop into cancer. Most polyps identified at screening colonoscopy are amenable to conventional forceps or snare polypectomy.[7] However, approximately 10% to 15% of polyps encountered at colonoscopy may be considered difficult because of their size, location, and/or morphology.[8] These difficult polyps are the topic of this article.

Disclosures: Dr M.J. Pidala is a proctor for Intuitive Surgical. Dr M.V. Cusick has nothing to disclose.
[a] Colon & Rectal Surgery, University of Texas/McGovern Medical School, 800 Peakwood Drive, Suite 2C, Houston, TX 77090, USA; [b] Colon & Rectal Surgery, University of Texas/McGovern Medical School, Smith Tower, Suite 2307, 6550 Fannin Street, Houston, TX 77030, USA
* Corresponding author.
E-mail address: mark.j.pidala@uth.tmc.edu

Surg Clin N Am 97 (2017) 515–527
http://dx.doi.org/10.1016/j.suc.2017.01.003
0039-6109/17/© 2017 Elsevier Inc. All rights reserved.

surgical.theclinics.com

DEFINITION OF A DIFFICULT POLYP

The definition of the difficult polyp is not well established. As implied in the name, these polyps are difficult to remove and often pose a challenge to endoscopists. As a result, patients with difficult polyps frequently require referral to a more experienced endoscopist or surgeon. These polyps are typically defined by their size, morphology, and/or location (**Box 1**). Difficult polyps are macroscopically benign, generally greater than 20 mm in size, and frequently have a flat or sessile morphology.[9] Most are found in the right colon, where the thinner colonic wall adds a degree of complexity to polypectomy.[10,11] These polyps may also pose a challenge when they are found wrapped around haustral folds or around sharp bends that are difficult to access.[8,12,13] The term giant polyp has been used to describe polyps greater than 30 mm.[14,15] Large pedunculated polyps, most often encountered in the left colon and sigmoid, also present difficulties because their removal carries increased risk of bleeding from larger vessels within the stalk.[16,17]

In practice, what constitutes a "difficult" polyp is very subjective.[18] What may appear difficult for one endoscopist may be routine for another.[19,20] As a result, any polyp referred to another physician for removal following an initial colonoscopy may be considered "difficult." These referrals are based on the endoscopist's comfort, level of experience, equipment availability, and support structure. In today's medicolegal climate, some endoscopists are unwilling to accept the risk, albeit small, of removing these larger lesions due to their increased risk of complications.[21,22] In addition, it has been shown that the physician work required to remove these difficult polyps (>20 mm) is more than twice that for more routine polyps (<20 mm), despite minimal or no impact on reimbursement.[23] As there is ongoing pressure on physicians to maintain higher case volumes, busy endoscopists may be reluctant to manage these more difficult lesions.

Premalignant Polyps Versus Invasive Cancers

The initial goal of the endoscopic evaluation of any colorectal polyp is to localize it and determine if it contains an invasive malignancy. Histologic predictors of malignancy include polyp size[24] and villous histology.[25–28] Macroscopic signs include ulceration, induration, friability, and fixation to the colonic wall. High-grade dysplasia on initial biopsy has also been shown to be an indicator of a potential underlying invasive cancer (**Box 2**).[11,25,26,29,30]

A saline lift not only assists with polypectomy and limits associated bleeding but can also be used to identify invasive cancers. Following submucosal injection, benign adenomas are lifted off the muscularis propria. On the contrary, cancers often have fibrosis and desmoplastic reaction and will not lift with saline injection.[31] Although

---

Box 1
Features of the difficult colorectal polyp

1. Macroscopically benign
2. Large (typically >20 mm)
3. Flat or sessile
4. Located around folds or kinks
5. Most in right colon or cecum
6. Large pedunculated polyps with thick stalk

> **Box 2**
> **Endoscopic signs of malignancy**
>
> - Induration
> - Friability
> - Fixity
> - Ulceration
> - Non-lifting sign

nonlifting may also occur secondary to scar from prior biopsy, the sign may be used in conjunction with other features to help predict whether a polyp harbors invasive malignancy.

Several detailed classification systems have been developed to further enhance the endoscopists' ability to determine benign from malignant lesions.[32–34] These systems stratify the risk of underlying malignancy by assessing mucosal irregularities and various mucosal pit patterns using image-enhancing technologies, such as magnified endoscopy, chromoendoscopy, and narrow band imaging.[35–37] These systems are not typically used in the United States, and their clinical utility is uncertain.

Despite a thorough endoscopic and histologic evaluation, 6% to 12% of difficult "premalignant" polyps may still contain invasive carcinoma.[10,11,13,14] However, malignant polyps without high-risk histologic criteria may be amenable to endoscopic resection alone for cure.[38–40] These high-risk criteria include poorly differentiated lesions, the presence of lymphovascular invasion, or surgical margins less than 2 mm.[30]

Flat, sessile polyps harboring invasive malignancy were historically thought to be associated with a high risk of nodal metastasis as well and have been typically treated with subsequent colectomy.[41,42] Based on work by Kudo,[43] flat lesions with malignant invasion limited to the superficial third or 1000 μm of the submucosa have been associated with lymph node metastasis of 0% to 3%.[44,45] As a result, flat polyps with malignant invasion limited to the superficial third of the submucosa (<1000 μm) and no other high-risk histologic features may be treated with en bloc endoscopic resection alone.[42,43,46,47] Malignant polyps removed by piecemeal polypectomy do not allow for adequate pathologic assessment of resection margins and should be referred for surgical evaluation.

Polyps Treated with Colectomy

Two recent studies focused on the final pathology of polyps not amenable to endoscopic removal that resulted in a colectomy.[25,26] A 2010 study from Washington University[25] found that 22/165 (13.3%) had an invasive cancer on final pathology, whereas a 2012 study from the Mayo Clinic[26] found that 133/750 (17.7%) unresectable polyps harbored a malignancy, of which 23% were node positive. Of note, both studies found that high-grade dysplasia was a strong predictor of malignancy, with 32% to 39% of these polyps ultimately being found to contain cancer on final pathology.

NATURAL HISTORY OF UNTREATED POLYPS

In the modern era, most colon polyps are excised endoscopically or surgically, not only to prevent future growth but also to ensure diagnostic accuracy. As a result, little is known about the natural history of untreated colorectal polyps, and most information must be gathered from studies that predated the widespread adoption of flexible endoscopy. A 1963 study analyzed more than 20,000 barium enemas and found 303 patients with polyps greater than a centimeter in size.[48] Patients were followed with serial contrast enemas for up to 128 months (mean = 30 months), and the investigators found that 20 polyps (6.6%) developed into cancer. The investigators concluded that the rates of growth for most polyps were "exceedingly slow," and most benign adenomatous polyps could not grow into cancer throughout an average person's lifetime. Even the fastest growing cancers reported in this study had doubling times as long as 1155 days.

A similar study from the Mayo Clinic, which predated their experience with endoscopy, was published in 1987, where 226 patients with polyps greater than 1 cm were followed with contrast enemas for a mean of 68 months (range 12–229).[49] Polyp growth was detected in only 37% of polyps, and invasive cancer was found in 9.3% at a mean of 108 months (range 24–225). The investigators estimated that the cumulative risk of malignancy at the site of the index polyp to be 2.5% at 5 years, 8% at 10 years, and 24% at 20 years. This slow rate of growth must be taken into account when recommending therapy for elderly patients or patients with significant life limiting comorbidities.

TREATMENT OPTIONS FOR DIFFICULT COLORECTAL POLYPS
Important Considerations

When considering intervention for a difficult polyp, the physician must ensure that the treatment causes less harm than good. If a polyp is thought to be premalignant, then any intervention is essentially prophylactic in nature. Therefore, a strong understanding of the polyp's natural history, as previously outlined, must be understood and weighed against the risks of intervention. Patient age and comorbidities should impact decision making, and the treatment of a frail, elderly patient with a difficult polyp may be very different from a younger, healthier patient.

Another consideration is whether the surgery is truly "prophylactic." As previously mentioned, many advanced polyps actually contain an invasive malignancy despite benign histology from the original biopsies. In addition, some polyps may be symptomatic, and removal will not only prevent growth but also alleviate problems such as bleeding and mucus secretion.

Polyp number and location are also important. Multiple polyps may require more invasive management than a single polyp, especially if in noncontiguous locations. Regarding location, the cecum is large and thin walled and thus more prone to perforation with advanced polypectomy. Right colectomy is also the simplest and safest location for a laparoscopic colectomy. The rectum, on the other hand, allows for local excision, plus or minus advanced techniques such as transanal endoscopic microsurgery (TEM), and tends to be more forgiving when deeper endoscopic resections are warranted. At the same time, proctectomy has significant functional implications, and a higher risk profile when compared with right colectomy.

Conventional Snare Polypectomy

Because most difficult polyps are benign, endoscopic excision should be performed whenever possible rather than major abdominopelvic surgery. When a difficult polyp exists, the first step is often a repeat colonoscopy by an endoscopist experienced in complex polypectomy,[7,8,50] as endoscopic excision is associated with significantly lower morbidity and cost when compared with laparoscopic colectomy.[51–53]

Conventional snare polypectomy for large difficult polyps has been reported to be safe and feasible. Binmoeller and colleagues[14] reported successful snare polypectomy without submucosal injections in 176 polyps greater than 30 mm. Malignancy was noted in 12% of polyps, and bleeding complications occurred in 24%. There were no perforations and no surgeries performed for complications. Other reports have demonstrated similar success at removing difficult polyps with conventional snare excision.[16,54,55]

Church,[56] Voloyiannis and colleagues,[57] and Lipof and colleagues[21] reported on patients with difficult polyps referred directly to the colorectal surgeon for resection. In all 3 studies, patients underwent repeat colonoscopy by the colorectal surgeon before any surgical resection. Successful snare polypectomy and avoidance of surgery were achieved in 32% to 74% of patients (**Table 1**).

Endoscopic Mucosal Resection

Advanced endoscopic resection techniques are indicated for difficult polyps that are not amenable to simple snaring. Injection-assisted endoscopic mucosal resection (EMR) or "saline lift polypectomy" was first described for rigid sigmoidoscopy in 1955 and adopted to flexible endoscopy in 1973.[58,59] A solution is injected into the submucosal space creating a cushion that allows for snare excision of the overlying mucosa. The lifting allows for better capture of the offending mucosa and protects the deeper muscular layer of the colonic wall from thermal injury. Ideally, the abnormal mucosa is resected with a single snare excision. Alternatively, multiple injections and piecemeal resection may be necessary to completely remove the specimen. Additional techniques to assist in complete resection during EMR have been described, including cap-assisted EMR and suction-assisted EMR. These techniques use a cap that is positioned at the end of the endoscope and allows for suctioning of the desired mucosa into the cap before excision.[59]

Various injection solutions have been used for EMR, and the choice is based on personal experience and preference of the endoscopist. An ideal solution should be inexpensive, readily available, nontoxic, and easy to inject while providing a sustained cushion for resection. There are currently no US Food and Drug Administration-approved injection solutions for EMR, but frequently, normal saline, hyaluronic acid, hydroxypropyl methylcellulose, succinylated gelatin, glycerol, and fibrinogen solutions are used. Dilute epinephrine (1:100,000–1:200,000) is often added to the injection solution to minimize bleeding and delay the reabsorption of the cushion.[59,60] Some endoscopists prefer to add staining dyes, such as indigo carmine or methylene blue, to the injection solution to help discern the margins of

Table 1
Impact of repeat colonoscopy and attempted snare polypectomy to avoid surgery on patients with difficult polyps referred for resection to colorectal surgery service

Author, Year	N	Size	Successful Polypectomy, %	Perforation	Bleeding
Church,[56] 2003	58	Median 45 mm	74	1 (1.7%) postpolypectomy syndrome	5.1%
Voloyiannis et al,[57] 2008	172	Mean 26 mm	59	2 (1%)	5%
Lipof et al,[21] 2005	71	Mean 24 mm	32	Not reported	Not reported

Data from Refs.[21,56,57]

the target lesion. The coloration of the deeper layers is thought to aid in intraprocedural identification of the muscularis propria, and any associated muscular injury or perforation.[59,61,62]

When performing EMR, en bloc resection is preferred to piecemeal polypectomy. En bloc resection allows for more accurate histologic evaluation of the entire specimen and is associated with lower recurrence rates.[63] A meta-analysis by Belderbos and colleagues[64] evaluated 33 studies and noted an overall recurrence rate for EMR resections to be 15%. The recurrence rate is 3% for en bloc resection and 20% for piecemeal resection.

Bleeding is the most common complication after EMR, with reported intraprocedural rates varying from 11% to 22%.[59,63,65] The risk of intraprocedural bleeding is associated with large polyps, minimally elevated sessile polyps, polyps with villous or tubulovillous histology, and EMR performed at low-volume centers. This type of bleeding is typically managed successfully during the procedure with the use of endoclips, coagulation forceps, or coagulation with the snare tip.[63] Postprocedural bleeding rates have been reported to range between 2% and 11%, with clinically significant bleeding reported in 6%.[59,63,65] The risk of postprocedure bleeding is increased with more proximal lesions, larger polyp size, and intraprocedural difficulty or complication.[65]

The risk of colonic perforation during or after EMR is low, with reported rates of 1% to 2%.[63,66] Early recognition of small perforation can be managed with endoclips.[59,63] Late recognition or delayed perforations typically require surgical intervention.

Endoscopic Submucosal Dissection

Endoscopic submucosal dissection (ESD) was first described in 1988 for the resection of gastric lesions and adopted for the treatment of colonic lesions in early 1990s.[67] ESD involves a specialized endoscopic knife, which dissects the polyp off the muscularis propria following submucosal lifting. Compared with EMR, ESD allows for resection of larger, deeper lesions for curative intent.

The initial step in ESD includes marking the lesion to be resected and injecting a lifting agent into the submucosa at its periphery. Using the endoscopic knife, the mucosa is incised circumferentially. Additional submucosal injections are performed as necessary to lift the central portion of the lesion to allow for complete resection. There are many different commercially available devices available to perform ESD. Most of those approved by the US Food and Drug Administration are manufactured by Olympus (Olympus America, Center Valley, PA, USA) and ERBE (ERBE USA, Marietta, GA, USA). In addition to the cutting tool, hemostatic forceps are frequently used to control intraprocedural bleeding. Intraprocedural bleeding, deep resections, and small perforations recognized during the procedure can be closed with endoscopically available clips.

De Ceglie and colleagues[66] performed a systematic review of 66 studies comparing EMR and ESD, and the findings are summarized in **Table 2**. Several other meta-analyses have compared ESD with EMR, and all have demonstrated that ESD has a higher en bloc resection rate and lower local recurrence rate than EMR.[68–70] Despite these advantages, however, ESD was reported to be more time consuming and more often required postprocedural hospitalization. In addition, ESD was also associated with higher risk of perforation (4.8%–10%).[63,66,68]

Bleeding is once again the most often encountered intraprocedural complication associated with ESD and is reported to range from 10% to 22%.[69] When a perforation is encountered, the endoscopist should ensure the defect remains in the field of vision and clear of fluid. Endoscopic clips can be placed to seal the defect. If multiple clips

Table 2
Review comparing more than 17,900 endoscopically resected lesions by endoscopic mucosal resection and endoscopic submucosal dissection

	EMR, %	ESD, %
En-bloc resection rate	62.8 (6793/10,803)	90.5 (5500/6077)
Complete resection rate	92 (9707/10,560)	82.1 (3743/4558)
Bleeding	2.3 (270/11,873)	2.0 (124/6077)
Perforation	0.9 (109/11,873)	4.8 (296/6077)
Recurrence rate	10.4 (765/7303) overall	1.2 (50/3910) overall
	12.1 (131/1085) for piecemeal	1.2 (30/2562) for piecemeal
	3.0 (36/1187) for en bloc	0.2 (5/2562) for en bloc

Data from De Ceglie A, Hassan C, Mangiavillano B, et al. Endoscopic mucosal resection and endoscopic submucosal dissection for colorectal lesions: a systematic review. Crit Rev Oncol Hematol 2016;104:138–55.

are required, placement should be initiated from the lateral edge of the defect to ensure a tension-free closure. Although stricture formation after ESD is reported after esophageal and gastric procedures, stricture after colorectal ESD has not been reported.

Combined Endoscopic and Laparoscopic Surgery

Colon resection has historically been the treatment of choice for benign polyps that could not be managed endoscopically,[25,71,72] but this premise has been recently challenged. A combined endoscopic and laparoscopic approach aims to marry the benefits of both techniques in order to safely remove precancerous polyps without a formal resection. This technique was initially described in 1993 by Drs Beck and Karulf[73] and has since undergone several modifications.

During this procedure, laparoscopic mobilization of the involved colonic segment is performed followed by colonoscopic snare polypectomy. The laparoscopist monitors the serosal side of the colon during the procedure and assists the endoscopist by moving and manipulating the colon to facilitate polypectomy. If concern develops for full-thickness burn or perforation, the site is repaired with laparoscopic suturing. Endoluminal insufflation often helps inspect the suture line for leaks.

Laparoscopic mobilization of the segment of colon harboring the difficult polyp helps the endoscopist better visualize and remove difficult polyps that initially may have been around folds or tight turns. In addition, the surgeon can use laparoscopic instruments to push on the serosal aspect of the colon to "present" the polyp to the endoscopist for polypectomy.[74–76] Submucosal fluid injection to lift the polyp off the underlying muscle may aid polypectomy. If necessary, a colotomy and full-thickness excision can be performed. These combined endoscopic and laparoscopic techniques have been successful in removing 69% to 87% of benign-appearing polyps not amenable to routine snare polypectomy.[75–83]

Another variation of combined endoscopic and laparoscopic surgery uses endoscopy to assist with a limited laparoscopic wedge resection of the colon.[73,74,78] This technique is best used for large lesions in the tip of the cecum or around the appendiceal orifice. The cecum can be mobilized laparoscopically and surgically stapled off while under direct luminal visualization by the endoscopist. The colonoscopic view can be used to monitor the resection margin as well as intubate the ileocecal valve to assure luminal patency during cecectomy.

One of the drawbacks to laparoscopic surgery in conjunction with colonoscopy is the difficulty with visualization and manipulation of the distended colon resulting from endoscopic air insufflation.[84] Because CO_2 is rapidly absorbed from the colonic lumen, the extent and duration of colonic distension are decreased, and this is the preferred method of insufflation for endolaparoscopic cases, offering the laparoscopic surgeon better visualization and safer manipulation of the operative field.[85,86]

Combined endolaparoscopic surgery is still in evolution, and the outcomes of relevant case series are summarized in **Table 3**. When compared with segmental resection, successful combined endoscopic and laparoscopic surgery is associated with lower morbidity, lower cost, and shorter length of hospital stay.[51,81] Success rates range from 67% to 87%, with recurrence rates of 0% to 13%.[75,76,79,81]

Invasive cancer has been reported in combined endoscopic and laparoscopic procedures between 0% and 11%.[75,76,78–81] Some have recommended immediate frozen section evaluation of the polyp at the time of surgery with progression to oncologic resection for those demonstrating invasive cancer.[74,75,77] Others have advocated a more selective approach to frozen section examinations in these cases, because of the low incidence of invasive malignancy, and the time and cost involved in frozen section.[79,83] Ultimately, patients diagnosed with invasive cancer and high-risk features should undergo colectomy.

Transanal Minimally Invasive Surgery and Transanal Endoscopic Microsurgery

For difficult polyps located in the rectum, transanal excision is often the best approach. Transanal minimally invasive surgery and TEM are safe and effective techniques for removal of rectal polyps. These techniques are discussed in detail in D. Owen Young and Anjali S. Kumar's article, "Local Excision of Rectal Cancer," in this issue.

Surgical Resection

Historically, surgical resection has been the primary therapy for benign polyps not amenable to endoscopic removal. With the development of advanced endoscopic procedures and combined endoscopic and laparoscopic techniques, surgical

Table 3
Select series of combined endoscopic and laparoscopic surgery for difficult colon polyps

Author, Year	N	Successful Polyp Removal, %	Invasive Cancer, %	Complications, %	Recurrence
Wilhelm et al,[80] 2009	146	82	11	25	0.9%
Wood et al,[77] 2011	13	69	7.7	15	Not reported
Lee et al,[79] 2013	75	74	6.7	9.2	10%
Crawford et al,[76] 2015	30	67	3.3	10	3.3%
Yan et al,[75] 2011	23	87	0	0	13%
Franklin et al,[78] 2007	110	83	9	0	Not reported
Goh et al,[81] 2014	30	73	6.7	13.3	0%
Cruz et al,[87] 2011	25	76	4	8	Not reported

Data from Refs.[75–81,87]

resection for difficult colorectal polyps should be reserved for failure or lack of availability of these less invasive approaches. When colon resection is required, a formal oncologic resection with high ligation of the feeding artery has been recommended because of the previously mentioned high incidence of invasive cancers. Most resections can be performed laparoscopically and are generally safe and well tolerated. Despite significant technical advancements in recent years, segmental colectomy is often still required to safely remove complex polyps and should remain an important tool in the surgeon's armamentarium.

SUMMARY

Advances in technology along with an improved understanding of the natural history of colonic polyps have opened the doors for many new techniques for the management of difficult polyps. Many patient-specific and polyp-specific factors must be considered. In the modern era, most premalignant polyps can be completely removed without invasive surgery. However, surgical resection is still appropriate for the most difficult lesions.

REFERENCES

1. Muto T, Bussey HJR, Morson BC. The evolution of cancer of the colon and rectum. Cancer 1975;36:2251–70.
2. Morson B. President's address. The polyp-cancer sequence in the large bowel. Proc R Soc Med 1977;67:451–7.
3. Winawer SJ, Zauber AG. The advanced adenoma as the primary target of screening. Gastrointest Endosc Clin N Am 2002;12:1–9.
4. Winawer SJ, Zauber AG, Ho MN, et al. Prevention of colorectal cancer by colonoscopic polypectomy. The National Polyp Study Workgroup. N Engl J Med 1993; 329:1977–81.
5. Zauber AG, Winawer SJ, O'Brien MJ, et al. Colonoscopic polypectomy and long-term prevention of colorectal-cancer deaths. N Engl J Med 2012;366:687–96.
6. Nishihara R, Wu K, Lochhead P, et al. Long-term colorectal-cancer incidence and mortality after lower endoscopy. N Engl J Med 2013;369:1095–105.
7. Hewett DG. Colonoscopic polypectomy: current techniques and controversies. Gastroenterol Clin North Am 2013;42:443–58.
8. Gallegos-Orozco JF, Gurudu SR. Complex colon polypectomy. Gastroenterol Hepatol 2010;6:375–82.
9. Waye JD. Advanced polypectomy. Gastrointest Endosc Clin N Am 2005;15: 733–56.
10. Conio M, Repici A, Demarquay JF, et al. EMR of large sessile colorectal polyps. Gastrointest Endosc 2004;60:234–41.
11. Gorgun E, Benlice C, Church JM. Does cancer risk in colonic polyps unsuitable for polypectomy support the need for advanced endoscopic resections? J Am Coll Surg 2016;223:478–84.
12. Brooker JC, Saunders BP, Shah SG, et al. Endoscopic resection of large sessile colonic polyps by specialist and non-specialist endoscopists. Br J Surg 2002;89: 1020–4.
13. Church JM. Experience in the endoscopic management of large colonic polyps. ANZ J Surg 2003;73:988–95.
14. Binmoeller KF, Bohnacker S, Seifert H, et al. Endoscopic snare excision of "giant" colorectal polyps. Gastrointest Endosc 1996;43:183–8.

15. Dell'Abate P, Iosca A, Galimberti A, et al. Endoscopic treatment of colorectal benign-appearing lesions 3 cm or larger: techniques and outcomes. Dis Colon Rectum 2001;44:112–8.

16. Doniec JM, Lohnert MS, Schniewind B, et al. Endoscopic removal of large colorectal polyps: prevention of unnecessary surgery? Dis Colon Rectum 2003;46:340–8.

17. Kouklakis G, Mpoumponaris A, Gatopoulou A, et al. Endoscopic resection of large pedunculated colonic polyps and risk of postpolypectomy bleeding with adrenaline injection versus endoloop and hemoclip: a prospective, randomized study. Surg Endosc 2009;23:2732–7.

18. Tholoor S, Tsagkournis O, Basford P, et al. Managing difficult polyps: techniques and pitfalls. Ann Gastroenterol 2013;26:114–21.

19. Monkemuller K, Neumann H, Fry LC, et al. Polypectomy techniques for difficult colon polyps. Dig Dis 2008;26:342–6.

20. Vormbrock K, Monkemuller K. Difficult colon polypectomy. World J Gastrointest Endosc 2012;16:269–80.

21. Lipof T, Bartus C, Sardella W, et al. Preoperative colonoscopy decreases the need for laparoscopic management of colonic polyps. Dis Colon Rectum 2005;48:1076–80.

22. Sonnenberg A, Boardman CR. Costs of fear. Am J Gastroenterol 2013;108:173–5.

23. Overhiser AJ, Rex DK. Work and resources needed for endoscopic resection of large sessile colorectal polyps. Clin Gastroenterol Hepatol 2007;5:1076–9.

24. Galandiuk S, Fazio VW, Jagelman DG, et al. Villous and tubulovillous adenomas of the colon and rectum. A retrospective review, 1964-1985. Am J Surg 1987;153:41–7.

25. Loungnarath R, Mutch MG, Birnbaum EH, et al. Laparoscopic colectomy using cancer principles is appropriate for colonoscopically unresectable adenomas of the colon. Dis Colon Rectum 2010;53:1017–22.

26. Bertelson NL, Kalkbrenner KA, Merchea A, et al. Colectomy for endoscopically unresectable polyps: how often is it cancer? Dis Colon Rectum 2012;55(11):1111–6.

27. Shinya H, Wolff WI. Morphology, anatomic distribution and cancer potential of colonic polyps. Ann Surg 1979;190:679–83.

28. O'Brien MJ, Winawer SJ, Zauber AG, et al. The National Polyp Study. Patient and polyp characteristics associated with high-grade dysplasia in colorectal adenomas. Gastroenterology 1990;98:371–9.

29. McDonald JM, Moonka R, Bell RH Jr. Pathologic risk factors of occult malignancy in endoscopically unresectable colonic adenomas. Am J Surg 1999;177:384–7.

30. Ramirez M, Schierling S, Papaconstantinou HT, et al. Management of the malignant polyp. Clin Colon Rectal Surg 2008;21:286–90.

31. Uno Y, Munakata A. The non-lifting sign of invasive colon cancer. Gastrointest Endosc 1994;40:485–9.

32. Participants in Paris Workshop. The Paris endoscopic classification of superficial neoplastic lesions: esophagus, stomach, and colon: November 30 to December 1, 2002. Gastrointest Endosc 2003;58:S3–43.

33. Kudo SE, Lambert R, Allen JI, et al. Nonpolypoid neoplastic lesions of the colorectal mucosa. Gastrointest Endosc 2008;68:S3–47.

34. Hayashi N, Tanaka S, Hewett DG, et al. Endoscopic prediction of deep submucosal invasive carcinoma: validation of the narrow-band imaging international colorectal endoscopic (NICE) classification. Gastrointest Endosc 2013;78:625–32.

35. Kanao H, Tanaka S, Oka S, et al. Clinical significance of type V(I) pit pattern sub-classification in determining the depth of invasion of colorectal neoplasms. World J Gastroenterol 2008;14:211–7.

36. Sanchez-Yague A, Kaltencach T, Raju G, et al. Advanced endoscopic resection of colorectal lesions. Gastroenterol Clin North Am 2013;42:459–77.

37. Saitoh Y, Obara T, Watari J, et al. Invasion depth diagnosis of depressed type early colorectal cancers by combined use of videoendsocopy and chromoendo-scopy. Gastrointest Endosc 1998;48:362–70.

38. Seitz U, Bohnacker S, Seewald S, et al. Is endoscopic polypectomy an adequate therapy for malignant colorectal adenomas? Presentation of 114 patients and review of the literature. Dis Colon Rectum 2004;47:1789–96.

39. Aarons CB, Shanmugan S, Bleier JI. Management of malignant colon polyps: current status and controversies. World J Gastroenterol 2014;20:16178–83.

40. Hall JF. Management of malignant adenomas. Clin Colon Rectal Surg 2015;28:215–9.

41. Nivatvongs S, Rojanasakul A, Reiman H, et al. The risk of lymph node metastasis in colorectal polyps with invasive adenocarcinoma. Dis Colon Rectum 1991;34:323–8.

42. Nivatvongs S. Surgical management of malignant colorectal polyps. Surg Clin North Am 2002;82:959–66.

43. Kudo S. Endoscopic mucosal resection of flat and depressed types of early colorectal cancer. Endoscopy 1993;25:455–61.

44. Nascimbeni R, Burgart L, Nivatvongs S, et al. Risk of lymph node metastasis in T1 carcinoma of the colon and rectum. Dis Colon Rectum 2002;45:200–6.

45. Kikuchi R, Takano M, Takagi K, et al. Management of early invasive colorectal cancer: risk of recurrence and clinical guidelines. Dis Colon Rectum 1995;38:1286–95.

46. Kitajima K, Fujimori T, Fujii S, et al. Correlations between lymph node metastasis and depth of submucosal invasion in submucosal invasive colorectal carcinoma: a Japanese collaborative study. J Gastroenterol 2004;39:534–43.

47. Repici A, Pellicano R, Strangio G, et al. Endoscopic mucosal resection for early colorectal neoplasia: pathologic basis, procedures, and outcomes. Dis Colon Rectum 2009;52:1502–15.

48. Welin S, Youker J, Spratt JS Jr. The rates and patterns of growth of 375 tumors of the large intestine and rectum observed serially by double contrast enema study (Malmoe technique). Am J Roentgenol Radium Ther Nucl Med 1963;90:673–87.

49. Stryker SJ, Wolff BG, Culp CE, et al. Natural history of untreated colonic polyps. Gastroenterol 1987;93:1009–13.

50. Aziz Aadam A, Wani S, Kahi C, et al. Physician assessment and management of complex colon polyps: a multicenter video-based survey study. Am J Gastroenterol 2014;109:1312–24.

51. Church J, Erkan A. Scope or scalpel? A matched study of the treatment of large colorectal polyps. ANZ J Surg 2016. http://dx.doi.org/10.1111/ans.13675.

52. Law R, Das A, Gregory D, et al. Endoscopic resection is cost-effective compared with laparoscopic resection in the management of complex colon polyps: an economic analysis. Gastrointest Endosc 2016;83:1248–57.

53. Swan MP, Bourke MJ, Alexander S, et al. Large refractory colonic polyps: is it time to change our practice? A prospective study of the clinical and economic impact of a tertiary referral colonic mucosal resection and polypectomy service (with videos). Gastrointest Endosc 2009;70:1128–36.

54. Nivatvongs S, Snover DC, Fang DT. Piecemeal snare excision of large sessile colon and rectal polyps: is it adequate? Gastrointest Endosc 1984;30:18–20.

55. Bedogni G, Bertoni G, Ricci E, et al. Colonoscopic excision of large and giant colorectal polyps: technical implications and results over eight years. Dis Colon Rectum 1986;29:831–5.

56. Church J. Avoiding surgery in patients with colorectal polyps. Dis Colon Rectum 2003;46:1513–6.

57. Voloyiannis T, Snyder MJ, Bailey HR, et al. Management of the difficult colon polyp referred for resection: resect or rescope? Dis Colon Rectum 2008;51: 292–5 [Erratum appears in Dis Colon Rectum 2008;51:1300].

58. Rosenberg N. Submucosal saline wheal as safety factor in fulguration of rectal and sigmoidal polypi. AMA Arch Surg 1995;70:120–2.

59. ASGE Technology Committee, Hwang JH, Konda V, et al. Endoscopic mucosal resection. Gastrointest Endosc 2015;82:215–26.

60. Fujishiro M, Yahagi N, Kashimura K, et al. Comparison of various submucosal injection solutions for maintaining mucosal elevation during endoscopic mucosal resection. Endoscopy 2004;36:579–83.

61. Holt BA, Javasekeran V, Sonson R, et al. Topical submucosal chromoendoscopy defines the level of resection in colonic EMR and may improve procedural safety (with video). Gastrointest Endosc 2013;77:949–53.

62. Binmoeller KF, Weilert F, Shah J, et al. "Underwater" EMR without submucosal injection for large sessile colorectal polyps (with video). Gastrointest Endosc 2012; 75:1086–91.

63. Klein A, Bourke MJ. Advanced polypectomy and resection techniques. Gastrointest Endosc Clin N Am 2015;25:303–33.

64. Belderbos TD, Leenders M, Moons LM, et al. Local recurrence after endoscopic mucosal resection of nonpedunculated colorectal lesions: systematic review and meta-analysis. Endoscopy 2014;46:388–402.

65. Burgess NG, Metz AJ, Williams SJ, et al. Risk factors for intraprocedural and clinically significant delayed bleeding after wide-field endoscopic mucosal resection of large colonic lesions. Clin Gastroenterol Hepatol 2014;12:651–61.

66. De Ceglie A, Hassan C, Mangiavillano B, et al. Endoscopic mucosal resection and endoscopic submucosal dissection for colorectal lesions: a systematic review. Crit Rev Oncol Hematol 2016;104:138–55.

67. Hirao M, Masuda K, Asanuma T, et al. Endoscopic resection of early gastric cancer and other tumors with local injection of hypertonic saline-epinephrine. Gastrointest Endosc 1988;34:264–9.

68. Saito Y, Fukuzawa M, Matsuda T, et al. Clinical outcome of endoscopic submucosal dissection versus endoscopic mucosal resection of large colorectal tumors as determined by curative resection. Surg Endosc 2010;24:343–52.

69. Wang J, Zhang XH, Ge J, et al. Endoscopic submucosal dissection vs endoscopic mucosal resection for colorectal tumors: a meta-analysis. World J Gastroenterol 2014;20:8282–6.

70. Fujiya M, Tanaka K, Dokoshi T, et al. Efficacy and adverse events of EMR and endoscopic submucosal dissection for the treatment of colon neoplasms: a meta-analysis of studies comparing EMR and endoscopic submucosal dissection. Gastrointest Endosc 2015;81:583–95.

71. Pokala N, Delaney CP, Kiran RP, et al. Outcome of laparoscopic colectomy for polyps not suitable for endoscopic resection. Surg Endosc 2007;21:400–3.

72. Lascarides C, Buscaglia JM, Denoya PI, et al. Laparoscopic right colectomy vs laparoscopic-assisted colonoscopic polypectomy for endoscopically unresectable polyps: a randomized controlled trial. Colorectal Dis 2016;18(11):1050–6.
73. Beck DE, Karulf RE. Laparoscopic-assisted full thickness endoscopic polypectomy. Dis Colon Rectum 1993;36:693–5.
74. Franklin ME, Diaz-E JA, Abrego D, et al. Laparoscopic-assisted colonoscopic polypectomy: the Texas Endosurgery Institute experience. Dis Colon Rectum 2000;43:1246–9.
75. Yan J, Koiana T, Lee S, et al. Treatment for right colon polyps not removable using standard colonoscopy: combined laparoscopic-colonoscopic approach. Dis Colon Rectum 2011;54:753–8.
76. Crawford AB, Yang I, Wu RC, et al. Dynamic article: combined endoscopic-laparoscopic surgery for complex colonic polyps: postoperative outcomes and video demonstration of 3 key operative techniques. Dis Colon Rectum 2015;58: 363–9.
77. Wood JJ, Lord AC, Wheeler JM, et al. Laparo-endoscopic resection for extensive and inaccessible colorectal polyps: a feasible and safe procedure. Ann R Coll Surg Engl 2011;93:241–5.
78. Franklin ME, Leyva-Alvizo A, Abrego-Medina D, et al. Laparoscopically monitored colonoscopic polypectomy: an established form of endoluminal therapy for colorectal polyps. Surg Endosc 2007;21:1650–3.
79. Lee SW, Garrett KA, Shin JH, et al. Dynamic article: long-term outcomes of patients undergoing combined endolaparoscopic surgery for benign colon polyps. Dis Colon Rectum 2013;56:869–73.
80. Wilhelm D, von Delius S, Weber L, et al. Combined laparoscopic-endoscopic resections of colorectal polyps: 10-year experience and follow-up. Surg Endosc 2009;23:688–93.
81. Goh C, Burke JP, McNamara DA, et al. Endolaparoscopic removal of colonic polyps. Colorectal Dis 2014;16:271–5.
82. Fukunaga Y, Tamegai Y, Chino A, et al. New technique of en bloc resection of colorectal tumor using laparoscopy and endoscopy cooperatively (laparoscopy and endoscopy cooperative surgery-colorectal). Dis Colon Rectum 2014;57: 267–71.
83. Lin AY, O'Mahoney PR, Milsom JW, et al. Dynamic article: full-thickness excision for benign colon polyps using combined endoscopic laparoscopic surgery. Dis Colon Rectum 2016;59:16–21.
84. Kim SH, Milsom JW, Church JM, et al. Perioperative tumor localization for laparoscopic colorectal surgery. Surg Endosc 1997;11:1013–6.
85. Sajid MD, Caswell J, Bhatti MI, et al. Carbon dioxide insufflation vs conventional air insufflation for colonoscopy: a systemic review and meta-analysis of published randomized controlled trials. Colorectal Dis 2015;17:111–23.
86. Nakajima K, Lee SW, Sonoda T, et al. Intraoperative carbon dioxide colonoscopy: a safe insufflation alternative for locating colonic lesions during laparoscopic surgery. Surg Endosc 2005;19:321–5.
87. Cruz RA, Ragupathi M, Pedraza R, et al. Minimally invasive approaches for the management of "difficult" colonic polyps. Diagn Ther Endosc 2011;2011:1–5.

Emergency Presentations of Colorectal Cancer

Canaan Baer, MD[a],*, Raman Menon, MD[a], Sarah Bastawrous, DO[b],
Amir Bastawrous, MD, MBA[a]

KEYWORDS

- Emergency • Colorectal • Carcinoma • Obstruction • Perforation • Bleeding
- Endoluminal stent

KEY POINTS

- Proximal large bowel obstructions are typically treated with resection and anastomosis, whereas distal obstructions have more treatment options and require more catering to the individual situation.
- Obstructing rectal cancer is treated with proximal diversion, allowing for appropriate neoadjuvant therapy before oncologic resection.
- The approach to perforated cancers depends on the degree of peritoneal contamination and associated sepsis.
- Massive hemorrhage is uncommon in colorectal cancer and is treated similar to benign sources of colonic hemorrhage.

INTRODUCTION

Despite increased screening efforts, up to 33% of patients with colorectal cancer will present with symptoms requiring acute or emergent surgical intervention.[1,2] Common emergency presentations include large bowel obstruction, perforation, and hemorrhage. Rates of morbidity, mortality, and stoma formation are higher for patients requiring emergent intervention compared with those managed electively.[3,4] Worse outcomes are felt to be not only related to the emergency itself but also to baseline differences in the 2 patient populations, with emergency patients having more physiologic derangements, dehydration and electrolytes abnormalities, poor nutrition, and neglected comorbidities.

Tumor biology may also play a role in their presentation and outcome. Cancers resected emergently are typically of a more advanced T stage, higher histologic grade,

Disclosures: Dr A. Bastawrous received an honorarium from Intuitive Surgical and Cubist Pharmaceuticals. Dr C. Baer received a grant from the Foundation for Surgical Fellowships.
[a] Colon and Rectal Clinic, Swedish Medical Center, 1101 Madison, Suite 500, Seattle, WA 98104, USA; [b] Department of Radiology, Puget Sound Veteran's Affairs Administration Hospital, University of Washington, 1660 South Columbian Way, Seattle, WA 98108, USA
* Corresponding author.
E-mail address: canaan.baer@swedish.org

and more likely to exhibit lymphovascular invasion.[5-7] Concomitant liver metastases are common as well.[7-9] If forced to operate at the patient's index presentation, the diagnosis and accurate staging information may be unavailable or incomplete. When initial findings suggest widely metastatic disease, the necessity for emergent interventions may have lasting implications on the eligibility for systemic chemotherapy.

The complexities of patients presenting with limited information and suboptimal physiology require individualization of surgical management. The tenets of oncologic resection for colorectal cancer surgery include wide radial, proximal, and distal margins and high ligation of the lymphovascular pedicle for extended lymphadenectomy (>12 nodes). These oncologic principles should be upheld even in cases of emergency surgery for symptomatic colorectal cancers.

The Clinical Practice Guidelines Committee of the American Society of Colon and Rectal Surgeons defines goals of treatment of colon cancer–related emergencies to include the following: (1) avert the immediate negative impact of the complication; (2) achieve the best possible tumor control; (3) ensure timely recovery to permit initiation of appropriate adjuvant or systemic treatment.[10] In this article, the authors look at specific emergency scenarios and the surgical options to achieve those goals.

LARGE BOWEL OBSTRUCTION

Obstruction is a common symptom of colorectal cancer, with an incidence range of 15% to 29%.[11] Obstruction is also the most common indication for emergency surgery for colorectal cancer, making up 77% of emergencies in a recent series.[3] Similarly, colonic malignancy is the most common cause of large bowel obstruction in adults.[1,12,13] As such, surgery for large bowel obstruction presenting acutely should be performed in an oncologic fashion, even if a formal diagnosis of malignancy has not yet been made. Patients presenting with obstruction and no evidence of metastatic disease should be operated on with curative intent.[1]

The presentation of complete bowel obstruction from a colon cancer is typically delayed by a gradual onset of symptoms. Patients may report increasing difficulty with bowel movements or self-medicating with over-the-counter laxatives. They may have developed significant abdominal distension before complete obstipation results in a need for emergency medical attention. Such an insidious onset can result in fairly stable physiology in patients presenting with malignant obstructions. Severe dehydration and electrolyte abnormalities are typically late signs. In some cases, symptoms can be sudden in onset, with severe persistent colicky abdominal pain.[14]

Computed tomography (CT) has become the imaging modality of choice for patients presenting with symptoms concerning for colonic obstruction. It is readily available in emergency departments and can localize an obstructing lesion with a sensitivity of 96% and specificity of 93%.[15,16] Particularly with the use of a triple-contrast protocol (oral, rectal, and intravenous [IV]), CT can make an accurate diagnosis in nearly 89% of cases. CT also offers accurate staging information of both locoregional and distant disease spread[15-17] (Fig. 1).

Although less commonly used in current practice, hydrosoluble contrast enema is also a valuable imaging technique. Sensitivity and specificity in colonic obstructions are 80% and 100%, respectively.[15-17] In a stool-filled colon, CT may not be able to identify a small intraluminal lesion that is readily apparent on contrast enema[16] (Fig. 2).

Colonoscopy is often not available or appropriate in the emergency setting, and patients presenting in extremis may require surgical intervention before an endoscopic evaluation can be arranged. When feasible, colonoscopy offers the ability to identify

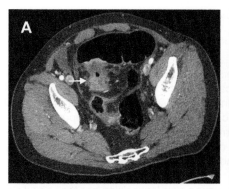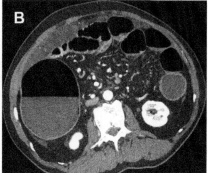

Fig. 1. (*A*) Axial CT images with IV contrast in a patient with an obstructing sigmoid adeno-carcinoma (*arrow*). (*B*) There is marked dilatation of the cecum with an air fluid level. Note omental caking due to metastases.

and localize an obstructing lesion as well as to confirm a diagnosis with tissue sampling. Colonoscopy also offers the potential for relief of obstructions with placement of endoluminal stents, to be discussed in more detail later. When encountered outside of the emergency setting, lacking corollary symptoms, a lesion that cannot be traversed with a standard colonoscope (diameter 11.8–13.0 mm) is much more likely to require an emergency operation, with a hazard ratio of 6.9 (1.6–29.7).[4] This finding warrants an expedited referral to a surgical specialist.

Obstructing colon cancers can be defined as occurring either proximal or distal to the splenic flexure, with site of disease having a significant impact on treatment options. The left colon is more prone to obstruction, most commonly in the sigmoid.[18] Reasons for this include a tendency toward morphologically more annular lesions, a relatively narrow colonic luminal diameter, and a thicker stool consistency.[19] The

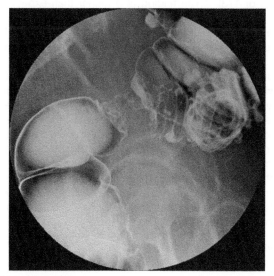

Fig. 2. Hydrosoluble contrast enema reveals a 4-cm annular carcinoma at the rectosigmoid junction.

larger diameter of the right colon means that obstructions are less common, typically involving very bulky tumors.

Proximal Obstructions

Because of the larger diameter of the cecum and ascending colon, right-sided obstructions are less common and historically thought to represent bulky tumors of more advanced stage. Early studies found lower disease-free survival in proximal obstructing cancers compared with distal cancers, independent of perioperative complications or the presence of lymph node metastases.[19] A more recent analysis, however, looked at 377 patients undergoing colectomy for obstructing cancers, evenly split between proximal and distal sites, and found no difference in rates of recurrence or 3-year survival.[20]

In general, proximal colonic obstructions have a simpler decision tree than distal obstructions. Resection is often viewed as less technically demanding and most patients can undergo an ileocolonic anastomosis, which is lower risk for complications when compared to colocolonic or colorectal anastomoses. Reasons for this anastomosis being more favorable include a more reliable blood supply and a lower incidence of significant proximal bowel dilation and size mismatch.

Oncologic resection with primary anastomosis for right colon cancers has long been advocated as safe and definitive surgical management in all but the frailest of patients, with fewer anastomotic complications compared with distal resections.[8] The leak rate after right hemicolectomy or extended right colectomy, even in emergency settings, is estimated at 2.8% to 4.6%, leading many to pursue this approach even in high-risk patients.[17] This rate is somewhat higher than the reported leak rate for an elective right colectomy in the range of 1% to 2%.

Other studies, however, have documented higher rates of complications. A recent review of 87 emergency colectomies included 43 proximal cancers. Anastomotic dehiscence after right hemicolectomy occurred in 12% (4 of 33). Two additional patients had resection of the transverse colon only with primary colocolonic anastomosis; 1 leaked.[3] In another large study, the leak rate after right colectomy was as high as 16.4% (28 of 173).[20] The finding of a higher-than-expected leak rate after right colectomies has led some investigators to advocate the benefits of a protective or terminal stoma in a subset of high-risk patients.[21] Specific criteria have yet to be defined. In these cases, attempt should still be made for definitive oncologic resection.

The operative approach to an obstructing ascending colon tumor is typically a right hemicolectomy with high ligation of the ileocolic artery and the right branch of the middle colic artery, and an ileo-transverse anastomosis. When tumors are present in the mid to distal transverse colon, a proper oncologic resection includes high ligation of the middle colic artery. When this is required, there is vascular compromise of the "watershed" splenic flexure, and the best approach is an "extended right colectomy," including resection of the splenic flexure and an ileo-descending anastomosis. Of note, whenever the patient's baseline condition or the intraoperative variables lead to a high risk of anastomotic leak, the safest approach is resection with an end ileostomy. For patients with more equivocal presentations, ileocolonic anastomosis with a proximal loop ileostomy may be appropriate.

Distal Obstructions

Because of narrow bowel diameter and thicker stool consistency, the descending and sigmoid colon are common sites for obstructing colon carcinomas. Compared with proximal lesions, there are considerably more options available to the surgeon addressing such a patient. Although it is widely acknowledged that the specific approach must be tailored to each individual patient, surgeon expertise, and available resources, there remains significant controversy on the optimal emergency management of obstructing distal colon cancers. These options are outlined and compared in a 2010 guideline statement from the World Society for Emergency Surgery (WSES) and Peritoneum and Surgery Society.[22]

Loop colostomy

Loop colostomy is an established component of the surgical treatment options for obstructing distal carcinomas, with the intent of providing definitive oncologic resection in a staged approach. The obstruction is thus managed in the first stage with creation of a proximal loop colostomy. In the second stage, the tumor is resected and the stoma reversed. Alternatively, colostomy reversal can be performed as a third stage. Depending on patient- and tumors-specific factors, the transverse or descending colon can be used. In general, a loop ileostomy is discouraged, because the presence of a competent ileocecal valve may prevent adequate alleviation of the distal obstruction.

The appeal of this staged approach is that it minimizes operative time and surgical trauma during the acute presentation when physiologic derangements and tissue integrity are suboptimal. The initial colostomy may even be performed with only local analgesia in some cases.[15] It also reduces the risk of contamination from unprepared bowel and allows for complete staging and multidisciplinary review before definitive treatment.[22] However, loop colostomies are often associated with high complication rates, including stomal prolapse, hernia, and dehydration, and the approach does not allow for an oncologic resection.

Loop colostomy is a safe option best suited to patients who are too frail to endure a resectional procedure. Loop colostomy may also be appropriate when the cancer is locally advanced and invading adjacent organs, limiting the feasibility of a proper oncologic resection in an emergency situation.

Hartmann resection

The classic Hartmann procedure involves resection of the primary lesion with creation of an end colostomy and closing the distal colon/rectum. Large reviews have established the feasibility of emergency resection following standard oncologic principles of high ligation of the vascular pedicle, retrieval of at least 12 regional lymph nodes, and en bloc resection of adjacent tissues for negative margins.[3,23] Like a loop colostomy, this approach mitigates the risk of anastomotic leak. Hartmann resection is currently the most common operation performed for distal colon carcinomas presenting emergently, especially by general surgeons.[15,24,25]

Despite the longer operative time for a formal resection, literature has not shown any worse short- or long-term outcomes in patients undergoing formal Hartmann resection compared with the staged approach. A randomized study by Kronborg[26] showed no difference in mortality, recurrence rate, and cancer-specific survival between colostomy or Hartmann procedure in emergency presentations. The only difference found in this study was a longer hospital stay in the staged approach due to the need for multiple subsequent operations. Of note, this study has been criticized for its long accrual period, incomplete follow-up, and heterogenous underlying pathology. A Cochrane systematic review in 2004, which did not include the Kronborg study due to methodological flaws, nevertheless made the same conclusions.[27] WSES guidelines conclude that colostomy (staged approach) should be reserved for "damage control" situations, unresectable tumors, and cases where multimodal treatment is anticipated before formal resection.[22]

A contradictory conclusion was made by another recent randomized controlled trial (RCT), which found no difference in outcomes, including transfusion rates or duration of hospitalization between a staged approach and Hartmann resection.[28] The investigators of this study argue rather that colostomy for staged approach is ideal for younger, healthier patients who will tolerate definitive surgery in as little as 2 to 3 weeks when less bowel distention and inflammation may allow for a technically easier and more oncologically sound resection.[28] Nevertheless, most investigators agree that Hartmann resection is the procedure of choice for older patients with high American Society of Anesthesiologists (ASA) scores, advanced obstructions, and proximal bowel distention, and whose underlying medical comorbidities might preclude definitive surgery in a staged fashion.[15,22,26–28]

The main disadvantage of a Hartmann resection is the residual stoma. Among patients with colon cancer, the rate of Hartmann reversal is only 20% for reasons including advanced disease, complications from treatment, and poor performance status.[29,30] Operations to restore intestinal continuity are also associated with significant morbidity and mortality.[15] Stomas are not without their own complications, and rates increase the longer they are in place, adversely affecting quality of life.[31,32]

Single-stage primary resection and anastomosis

For many years, a single-stage oncologic resection with primary anastomosis was considered too high of a risk in the emergency setting. Concerns included further physiologic derangement to a critically ill patient, increased extent of surgery and operating room time, difficulty manipulating and mobilizing a distended colon, and potential for contamination of the peritoneal cavity. Patients may be severely malnourished due to reduced oral intake before presenting with obstruction, and proceeding with an operation before nutritional optimization may increase their risk for postoperative complications, especially if the condition of proximal bowel is dilated, ischemic, or otherwise suboptimal for an anastomosis. Of utmost importance are the complications from an anastomotic leak, which can be catastrophic and forestall adjuvant systemic chemotherapy when indicated.

Large studies, however, have established the feasibility of primary resection and anastomosis (PRA) in appropriately selected patients. Resection with primary anastomosis can reduce length of stay and reduce number of operations with similar rates of morbidity and mortality. Nonrandomized reviews and retrospective data have shown the rate of anastomotic leak in emergency settings to be 2.2% to 12%, which is similar to rates in elective colon resection of 1.9% to 8%.[22] Thus, even in acutely symptomatic distal colon carcinomas, PRA is recommended in the position statement from the Association of Coloproctologists of Great Britain and Ireland.[31,33]

Appropriate patient selection is critical to success in this inherently high-risk environment. Specific factors that have been associated with poor outcomes in obstructing colon cancer operations include age greater than 70, ASA grades III–IV, preoperative renal failure, surgery within 24 hours of presentation, and advanced cancer stage.[21,29,33] Any of these factors may argue for either a Hartmann resection with end colostomy or potentially a primary anastomosis with a protecting loop ileostomy.

Total abdominal colectomy

Total abdominal colectomy with ileorectal anastomosis (TAC/IRA) is another option for select patients. It also removes the distended and potentially ischemic proximal colon, resecting back to healthy terminal ileum for a primary anastomosis. This approach is particularly appropriate in cases with suspected synchronous tumors or hereditary colorectal cancer syndromes. Another very important indication for TAC/IRA is cecal perforation or impending perforation, which is common in advanced distal obstructions. In general, a double resection to remove the cecum and the distal tumor separately, leaving the transverse colon intact, is not recommended.

A small randomized trial compared outcomes from subtotal colectomy to segmental resection (PRA) and found no difference in hospital mortality or complication rates. Segmental colectomies in this study included intraoperative colonic irrigation. At 4 months, however, the subtotal colectomy patients reported more frequent bowel movements and more presentations with bowel problems than in the PRA group. The investigators concluded that subtotal colectomy should be reserved for cases of synchronous lesions or when the integrity and viability of proximal colon is questioned.[34]

Self-expanding metal stents

Self-expandable metal stents (SEMS) represent a nonoperative modality to address distal colonic malignant obstructions. These stents were first developed in the 1990s for palliation of obstructions from unresectable tumors or in patients deemed poor candidates for resectional surgery.[24,35,36] Stents are also used as a temporizing "bridge to surgery" with the goal of enabling elective, possibly laparoscopic, resection.

SEMS involve the endoscopic placement of a guide wire across the obstructing lesion, often with the assistance of fluoroscopy, followed by an uncovered, self-expanding metal stent. Balloon dilation is not typically necessary. Once the stent has been deployed, success is confirmed by a rush of air and fluid past the obstruction (**Fig. 3**). If desired, the endoscope can typically be advanced through the stent to visualize the proximal colon. Although stenting is technically feasible for all areas of the colon, it has been more successful and better studied for left-sided lesions.

Stenting is an attractive alternative to emergency surgery. Proponents argue that stenting can allow for the managing team to stabilize the patient, correct dehydration and other electrolyte imbalances, optimize medical comorbidities and nutritional status, complete oncologic staging, and involve a multidisciplinary team. Early studies supporting the use of SEMS in this context argued that as a bridge to surgery, stents could reduce morbidity and mortality and lower stoma rates compared with surgery alone.[35,37–41]

Not all reported data, however, have supported these initial claims. For example, a recent observational study compared surgery to SEMS as a bridge to surgery. Despite high rates of technical success with stent placement (91%) and relatively low rates of complications (microperforation rate 13%), there was no difference in perioperative mortality and no difference in rates of primary anastomosis or stoma creation.[31]

In a large systematic review and meta-analysis, the rate of clinical success relieving obstruction with SEMS was only 52.5% overall, compared with 99% with surgery. Morbidity and mortality were again similar between groups; however, the rates of primary anastomosis were surprisingly low in the bridge-to-surgery group, only 64.9% compared with 55% in the surgery-first group, not statistically different. Anastomotic leak rates were slightly better in the stented patients, but also not significant.[42]

Stent deployment is not without risk. In fact, of the 6 RCTs comparing SEMS to upfront surgery in distal obstructing cancers, half closed enrollment early due to high rates of stent-related complications, most notably perforation during deployment.[15,35] Other complications include failure to relieve the obstruction, migration, and subsequent stent occlusion. Tumor perforation during stent deployment likely

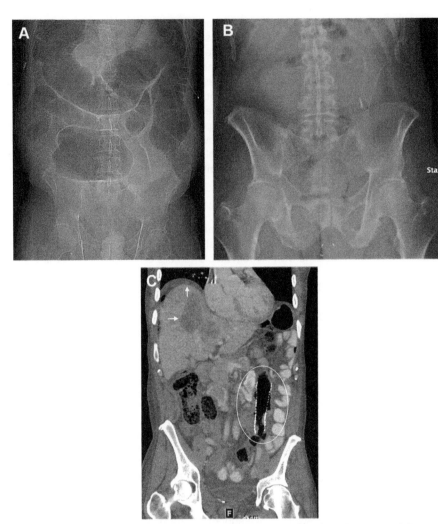

Fig. 3. Anterior posterior upright radiograph (*A*) before and (*B*) after placement of descending colon metal stent for decompression of obstructing colon cancer (*C*). Coronal CT image shows stent in descending colon. Note liver and peritoneal metastatic lesions (*arrow*).

mandates emergency surgery. Peritoneal spillage adds additional physiologic stress to the patient and may limit the surgical options in the setting of feculent peritonitis.

Some authors argue that even following uncomplicated deployment, the local trauma from a stent may encourage tumor cell dissemination and worsen oncologic outcomes.[43] A retrospective comparative study using SEMS as a bridge to surgery found a significantly lower overall 5-year survival in the SEMS group compared with surgery alone (25% vs 62%, respectively). Cancer-specific mortality was also higher in the SEMS group (48% vs 21% for surgery only). There were also nonsignificant benefits for the surgery-only group in disease-free survival, recurrence rates, and mean time to recurrence. In fact, in the study's multivariate analysis, stent insertion was the only modifiable factor affecting the poor outcomes in that arm.[44]

In general, success rates are higher and complication rates lower in SEMS case series involving experienced endoscopists. However, further studies are needed before SEMS is considered the standard for malignant bowel obstructions. In the presence of metastatic disease or short life expectancy, stents may prevent a morbid operation and allow quicker initiation or continuation of systemic chemotherapy. SEMS should only be performed by endoscopists with adequate expertise to limit complication rates.

Obstructing Rectal Cancer

Rectal bleeding and a change in stool appearance are the most common symptoms of rectal cancer.[45] Many early asymptomatic rectal cancers will be found on screening endoscopy, but a rectal cancer presenting with acute obstructive symptoms is typically of a locally advanced stage.

The additional challenges and morbidity associated with pelvic surgery weigh in the decision making for acutely symptomatic rectal cancers. Optimal oncologic resection should include total mesorectal excision. In the elective setting, neoadjuvant chemoradiation has become the standard of care for T3 or node-positive rectal cancers in the United States. Compared with the previous discussion of colon cancers, there is more enthusiasm for measures that safely temporize acute symptoms of rectal cancer to allow for complete staging and initiation of neoadjuvant treatment.

Loop ileostomy or colostomy

In patients with obstructing mid and low rectal cancers without findings of metastatic spread, simple diversion provides the opportunity to complete staging and give neoadjuvant chemoradiation with a staged oncologic resection for curative intent. Loop colostomy allows for decompression as well as access to the proximal colon for assessment of proximal synchronous lesions. However, it may limit opportunities for reconstructing bowel continuity with an eventual low anterior resection by sacrificing bowel length or blood supply to the future anastomosis. A loop ileostomy often works better for these patients, although it is associated with a small risk of a closed loop obstruction when a competent ileocecal valve exists. In the setting where sphincter preservation is clearly not an option, a loop colostomy is more fitting.

Hartmann resection

In the case of obstructing carcinomas of the upper rectum, a Hartmann procedure may be chosen, providing definitive resection without the added risks of an anastomosis. Indeed, this option may be appropriate for older patients with more comorbidities, even in the absence of acute obstruction. Patients should be aware that colostomy reversal in this setting is extremely uncommon.

Self-expandable metal stents

As described above for distal colon cancers, the use of SEMS for obstructing rectal cancers is most appropriate in patients with widely metastatic disease who will benefit most from systemic chemotherapy, or who are too physiologically stressed to tolerate a low anterior resection or abdominal perineal resection. The risk of tumor perforation during placement limits their use in treatment plans with curative intent.[1] Importantly, placement of rectal stents carries significant risk of distal migration and severe tenesmus from pressure on the upper anal sphincter mechanism. Therefore, SEMS is limited to lesions in the upper rectum.

PERFORATION

Perforation is the second most common reason for urgent or emergent surgery associated with colorectal carcinoma, with an incidence of 2.6% to 12%.[46,47] Perforations most commonly occur at the site of the primary tumor, due to necrosis and friable tissue. Depending on the location, these may progress to either free or contained perforations. Perforation can also occur proximal to an obstructing carcinoma. Increasing pressure and distension from a complete distal obstruction follow the Law of Laplace, which can ultimately result in ischemia of the proximal bowel and perforations at remote proximal sites. The cecum is the most common site of this type of diastatic perforation.[6] This clinical presentation has been recognized as an independent prognostic factor for morbidity and mortality.[7]

An obstructing cancer increases the risk of perforation, with rates of 12% to 19%.[48] Perforation is reported to be the most lethal complication of colorectal carcinoma. In some studies, mortality associated with secondary peritonitis from perforation is as high as 30% to 50%.[1,49]

Free Perforation

Free perforation with spillage into the peritoneum is suggested by the classic findings of generalized peritonitis, including involuntary guarding and rebound tenderness. CT imaging may show free air, free fluid, air at the site of perforation, pneumatosis intestinalis, or portal venous air. In the diagnosis of a perforation from colorectal carcinoma, CT has a sensitivity of 95% to 98%, specificity of 95% to 97%, and accuracy of 95%[1] (**Fig. 4**).

Colorectal perforation seeding the peritoneal cavity is a surgical emergency with poor outcomes. These patients can rapidly progress into septic shock, disseminated intravascular coagulation, multisystem organ failure, and death. Although emergent surgical intervention is often required, outcomes have been generally poor, with mortalities ranging in older studies from 6% to 33%.[50–52] Even the most recent series highlighting advanced critical care management, by Yamamoto and colleagues,[50] still report a mortality of 12%. Risk factors included older age and low preoperative blood pressure. Before any operation in the setting of a perforated colorectal cancer, patients and families should be thoroughly counseled regarding the poor prognosis.

The surgical approach is typically open exploration and thorough washout with identification of the diseased and perforated site. Even without the established diagnosis of malignancy, resection of the perforated site should adhere to the principles of oncologic resection with extended lymphadenectomy for accurate pathologic staging. Despite the poor perioperative mortalities, patients presenting with perforation from a colorectal cancer, without findings of widely metastatic lesions, should still be managed with a curative intent. Tumor perforation upstages the lesion's T stage to T4, but does not directly impact the M stage. Oncologic resection typically concludes with creation of an end stoma. Primary anastomosis may be considered in the carefully selected patient, provided that the anastomosis is protected with a diverting ileostomy.[29]

When they cause perforation, lesions proximal to the splenic flexure are twice as likely to result in peritonitis than to form a localized abscess.[53] Poorly contained leaks should also be expected with this is also true of the diastatic perforations mentioned above, wherein a distal obstructing carcinoma results in ischemia and perforation of the proximal bowel, most commonly the cecum. Subtotal colectomy is the operation of choice in these settings. An ileocolic or ileorectal anastomosis may be considered in low-risk patients.[46]

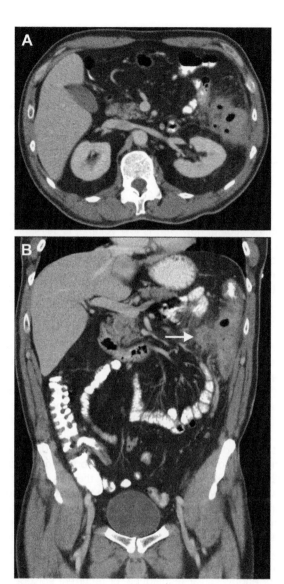

Fig. 4. (A) Axial and (B) coronal CT images show a left colon soft tissue mass with marked narrowing of the lumen with circumferential wall thickening and infiltration of the surrounding pericolonic fat compatible with localized perforation. Note adjacent pericolonic abscess (*arrow*).

Abscess

Contained perforations may present with localized tenderness. Imaging may reveal a phlegmon or abscess, which is more common than free perforation in descending and sigmoid colon lesions.[53] Many cases of perforated colorectal cancer presenting as abscess are not diagnosed preoperatively and can mimic diverticulitis or appendicitis on CT imaging.[46,53]

The role for percutaneous drainage of contained perforations from a carcinoma differs from that of benign diseases. In the presence of widely metastatic disease, treatment with antibiotics and percutaneous drainage avoids the morbidity of an operation. In some cases, however, drawn out infectious complications can forestall systemic chemotherapy. In the absence of widely disseminated disease, percutaneous drainage of a contained perforation may result in seeding tumor cells along the drainage tract rendering the disease metastatic.[53] When a malignancy is suspected, drains should be placed in a manner where the skin and drain tract can be later resected en bloc with the cancer. Definitive surgical management involves en bloc resection of the mass and any invaded adjacent organs and/or percutaneous drains whenever technically feasible.[1]

BLEEDING

Gastrointestinal bleeding is reported in up to 50% of patients with colorectal cancer.[1,54] Most of this bleeding, however, is low volume, is self-limited, and does not require emergent surgical intervention. Bleeding is often an early symptom of a colorectal cancer associated with lower risk of advanced stage at diagnosis, and a shorter delay in presentation. Unlike the insidious onset of an obstructing cancer, patients often remember to the day when bleeding began.[45] Bleeding is complicated by the fact that most acute tumor bleeding is likely in the setting of chronic anemia of cancer and blood loss from the tumor.

Acute massive gastrointestinal bleeding from a colorectal carcinoma is rare. The initial management is aimed at resuscitation, establishing large-bore IV access, and stabilization with crystalloid and correction of underlying coagulopathy or other metabolic abnormalities.

In the clinically stable patient, efforts to localize the source of bleeding should be sought before surgical treatment whenever possible.[1] Endoscopy will identify the source in 74% to 89% of cases, although this technique may be limited in the unprepared colon.[55,56] Tagged red blood cell scan is less sensitive, localizing the source in 26% to 72%, but it does detect bleeding at rates as low as 0.1 mL/min, making it a potential screening test before angioembolization. Embolization has documented success rates of 42% to 86%; however, it carries the risk of worsening intestinal ischemia.[1,55] This option may be more attractive in the setting of metastatic disease to avoid laparotomy and associated delays in systemic chemotherapy.

Surgery is the most effective and definitive approach for a hemorrhaging colorectal cancer. Some general indications for surgical intervention include hemodynamic instability despite transfusion of more than 6 units of blood products, slow bleeding requiring more than 3 units of blood products per day, inability to stop hemorrhage with endoscopic or endovascular techniques, or recurrent episodes of hemorrhagic shock.[57]

When the site has been localized, resection should adhere to oncologic principles with curative intent. The decision to form a stoma or perform a PRA with or without proximal diversion should be carefully considered in light of any anemia, coagulopathy, and unstable hemodynamics that often accompany the bleeding patient.

MINIMALLY INVASIVE PLATFORMS

Emergency laparoscopic colectomy for symptomatic colorectal cancer has been described in several case series and case-control studies. Laparoscopy typically requires longer operative times, but is associated with lower blood loss, shorter hospital stay, and similar morbidities and mortalities when compared with open surgery. Rates of conversion to open surgery range from 0% to 17% in emergency colectomies.[58]

Appropriate patient selection is central to the safety and feasibility of minimally invasive techniques in the emergency setting. Surgeon experience with elective laparoscopic colectomy techniques is prerequisite.

The first case report of emergency robotic colectomy was recently published for a hemorrhagic right-sided colon cancer, with good postoperative and oncologic outcomes.[58]

OUTCOMES

The feasibility of oncologic resections in the emergency setting has been well demonstrated. Teixeira and colleagues[3] documented R0 resection possible in up to 92% of emergency colectomies. Patients for whom R0 resection was not achieved had bulky T4 lesions or were unable to tolerate more radical en bloc resections. Adequate lymphadenectomy (>12 nodes) was documented in 71%.

The long-term and oncologic outcomes for colorectal cancers presenting with emergency complications are worse than their elective counterparts. A recent retrospective review from Ireland included 34% of colon resections performed emergently and collected long-term follow-up to assess oncologic outcomes. Emergency resections were more often T4 lesions (38% vs 13%) and more often lymph node positive (58% vs 38%). Perforation was the indication in 8%. Positive margins were found in 10% of emergency colectomies compared with only 1% of elective cases. With up to 5 years follow-up, the median survival for emergency presentations was only 59 months compared with 82 months for elective cases during the same time.[6] Other studies have shown similar results,[23,59] although exactly what is responsible for these worse outcomes is still debated.[60]

High rates of complications have been associated with urgent or emergent colectomy. One institution's retrospective review of 209 consecutive colectomies found higher rates of wound infections, wound dehiscence, and intra-abdominal abscess in emergency colectomies.[61] The rates of perioperative mortality for emergency colorectal cancer resections range from 5% to 34%.[62–64] The immediate threats to life will dictate how resources are allocated to the resuscitation and preoperative workup. The liberal use of stomas is advocated and demonstrated in most series.

SUMMARY

The management of emergency complications of colorectal carcinomas has changed over the past few decades. For proximal lesions, general consensus is that hemicolectomy with primary anastomosis is safe with an acceptably low leak rate. For distal obstructions, there is active investigation and controversy challenging practices both new and old. Single-stage resections and the use of endoluminal stents to temporize emergency presentations have allowed some surgical specialists to reduce the morbidities of stomas and multiple operations. Ultimately, the best management must be tailored to each specific scenario. In the treatment of emergency presentations of colorectal carcinoma, care must be individualized to the patient, the experience of the surgeon, and the resources available at the facility.

REFERENCES

1. Barnett A, Cedar A, Siddiqui F, et al. Colorectal cancer emergencies. J Gastrointest Cancer 2013;44(2):132–42.
2. Gunnarsson H, Holm T, Ekholm A, et al. Emergency presentation of colon cancer is most frequent during summer. Colorectal Dis 2011;13(6):663–8.

3. Teixeira F, Akaishi EH, Ushinohama AZ, et al. Can we respect the principles of oncologic resection in an emergency surgery to treat colon cancer? World J Emerg Surg 2015;10:5.

4. Chalieopanyarwong V, Boonpipattanapong T, Prechawittayakul P, et al. Endoscopic obstruction is associated with higher risk of acute events requiring emergency operation in colorectal cancer patients. World J Emerg Surg 2013;8:34.

5. Bayar B, Yilmaz KB, Akinci M, et al. An evaluation of treatment results of emergency versus elective surgery in colorectal cancer patients. Ulus Cerrahi Derg 2016;32:11–7.

6. Bass G, Fleming C, Conneely J, et al. Emergency first presentation of colorectal cancer predicts significantly poorer outcomes: a review of 356 consecutive Irish patients. Dis Colon Rectum 2009;52(4):678–84.

7. Alvarez JA, Baldonedo RF, Bear IG, et al. Presentation, treatment, and multivariate analysis of risk factors for obstructive and perforative colorectal carcinoma. Am J Surg 2005;190:376–82.

8. Phillips RK, Hittinger R, Fry JS, et al. Malignant large bowel obstruction. Br J Surg 1985;72:296–302.

9. Garcia-Valdecasas JC, Llovera JM, deLacy AM, et al. Obstructing colorectal carcinomas: prospective study. Dis Colon Rectum 1991;34(9):759–62.

10. Chang GJ, Kaiser AM, Mills S, et al. Practice parameters for the management of colon cancer. Dis Colon Rectum 2012;55:831–43.

11. Ohman U. Prognosis in patients with obstructing colorectal carcinoma. Am J Surg 1982;143:742–7.

12. De Dombal FT, Matharu SS, Staniland JR, et al. Presentation of cancer to the hospital as "acute abdominal pain". Br J Surg 1980;67:413–6.

13. Peterson M. Large intestine. In: Marx JA, Hockberger RS, Walls RM, editors. Rosen's emergency medicine: concepts and clinical practice. 6th edition. Philadelphia: Elsevier; 2006. p. 1332–4.

14. Gordon PH. Malignant neoplasms of the colon. In: Gordon PH, Nivatvongs S, editors. Principles and practice of surgery for the colon, rectum and anus. 3rd edition. New York: Informa Healthcare; 2007. p. 534–5.

15. Frago R, Ramirez E, Millan M, et al. Current management of acute malignant large bowel obstruction: a systematic review. Am J Surg 2014;207:127–38.

16. Frager D, Rovno HD, Baer JW, et al. Prospective evaluation of colonic obstruction with computed tomography. Abdom Imaging 1998;23(2):141–6.

17. Gainant A. Emergency management of acute colonic cancer obstruction. J Visc Surg 2012;149:e3–10.

18. Kleespies A, Fuessl KE, Seeliger H, et al. Determinants of morbidity and survival after elective non-curative resection of stage IV colon and rectal cancer. Int J Colorectal Dis 2009;24:1097–109.

19. Wolmark N, Wieand HS, Rockette HE, et al. The prognostic significance of tumour location and bowel obstruction in Dukes' B and C colorectal cancer. Ann Surg 1983;198:743–50.

20. Frago R, Biondo S, Millan M, et al. Differences between proximal and distal obstructing colonic cancer after curative surgery. Colorectal Dis 2011;13:e116–22.

21. Biondo S, Pares D, Frago R, et al. Large bowel obstruction: predictive factors for postoperative mortality. Dis Colon Rectum 2004;47:1889–97.

22. Ansaloni L, Andersson RE, Bazzoli F, et al. Guidelines in the management of obstructing cancer of the left colon: consensus conference of the World Society of Emergency Surgery (WSES) and Peritoneum and Surgery (PnS) Society. World J Emerg Surg 2010;5:29.

23. McArdle CS, Hole DJ. Emergency presentation of colorectal cancer is associated with poor 5-year survival. Br J Surg 2004;91(5):605–9.
24. Trompetas V. Emergency management of malignant acute left-sided colonic obstruction. Ann R Coll Surg Engl 2008;90:181–6.
25. Meyer F, Marusch F, Koch A, et al. Emergency operation in carcinomas of the left colon: value of Hartmann's procedure. Tech Coloproctol 2004;8(suppl):s226–9.
26. Kronborg O. Acute obstruction from tumour in the left colon without spread. A randomized trial of emergency colostomy versus resection. Int J Colorectal Dis 1995;10:1–5.
27. De Salvo GL, Gava C, Lise M, et al. Curative surgery for obstruction from primary left colorectal carcinoma: primary or staged resection? Cochrane Database Syst 2004;(2):CD002101.
28. Krstic S, Resanovic V, Alempijevic T, et al. Hartmann's procedure vs loop colostomy in the treatment of obstructive rectosigmoid cancer. World J Emerg Surg 2014;9:52.
29. Zorcolo L, Covotta L, Carlomagno N, et al. Safety of primary anastomosis in emergency colorectal surgery. Colorectal Dis 2003;5:262–9.
30. Desai DC, Brennan EJ, Reilly JF, et al. The utility of the Hartmann procedure. Am J Surg 1998;175:152–4.
31. Kavanagh DO, Nolan B, Judge C, et al. A comparative study of short- and medium-term outcomes comparing emergent surgery and stenting as a bridge to surgery in patients with acute malignant colonic obstruction. Dis Colon Rectum 2013;56:433–40.
32. Sprangers MA, Taal BG, Aaronson NK, et al. Quality of life in colorectal cancer. Stoma vs. nonstoma patients. Dis Colon Rectum 1995;38:361–9.
33. Tekkis PP, Kinsman R, Thompson MR, et al. The Association of Coloproctology of Great Britain and Ireland study of large bowel obstruction caused by colorectal cancer. Ann Surg 2004;204:76–81.
34. The SCOTIA Study Group. Single-stage treatment for malignant left-sided colonic obstruction: a prospective randomized clinical trial comparing subtotal colectomy with segmental resection following intraoperative irrigation. Br J Surg 1995;82:1622–7.
35. Kwak MS, Kim WS, Lee JM, et al. Does stenting as a bridge to surgery in left-sided colorectal cancer obstruction really worsen oncological outcomes? Dis Colon Rectum 2016;59:725–32.
36. Dohmoto M, Hünerbein M, Schlag PM. Palliative endoscopic therapy of rectal carcinoma. Eur J Cancer 1996;32a:25–9.
37. Khot UP, Lang AW, Murali K, et al. Systematic review of the efficacy and safety of colorectal stents. Br J Surg 2002;89:1096–102.
38. Cennamo V, Luigiano C, Coccolini F, et al. Meta-analysis of randomized trials comparing endoscopic stenting and surgical decompression for colorectal cancer obstruction. Int J Colorectal Dis 2013;28:855–63.
39. Sebastian S, Johnston S, Geoghegan T, et al. Pooled analysis of the efficacy and safety of self-expanding metal stenting in malignant colorectal obstruction. Am J Gastroenterol 2004;99:2051–7.
40. Matsuda A, Miyashita M, Matsumoto S, et al. Comparison of long-term outcomes of colonic stent as "bridge to surgery" and emergency surgery for malignant large-bowel obstruction: a meta-analysis. Ann Surg Oncol 2015;22:497–504.
41. Zhang Y, Shi J, Shi B, et al. Self-expanding metallic stent as a bridge to surgery versus emergency surgery for obstructive colorectal cancer: a meta-analysis. Surg Endosc 2012;26:110–9.

42. Cirocchi R, Farinella E, Trastulli S, et al. Safety and efficacy of endoscopic colonic stenting as a bridge to surgery in the management of intestinal obstruction due to left colon and rectal cancer: a systematic review and meta-analysis. Surg Oncol 2013;22(1):14–21.

43. Maruthachalam K, Lash GE, Shenton BK, et al. Tumour cell dissemination following endoscopic stent insertion. Br J Surg 2007;94:1151–4.

44. Sabbagh C, Browet F, Diouf M, et al. Is stenting as "a bridge to surgery" an oncologically safe strategy for the management of acute, left-sided, malignant, colonic obstruction? A comparative study with a propensity score analysis. Ann Surg 2013;258:107–15.

45. Korsgaard M, Pedersen L, Sorensen HT, et al. Reported symptoms, diagnostic delay and stage of colorectal cancer: a population-based study in Denmark. Colorectal Dis 2006;8:688–95.

46. Tsai HL, Hsieh JS, Yu FJ, et al. Perforated colonic cancer presenting as intra-abdominal abscess. Int J Colorectal Dis 2007;22(1):15–9.

47. Saegesser F, Sandblom P. Ischemic lesions of the distended colon. A complication of obstructive colorectal cancer. Am J Surg 1975;129:309–15.

48. Umpleby HC, Williamson RCN. Survival in acute obstructing colorectal carcinoma. Dis Colon Rectum 1984;27:299–304.

49. Langell JT, Mulvihill SJ. Gastrointestinal perforation and the acute abdomen. Med Clin North Am 2008;92(3):599–625.

50. Yamamoto T, Kita R, Masui H, et al. Prediction of mortality in patients with colorectal perforation based on routinely available parameters: a retrospective study. World J Emerg Surg 2015;10:24.

51. Horiuchi A, Watanabe Y, Doi T, et al. Evaluation of prognostic factors and scoring system in colonic perforation. World J Gastroenterol 2007;13:3228–31.

52. Komatsu S, Shimomatsuya T, Nakajima M, et al. Prognostic factors and scoring system for survival in colonic perforation. Hepatogastroenterology 2005;52:761–4.

53. Yeo ES, Ng KH, Eu KW. Perforated colorectal cancer: an important differential diagnosis in all presumed diverticular abscesses. Ann Acad Med Singapore 2011;40(8):375–8.

54. Adelstein BA, Macaskill P, Chan SF, et al. Most bowel cancer symptoms do not indicate colorectal cancer and polyps: a systematic review. BMC Gastroenterol 2011;11:65.

55. Zuccaro G Jr. Management of the adult patient with acute lower gastrointestinal bleeding. Am J Gastroenterol 1998;93(8):1202–8.

56. Davila RE, Rajan E, Adler DG, et al. ASGE Guideline: the role of endoscopy in the patient with lower-GI bleeding. Gastrointest Endosc 2005;62(5):656–60.

57. Tavakkolizadeh A, Ashley S. Acute gastrointestinal hemorrhage. In: Townsend CM, Beauchamp RD, Evers BM, et al, editors. Sabiston textbook of surgery: the biological basis of modern surgical practice. 19th edition. Philadelphia: Elsevier; 2012. p. 1139–59.

58. Felli E, Brunetti F, Disabato M, et al. Robotic right colectomy for hemorrhagic right colon cancer: a case report and review of the literature of minimally invasive urgent colectomy. World J Emerg Surg 2014;9:32.

59. Oliphant R, Mansouri D, Nicholson GA, et al. Emergency presentation of node-negative colorectal cancer treated with curative surgery is associated with poorer short and longer-term survival. Int J Colorectal Dis 2014;29:591–8.

60. Weixler B, Warschkow R, Ramser M, et al. Urgent surgery after emergency presentation for colorectal cancer has no impact on overall and disease-free survival: a propensity score analysis. BMC Cancer 2016;16:208.

61. Kim J, Mittal R, Konyalian V, et al. Outcome analysis of patients undergoing colorectal resection for emergent and elective indications. Am Surg 2007;73:991–3.
62. Boyle DJ, Thorn C, Saini A, et al. Predictive factors for successful colonic stenting in acute large-bowel obstruction: a 15-year cohort analysis. Dis Colon Rectum 2015;58:358–62.
63. Breitenstein S, Rickenbacher A, Berdajs D, et al. Systematic evaluation of surgical strategies for acute malignant left-sided colonic obstruction. Br J Surg 2007; 94(12):1451–60.
64. Tan CJ, Dasari BV, Gardiner K. Systematic review and meta-analysis of randomized clinical trials of self-expanding metallic stents as a bridge to surgery versus emergency surgery for malignant left-sided large bowel obstruction. Br J Surg 2012;99:469–76.

Advances in Laparoscopic Colorectal Surgery

James Michael Parker, MD[a], Timothy F. Feldmann, MD[b], Kyle G. Cologne, MD[c],*

KEYWORDS

- Laparoscopy • Minimally invasive surgery • Colorectal cancer
- Hand-assisted laparoscopy • Learning curve

KEY POINTS

- Laparoscopic colorectal surgery is safe and oncologically equivalent to open surgery.
- Many short-term and long-term benefits exist for laparoscopic surgery when compared with open surgery.
- Several variations in surgical approach and technique exist, most of which have shown equivalent outcomes in the literature.
- Several patient-specific factors can have an impact on the efficacy of laparoscopic surgery but can be navigated with a safe, thoughtful approach.
- The learning curve for laparoscopic surgery is steep and often requires a strong foundation during surgical training.

INTRODUCTION

When laparoscopic colectomy was first introduced in 1991,[1,2] it did not experience the same level of enthusiasm among practitioners that was given to laparoscopic cholecystectomy. The procedure involved multiple quadrants and was more technically demanding than cholecystectomy. Early fears about port-site metastases[3,4] and potentially inferior oncologic outcomes prevented widespread adoption and ultimately resulted in the conduction of multiple high-quality randomized controlled trials that have now confirmed the safety and efficacy of laparoscopic surgery for colon cancer.[5–10] Current estimates suggest 59% of all elective colectomies are performed laparoscopically,[11] with slight variations based on diagnosis, geography, and hospital setting. Utilization tends to be higher among fellowship-trained colon and rectal surgeons.[12]

Disclosures: The authors have nothing to disclose.
[a] Department of Surgery, Middlesex Hospital Surgical Alliance, 520 Saybrook Road, Suite S-100, Middletown, CT 06457, USA; [b] Department of Surgery, Capital Medical Center, 3900 Capital Mall Drive Southwest, Olympia, WA 98502, USA; [c] Division of Colorectal Surgery, University of Southern California Keck School of Medicine, 1441 Eastlake Avenue, Suite 7418, Los Angeles, CA 90033, USA
* Corresponding author.
E-mail address: Kyle.Cologne@med.usc.edu

As understanding and experience have evolved, several technical improvements and adaptations have allowed for increased utilization of minimally invasive surgery (MIS). In addition to the more traditional straight multiport laparoscopic surgical (MLS) approaches, many surgeons use robotic-assisted surgery, hand-assisted laparoscopic surgical (HALS), and single-incision laparoscopic surgical (SILS) procedures, all of which fall under the MIS or laparoscopic umbrella. Each of these procedures, although unique, is governed by the same minimally invasive procedural codes (introduced in 2008) and thus reimbursement is no different among these options (including robotics). When compared with open surgery, all these variations in MIS technique maintain similar advantages, including shorter hospital length of stay, shorter duration of narcotic use, decreased pain scores, quicker return of bowel function, decreased rates of ileus, improved rates of surgical site infection, lower incisional hernia incidence (12.9 vs 2.4%), and decreased incidence of adhesive small bowel obstruction (6.1 vs 1.9%).[13–16] The choice between MLS, SILS, and HALS is made based on several surgeon-specific factors, such as personal preference, operative experience, equipment availability, and the skill level of the surgical assistant. Many patient factors also play a role, including prior abdominal surgery (PAS), body habitus, comorbidities, and desired cosmesis. Within each of these approaches, there is considerable variability in the operative steps, with the 2 main approaches medial-to-lateral dissection and lateral-to-medial dissection.

As outlined previously, laparoscopic surgery is oncologically equivalent to open surgery for colon cancer, but significant controversy still exists for the treatment of rectal cancer. In general, laparoscopic low anterior resections and abdominoperineal resections are more technically challenging than colectomy, and experts question whether or not MIS is appropriate for low pelvic cancers. This is discussed in greater detail in Rodrigo Oliva Perez and colleagues' article, "New Strategies in Rectal Cancer," in this issue.

This article provides a summary of the various approaches, including MLS, HALS, and SILS, for segmental colectomies and proctectomy. There is additional discussion of the learning curve for laparoscopic colorectal surgery, surgeon volume, and its relationship to outcomes. Furthermore, the surgical approach to difficult patients, such as those with obesity, prior radiation, or PAS, is discussed.

OPERATIVE STEPS
Patient Positioning

When positioning a patient, the first consideration is whether or not the surgeon requires access to the anus for examination or endoscopy or to allow for a circular stapled anastomosis. Therefore, whenever access to the anus is necessary, including left-sided resections and cases where colonoscopy may be necessary, the patient is placed in lithotomy stirrups, which gives access to the anus and also allows the surgeon and/or assistant to stand between the legs when technically advantageous. For right-sided resections, the patient may be placed supine, although many experts advocate for the use of lithotomy in all cases, because it allows for more versatility.

Laparoscopic colorectal surgery often requires work in multiple quadrants, so tucking both arms at the patient's side (with appropriate padding to prevent nerve injury) is best. Exaggerated Trendelenburg positioning and tilting are also needed at times, so care should be taken to secure the patient to the table and prevent movement during the case. A bean bag is often useful, although some surgeons prefer shoulder pads and tape to secure the patient to the table.

Instruments

Many simple and advanced instruments exist for complex laparoscopic surgery, and their use is often the result of surgeon preference and availability. For colorectal surgery, a high-quality camera is used. Some experts prefer a 0° camera to reduce the assistant's cognitive load, whereas others believe a 30° or 45° camera allows more versatility during a medial-to-lateral approach. Atraumatic graspers are used on the bowel with many acceptable reusable and disposable variants. A laparoscopic suction and irrigation device should be available, and it is best to incorporate this upfront rather than waiting until significant bleeding is experienced. Although most surgeons use monopolar electrocautery in some form, either as a hook or spatula or attached to laparoscopic scissors, the use of a bipolar vessel sealer is also encouraged and can eliminate the need for stapling devices, which require larger ports. Ultrasonic shears can also be used, but they are not able to ligate larger, named vessels, such as the inferior mesenteric artery (IMA), and there is significant lateral thermal spread with these devices, so care should be taken to avoid thermal injury to the bowel.

Ureteral stents can often be placed by urology and can assist with identification and preservation of the ureters during dissection. This is more useful on the left side, where the ureter travels close to the dissection and can be occasionally injured even in the most experienced hands. Ureteral stents are usually unnecessary for experienced surgeons but should be used often during a surgeon's early experience and continue to be useful for all surgeons during difficult cases, such as complicated diverticulitis.

Operative Steps

The first step in all cases is to achieve safe access to the abdomen and establish pneumoperitoneum. The abdomen is then thoroughly explored to identify adhesions, liver disease, spread of cancer, and relevant anatomic landmarks that have an impact on the case. If no problems are discovered, the omentum is then reflected cephalad over the stomach and liver to allow access to the colon and to allow the small bowel to be retracted out of the way.

Right Colectomy

The patient is placed in the Trendelenburg position with the left side tilted downward. The camera is usually placed above the umbilicus. Port placement is at the discretion of the surgeon but often includes two 5-mm ports for the surgeon (eg, left lower quadrant and suprapubic) and an optional 5-mm port for the assistant (eg, epigastric or left upper quadrant).

A medial-to-lateral dissection starts with placing the cecum on tension and retracting it toward the right lower quadrant, which almost always allows for identification of the ileocolic vessels. For most patients, the duodenum can also be visualized through the mesentery, located cephalad to the ileocolic vessels. An incision is made in the visceral peritoneum of the mesocolon, parallel and inferior to the ileocolic artery. Blunt dissection is then used to open the embryologic plane and separate the artery from the underlying duodenum. A high ligation of the ileocolic vessels is then performed with bipolar energy, the mesocolon is retracted anteriorly, and the medial-to-lateral dissection is continued laterally out to the abdominal wall over the top of Gerota fascia as well as cephalad until the hepatic flexure has been separated from the retroperitoneum. The duodenum and head of pancreas are visualized and kept free from harm during this dissection. The right branch of the middle colic artery is also ligated. Next, the terminal ileum is elevated off of the retroperitoneum, and the lateral colonic attachments are divided, connecting the lateral and medial dissection planes. The omentum is mobilized off the transverse colon, and the hepatic flexure is taken down in a medial-to-lateral fashion. After this, the mobilized and devascularized colon can be extracted through an incision in the abdominal wall for an extracorporeal anastomosis, or an intracorporeal anastomosis can be performed instead.

A laparoscopic lateral-to-medial dissection mirrors that of open surgery and includes medial colonic retraction with incision of the lateral attachments staying slightly medial to the line of Toldt to avoid dissection in the retroperitoneum. As the mobilization continues, care should be taken to identify the duodenum and avoid injury. Similar ligation of mesocolic vessels is performed, and similar options exist for specimen extraction and anastomosis.

Left Colectomy

The patient is placed in lithotomy stirrups and the Trendelenburg position, this time with the right side tilted downward. The camera is usually placed above the umbilicus. Port placement is at the discretion of the surgeon but often includes two 5-mm ports for the surgeon (eg, right lower quadrant and right upper quadrant or possibly suprapubic) and one to two 5-mm ports for the assistant (eg, left lower quadrant and/or left upper quadrant).

A medial-to-lateral dissection starts by elevating the rectosigmoid colon anteriorly, allowing for identification of the IMA and the sacral promontory. The visceral peritoneum of the mesocolon is incised medially at the level of the sacral promontory, allowing entrance into the presacral space. The IMA is elevated anteriorly, and blunt dissection is used to separate the artery from the underlying retroperitoneum. The left ureter must be identified and swept posterior to the dissection to avoid injury. A high ligation of the IMA is performed with bipolar energy, the left mesocolon is elevated anteriorly, and a medial-to-lateral dissection is continued over Gerota fascia to the abdominal wall. For pelvic cases, additional mescolic ligation, including the inferior mesenteric vein at the level of the ligament of Treitz, is necessary to obtain adequate colonic mobility. Next, the lateral attachments are divided to connect the lateral and medial dissection planes. The surgeon should have a low threshold for splenic flexure mobilization, which can be performed with a lateral or medial approach. Most experts recommend routine splenic flexure mobilization.

The site of distal transection is chosen based on pathology, the mesentery is divided, and a laparoscopic linear cutting stapler is used to divide the colon, typically via a 12-mm right lower quadrant incision. Many options exist for extraction, with perhaps the most appealing a low-transverse (Pfannenstiel) incision.

A lateral-to-medial dissection mirrors that of open surgery and includes medial tension on the colon and incision of the lateral attachments staying slightly medial to the line of Toldt to avoid dissection in the retroperitoneum. The left ureter is identified and preserved, and similar vessel ligation is performed.

Low Anterior Resection

A low anterior resection begins similar to a sigmoid colectomy, including mobilization of the left colon and ligation of the IMA. For pelvic cases, routine mobilization of the splenic flexure and routine ligation of the inferior mesenteric vein should be performed to allow adequate mobility.

The pelvic dissection is carried out in a manner similar to open surgery. For women, the uterus often requires elevation, which can be done with fixation suture through the anterior abdominal wall. The assistant elevates the rectum anterior and cephalad, and dissection begins posteriorly in the holy plane, with great care taken not to violate the fascia propria of the mesorectum. Dissection can usually be extended down to the level of the coccyx posteriorly, after which the lateral dissection is performed bilaterally. This takes a skilled assistant to operate the camera and provide retraction. The anterior dissection is performed last, and for female patients, it is often aided by a retractor within the vagina with anterior tension. Stapling in the deep pelvis is technically challenging, and often the best approach is a linear cutting stapler from a suprapubic port, with an anterior to posterior orientation and an assistant placing cephalad pressure on the perineum.

Conversion

It is important to mention that the quality of dissection and extent of colonic resection should never be compromised to finish the case laparoscopically. Whenever a surgeon determines that the case cannot continue safely in a laparoscopic fashion, immediate conversion to another technique is warranted. Conversion rates remain high for colorectal surgery, including 21% for the 2004 Clinical Outcomes of Surgical Therapy trial[5] and 12% in a more recent study.[11] Conversion from SILS to MLS or MLS to HALS is often useful and can allow a surgeon to safely complete the case with similar benefits to the patient.

SELECTION OF OPERATIVE APPROACH: MULTIPORT LAPAROSCOPIC SURGICAL, HAND-ASSISTED LAPAROSCOPIC SURGICAL, AND SINGLE-INCISION LAPAROSCOPIC SURGICAL

Multiport Laparoscopic Surgical

Straight laparoscopic approaches use multiple laparoscopic ports, with the largest incision that of a small specimen extraction port. This can be made in multiple locations, including a Pfannenstiel incision, lower midline, or the left lower quadrant using a muscle-splitting approach. The former 2 locations can be modified into a slightly larger incision to use one of several commercially available hand ports. This can be used for subsequent specimen extraction and extracorporeal anastomosis.

MLS often requires an experienced surgeon and a capable assistant to complete the case safely. It can be accomplished in a majority of cases, however, and is often the preferred approach for expert surgeons.

Hand-Assisted Laparoscopic Surgical

Depending on the size of a surgeon's hand, HALS may not alter the size of the patient's extraction site, or it may require an additional 2 cm to 3 cm of incision length. The decision to use HALS can be for a variety of reasons. For some surgeons, it is used during the early parts of the laparoscopic learning curve, allowing for tactile feedback and more dexterity during tissue manipulation. It is used by others to replace the need for an experienced assistant, which is often unavailable in certain environments. HALS is also useful as a tool for teaching resident surgeons, allowing for graduated autonomy while not sacrificing complete control of the case. Lastly, HALS is often used to complete a case that would otherwise not be amenable to laparoscopy, including cases with significant adhesions or inflammation, and surgery in morbidly obese individuals.

Bae and colleagues[17] demonstrated in a 2014 retrospective analysis of right colectomies that the HALS approach had similar short-term and oncologic outcomes compared with the traditional laparoscopic approach. The investigators noted that the HALS patients had more advanced disease, which may be a touted benefit but also a source of selection bias. In a 2015 case-matched study looking at oncologic outcomes, Gezen and colleagues[18] showed equivalence in disease-free survival (DFS) and overall survival (OS) among patients treated for adenocarcinoma of the rectum or sigmoid colon by an open, HALS, or MLS approach. The investigators note a shorter length of stay (LOS) in those who had traditional laparoscopy; however, the HALS patients had more preoperative cardiac and/or hypertensive disease.

The HALS approach is possible for all types of procedures, including proctectomy. Koh and colleagues[19] investigated abdominoperineal resection using the end-colostomy site for hand-access. With a small group of 6 patients, the investigators reported no conversions and a 6.8-day mean LOS with 1 parastomal hernia noted at 13.3-month mean follow-up. In addition to oncologic equivalence, other outcome measures are similar between HALS and MLS. In 2008, Sonoda and colleagues[20] showed similar postoperative rates of incisional hernia, small bowel obstruction, and wound infection between HALS and MLS patients after a 27-month median follow-up. Incisional hernias, in general, may be best prevented for left-sided resections by using the Pfannenstiel incision for extraction site and/or hand access rather than a lower midline incision.[21]

Hand-Assisted Laparoscopic Surgical Versus Open

In addition to comparing HALS and MLS patients directly, there are many comparisons between HALS and open surgical patients. In a 2015 case-matched study with more than 5 years of follow-up, Zhou and colleagues[22] showed that HALS patients had similar lymph node retrieval, margin positivity, locoregional recurrence, DFS, and OS in comparison with open surgical patients. The HALS patients had lower rates of wound infections, earlier tolerance of oral diet, and decreased LOS, which arguably justified the increased operative time. In a much larger case-matched review using the National Surgical Quality Improvement Program database, Benlice and colleagues[23] demonstrated that HALS patients had decreased overall morbidity, surgical site infections, urinary tract infections, ileus, reoperations, readmissions, and LOS in comparison with open surgical patients. This was noted after adjusting for baseline conditions, because the open surgical patients were demonstrably sicker. Finally, HALS for colorectal resection may give obese patients the opportunity for a safe minimally invasive operation, because Myers and colleagues[24] showed that HALS utilization was directly proportional to body mass index, with similar LOS, rate of reoperations, and 30-day mortality rates between the obese and nonobese patients.

Overall, touted benefits of a hand-assist approach include shorter operative times (compared with MLS), and a decreased learning curve – particularly for surgeons who are used to an open approach.[25] It allows a hybrid technique that includes tactile feedback while maintaining the benefits of a minimally invasive approach. Current evidence suggests it is equal to MLS for performing minimally invasive cancer surgery.

Although often found equivalent to MLS, some controversy exists for HALS, and Midura and colleagues'[26] retrospective review showed purely laparoscopic sigmoid colectomies had lower LOS and earlier return of bowel function in comparison to those patients having HALS or laparoscopic mobilization only. Therefore, it is safe to say that 1 technique cannot be universally applied to all patients, and a catered approach is better if the situation and surgeon expertise allows.

SINGLE-INCISION LAPAROSCOPIC SURGERY

SILS tends to be a more technically challenging approach to colectomy. This involves making a single, slightly larger incision and placing a single access port for dissection. There are several commercially available platforms for SILS with similar efficacy. The camera, instrument ports, and specimen extraction can be performed through this incision. Lack of triangulation, instrument collisions, and poor special visualization are the major challenges of this approach. Nonetheless, some investigators claim that patient benefits warrant the more technically challenging approach.

Papaconstantinou and colleagues[27] reported data comparing SILS, MLS, and HALS for right colectomy, showing benefit with SILS in regard to both postoperative pain scores and LOS. This experienced group demonstrated no significant difference in operative time, rate of conversion, or mean incision lengths between MLS and SILS. In addition, there may be no increased costs for the SILS approach as reported in 2014 case-matched study, where the investigators showed comparable costs between MLS and SILS patients with an finding of shorter operative times and, therefore, decreased anesthesia costs in the SILS patients.[28] An important review of publications on SILS colectomy, covering a 28-year period, demonstrated adequate lymph node harvest, negative margins in all patients, and respectably low morbidity and mortality rates. There was an overall 6.9% conversion rate but only a 1.6% rate of conversion to an open operation,[29] which likely speaks to the high level of surgeon expertise.

SILS studies are often retrospective and there may be a significant amount of selection bias in reporting of these small case series. Furthermore, they are most commonly performed by expert laparoscopists who are skilled in other forms of MIS. Therefore, the SILS technique has not been evaluated with the most rigorous methods and should only be attempted once other forms of MIS have been mastered, particularly for neoplastic indications.

Robotics Versus Laparoscopy

Robotic-assisted MIS has gained traction in recent years as an alternative to laparoscopy. It is extensively covered elsewhere this issue, so discussion in this article is limited to avoid duplication of efforts (See Slawomir Marecik and colleagues' article, "Robotic Colorectal Surgery for Neoplasia," in this issue). The oncologic outcomes, however, for robotic colorectal surgery have been shown equivalent to laparoscopy.[30]

PATIENT RISK FACTORS

Although patient factors may dictate the choice of operative technique, risk factors, including obesity, PAS, and previous pelvic radiation, are not a contraindication to a minimally invasive approach despite adding difficulty for the surgeon.

Obesity

Obesity has been shown to prolong operative times, increase conversion rates, and result in increased length of stay.[31,32] Much of the literature on this topic is the result of nonrandomized, retrospective trials and thus must be interpreted in light of potential bias. Several investigators have examined the effect of obesity on various approaches.

In general, laparoscopic surgery has been shown safe in obese patients. A 2014 retrospective case-matched study demonstrated no difference in short term outcomes between obese patients having a SILS colorectal operation and those obese patients having MLS. Each group (SILS vs MLS) had 37 patients and had similar conversion rates, operating time, hospital length of stay, reoperation, and readmission rates.[33] Mean body mass index was a modest, 34 in the obese group. Similar outcomes were reported for MLS in a 2014 case-matched study, with no difference in the rate of reoperation, intensive care admission, and readmission between obese and nonobese patients.[34] A 2016 systematic review compared 17,895 nonobese and 5754 obese patients, with no significant difference in postoperative morbidity, anastomotic leakage, reoperation rate, and mortality.[35] Although the obese patients had longer operative times, the lymph node harvests were equivalent overall, and 4 of the studies cited equivalence in OS and DFS.[35] A 2012 meta-analysis showed equivalent lymph node harvest and rate of reoperation for obese patients,[32] but the investigators recognized that some included studies showed increased postoperative morbidity related to cardiopulmonary and/or systemic complications. This may have some relation to the documented longer operative times and higher rates of conversion to an open approach in those patients with obesity.[32]

Although safe, laparoscopic colorectal surgery in obese patients is associated with a higher rate of conversion to open surgery (30% vs 12.7% in one recent study).[36] Longer operative times in obese patients are often noted as well,[31,37] and obese patients usually demonstrate higher rates of wound complications. This may influence surgeons to use HALS as a minimally invasive approach to obese patients, while accepting an open operation in those with PAS or advanced-stage disease and reserving MLS for those with lower-stage disease and virgin abdomens.[38]

As discussed previously, obese patients often have longer operative times, and they can be more difficult to position for surgery. Thus, it is not surprising that obesity has been shown an independent predictor for postoperative peripheral neuropathy in patients having laparoscopic colon surgery.[39]

In summary, obese patients can safely undergo laparoscopic colorectal surgery with similar or even increased advantages compared with normal-sized patients, but these surgeries are more technically challenging, and surgeons can expect longer operative times, increased postoperative morbidity, and a higher potential for conversion to an open operation. Therefore, these cases should be approached with a heightened awareness of the associated risks, and great care should be taken for patient positioning and the operative dissection. A hand-assisted approach can often be advantageous in these difficult patients. Overall, the minimally invasive approaches remain a viable option for obese patients without sacrificing important oncologic outcomes.

Prior Abdominal Surgery

As expected, patients with PAS present challenges to surgeons during any subsequent operation. There are multiple retrospective reviews comparing those patients with and without PAS. A 13-year retrospective cohort study was published by Yamamoto and colleagues[40] that showed patients with PAS having a higher rate of inadvertent enterotomy as well as prolonged recovery and ileus. Retrospective studies frequently report higher rates of wound infections, longer operative times with more frequent conversions, and occasionally higher rates of overall morbidity, but results tend to be mixed.[36,41,42] A recent meta-analysis evaluated 12 retrospective studies and determined that conversion rates and enterotomies were similar between patients with and without PAS.[43] It is likely, however, that differences in conversion rates depend on the extent and location of previous surgery.[44] The results in patients with prior operations for Crohn disease are also mixed and likely reflect the selection bias of different surgeons, with some more aggressive than others in attempting laparoscopic surgery with PAS.[45,46]

Patients requiring urgent or emergent surgery in the immediate postoperative period also technically count as having PAS. These patients often suffer from an anastomotic leak, and, depending on the leak location and severity, it is often feasible, and even preferable, to re-explore these patient laparoscopically. One recent retrospective study showed that laparoscopic reintervention resulted in a lower LOS, lower fascial dehiscence, and a lower mortality when compared with open reintervention.[47]

In summary, laparoscopic colorectal surgery in patients with PAS is safe and feasible but is often more difficult overall. In these situations, surgeons should focus on safe laparoscopic access, typically using a place and technique for access where adhesions are not anticipated, including the left upper quadrant. Published results for these patients are difficult to interpret because of selection bias.

Radiation

Radiated tissue leads to a diminished healing response compared with nonradiated tissue. Animal models support this because Franca and colleagues[48] showed a higher incidence of colorectal anastomotic dehiscence, using a rat model, in those receiving preoperative radiotherapy. Somewhat better outcomes were noted when the interval between radiotherapy and surgery was longer (8 weeks) than in a comparison group (4 weeks). Despite causing this disadvantage, radiation is useful to decrease recurrence in rectal cancer. Geisler and colleagues[49] looked specifically at laparoscopic colorectal surgical outcomes in the irradiated pelvis. Based on a retrospective review of 42 patients (11 having diverting stoma formation and 31 having a resection), there was a 10% conversion rate in the patients having a resection, with an overall average LOS of 5.5 days. Subset analysis noted 2 of 20 patients had an anastomotic leak, and fortunately both were proximally diverted and managed nonoperatively. The reason for radiation is not always for the neoadjuvant treatment of rectal cancer itself. As Buscail and colleagues[50] showed, the patients with prior radiation for prostate cancer (70 Gy) have worse outcomes that those with conventional neoadjuvant radiotherapy for rectal cancer (45 Gy), which supports the concept of considering defunctionalized anastomoses (with proximal stoma) or an end colostomy in this population.

From a staging point of view, the use of radiation correlates with fewer lymph nodes harvested, with results independent of tumor location and tumor stage.[51] Although this does not always have an impact on the plan of care postoperatively, the results help question the requirements regarding rectal cancer staging and the required number of lymph nodes. By knowing the possible effects of surgery in a radiated field, surgeons can ensure optimal oncologic dissection is performed and well vascularized anastomoses are created.

SURGEON VOLUME AND LEARNING CURVES

Technologic advances have led to a multitude of surgical approaches to colorectal disease. Each evolution in surgical technique leads to a new learning curve that must be ascended. This applies to laparoscopy as well as robotics. Even after the technique has been learned, some investigators believe a certain number of ongoing cases is needed to stay proficient. Reports on learning curve vary by the method used to calculate them. As part of some of the aforementioned randomized trials looking at outcomes for laparoscopic surgery, participants had to demonstrate successful performance of 20 procedures, because this was initially considered the learning curve. It was later determined that this was an underestimate. Subsequent study using cumulative sum analysis adjusted for case mix demonstrated that 55 procedures were necessary for right colectomy and 62 procedures for left colectomy to overcome the learning curve.[52] Specialized training programs in colorectal surgery may allow faster achievement of this goal. The learning curve for robotic procedures seems between 20 and 30 cases, during which time, procedures take significantly longer.[53]

To look at surgeon volume and its relationship with quality and cost outcomes, a retrospective study involving approximately 18,000 patients from the University HealthSystem Consortium was conducted. Results showed that high-volume surgeons, more than 11 colectomies for cancer per year, and medium-volume surgeons, 5 to 11 colectomies for cancer per year, were more likely to use laparoscopy for colon cancer resection than low-volume surgeons, less than 5 colectomies for cancer per year. Compared with operations done by low-volume surgeons, those done by high-volume surgeons had fewer postoperative complications, were less likely to require reoperation, and had direct costs that were nearly $927 lower per patient.[54] A much smaller single-surgeon retrospective review was done for SILS right colectomy, demonstrating significant improvement in operative times between the first 10 cases and the subsequent 10 cases.[55] Similarly, a publication from 2010 showed improvement in operative times for laparoscopic colectomy after the learning curve was completed, defined by the investigators as 40 cases, with no change in rate of conversion, complications, or direct costs during the study period.[56] With regard to the learning curve for total colectomy, Ozturk and colleagues[25] showed that early-experience HALS total colectomy has operative times similar to MLS total colectomy done by surgeons well beyond their learning curve, while having tremendously lower rate of conversion compared with MLS early in learning curve. The investigators conclude that the HALS approach may afford the novice surgeon the chance to complete a minimally invasive colorectal operation in an acceptable operative time.[26] Ozturk and colleagues[25] later showed that a statistically significant decrease in HALS operative time occurs after 50 cases without any change in quality-related outcomes.[57] Other investigators have demonstrated a longer learning curve of more than 100 cases to show an improvement. Pendlimari and colleagues[58] published data showing a statistically significant decrease in mean operating times from 263 to 185 minutes, based on various colorectal resections, with improvements in morbidity, infections, readmissions, and LOS noted after the learning curve.

Given that the learning curve begins in residency, a 2012 survey of colorectal residency graduates focused on a surgeon's comfort level in approaching minimally invasive segmental colectomies after completion of training. With a 51% response rate, the investigators concluded that 10 laparoscopic right colectomies and 30 laparoscopic left colectomies provided colorectal residents with a sufficient number of procedures "very comfortable" on entering practice. Given that 46% and 24% of residents did not reach that number of left and right colectomies, respectively, the investigators comment that the requirements of 50 laparoscopic resections may be adequate, but that further analysis regarding type of segmental colectomy is needed moving forward.[59]

Several barriers exist that limit a surgeon's ability to obtain and then maintain proficiency with laparoscopic colorectal surgery. Most partial colectomies are performed by general surgeons, with less than 12% performed by fellowship-trained colorectal surgeons.[60,61] The average general surgeon, however, performs approximately 11 colectomies per year,[60] with 14 colectomies placing surgeons in the 70th percentile and 23 colectomies placing them in the 90th percentile.[60] Therefore, obtaining proficiency may take as many as 5 years to 10 years of clinical practice. Furthermore, a perceived or realistic lack of hospital equipment and/or qualified surgical assistants may limit the use of laparoscopy in colorectal surgery,[62] which could have a negative impact on a learning curve.

There is certainly not a single number that identifies the moment at which one has passed the learning curve for a particular colorectal operation. It is likely based not only on the number of cases performed but also on the rate at which these cases are done. As more health care subspecialization occurs, colorectal specialists will increase their rate of nonemergent colectomies, at which point, more meaningful learning curve data will be obtained.

SUMMARY

Just as laparoscopy has become an important tool for surgeons in the treatment of neoplasia, open operations continue to play an important role in the treatment of more complex disease, and surgeons must base their approach on several patient-specific and disease-specific factors. Similarly, when a minimally invasive approach has been chosen, the use of MLS, HALS, and SILS must be catered to the situation, and 1 technique is not universally superior. Although a surgeon is ascending the learning curve for laparoscopic surgery, patients with favorable anatomy and disease states should be chosen with safety and oncologic equivalence as major priorities. Surgeons will likely continue to push the boundaries of MIS, and textbooks 20 years from now will contain new and advanced techniques that have been built off of current hard work and innovation.

REFERENCES

1. Jacobs M, Verdeja JC, Goldstein HS. Minimally invasive colon resection (laparoscopic colectomy). Surg Laparosc Endosc 1991;1(3):144–50.
2. Fowler DL, White SA. Laparoscopy-assisted sigmoid resection. Surg Laparosc Endosc 1991;1(3):183–8.
3. Johnstone PA, Rohde DC, Swartz SE, et al. Port site recurrences after laparoscopic and thoracoscopic procedures in malignancy. J Clin Oncol 1996;14(6):1950–6.
4. Alexander RJ, Jaques BC, Mitchell KG. Laparoscopically assisted colectomy and wound recurrence. Lancet 1993;341(8839):249–50.
5. Clinical Outcomes of Surgical Therapy Study Group. A comparison of laparoscopically assisted and open colectomy for colon cancer. N Engl J Med 2004;350(20):2050–9.
6. Veldkamp R, Kuhry E, Hop WC, et al. Laparoscopic surgery versus open surgery for colon cancer: short-term outcomes of a randomised trial. Lancet Oncol 2005;6(7):477–84.
7. Buunen M, Veldkamp R, Hop WC, et al. Survival after laparoscopic surgery versus open surgery for colon cancer: long-term outcome of a randomised clinical trial. Lancet Oncol 2009;10(1):44–52.
8. Guillou PJ, Quirke P, Thorpe H, et al. Short-term endpoints of conventional versus laparoscopic-assisted surgery in patients with colorectal cancer (MRC CLASICC trial): multicentre, randomised controlled trial. Lancet 2005;365(9472):1718–26.
9. Jayne DG, Thorpe HC, Copeland J, et al. Five-year follow-up of the Medical Research Council CLASICC trial of laparoscopically assisted versus open surgery for colorectal cancer. Br J Surg 2010;97(11):1638–45.
10. Jayne DG, Guillou PJ, Thorpe H, et al. Randomized trial of laparoscopic-assisted resection of colorectal carcinoma: 3-year results of the UK MRC CLASICC Trial Group. J Clin Oncol 2007;25(21):3061–8.
11. Moghadamyeghaneh Z, Carmichael JC, Mills S, et al. Variations in laparoscopic colectomy utilization in the United States. Dis Colon Rectum 2015;58(10):950–6.
12. Schoetz DJ Jr. Evolving practice patterns in colon and rectal surgery. J Am Coll Surg 2006;203(3):322–7.
13. Kuhry E, Schwenk W, Gaupset R, et al. Long-term outcome of laparoscopic surgery for colorectal cancer: a cochrane systematic review of randomised controlled trials. Cancer Treat Rev 2008;34(6):498–504.
14. Schwenk W, Haase O, Neudecker J, et al. Short term benefits for laparoscopic colorectal resection. Cochrane Database Syst Rev 2005;(3):CD003145.

15. Weeks JC, Nelson H, Gelber S, et al. Short-term quality-of-life outcomes following laparoscopic-assisted colectomy vs open colectomy for colon cancer: a randomized trial. JAMA 2002;287(3):321–8.

16. Duepree HJ, Senagore AJ, Delaney CP, et al. Does means of access affect the incidence of small bowel obstruction and ventral hernia after bowel resection? Laparoscopy versus laparotomy. J Am Coll Surg 2003;197(2):177–81.

17. Bae SU, Park JS, Choi YJ, et al. The role of hand-assisted laparoscopic surgery in a right hemicolectomy for right-sided colon cancer. Ann Coloproctol 2014;30(1):11–7.

18. Gezen FC, Aytac E, Costedio MM, et al. Hand-assisted versus straight-laparoscopic versus open proctosigmoidectomy for treatment of sigmoid and rectal cancer: a Case-Matched Study of 100 Patients. Perm J 2015;19(2):10–4.

19. Koh DC, Law CW, Kristian I, et al. Hand-assisted laparoscopic abdomino-perineal resection utilizing the planned end colostomy site. Tech Coloproctol 2010;14(2):201–6.

20. Sonoda T, Pandey S, Trencheva K, et al. Longterm complications of hand-assisted versus laparoscopic colectomy. J Am Coll Surg 2009;208(1):62–6.

21. DeSouza A, Domajnko B, Park J, et al. Incisional hernia, midline versus low transverse incision: what is the ideal incision for specimen extraction and hand-assisted laparoscopy? Surg Endosc 2011;25(4):1031–6.

22. Zhou X, Liu F, Lin C, et al. Hand-assisted laparoscopic surgery compared with open resection for mid and low rectal cancer: a case-matched study with long-term follow-up. World J Surg Oncol 2015;13:199.

23. Benlice C, Costedio M, Stocchi L, et al. Hand-assisted laparoscopic vs open colectomy: an assessment from the American College of Surgeons National Surgical Quality Improvement Program procedure-targeted cohort. Am J Surg 2016;212(5):808–13.

24. Myers EA, Feingold DL, Arnell TD, et al. The rate for the use of hand-assisted laparoscopic methods is directly proportional to body mass index. Surg Endosc 2014;28(1):108–15.

25. Ozturk E, Kiran RP, Remzi F, et al. Hand-assisted laparoscopic surgery may be a useful tool for surgeons early in the learning curve performing total abdominal colectomy. Colorectal Dis 2010;12(3):199–205.

26. Midura EF, Hanseman DJ, Davis BR, et al. Laparoscopic sigmoid colectomy: Are all laparoscopic techniques created equal? Surg Endosc 2016;30(8):3567–72.

27. Papaconstantinou HT, Sharp N, Thomas JS. Single-incision laparoscopic right colectomy: a case-matched comparison with standard laparoscopic and hand-assisted laparoscopic techniques. J Am Coll Surg 2011;213(1):72–80 [discussion: 80–2].

28. Sulu B, Gorgun E, Aytac E, et al. Comparison of hospital costs for single-port and conventional laparoscopic colorectal resection: a case-matched study. Tech Coloproctol 2014;18(9):835–9.

29. Makino T, Milsom JW, Lee SW. Feasibility and safety of single-incision laparoscopic colectomy: a systematic review. Ann Surg 2012;255(4):667–76.

30. Park JS, Choi GS, Lim KH, et al. Robotic-assisted versus laparoscopic surgery for low rectal cancer: case-matched analysis of short-term outcomes. Ann Surg Oncol 2010;17(12):3195–202.

31. Mustain WC, Davenport DL, Hourigan JS, et al. Obesity and laparoscopic colectomy: outcomes from the ACS-NSQIP database. Dis Colon Rectum 2012;55(4):429–35.

32. Makino T, Shukla PJ, Rubino F, et al. The impact of obesity on perioperative outcomes after laparoscopic colorectal resection. Ann Surg 2012;255(2):228–36.
33. Aytac E, Turina M, Gorgun E, et al. Single-port laparoscopic colorectal resections in obese patients are as safe and effective as conventional laparoscopy. Surg Endosc 2014;28(10):2884–9.
34. Estay C, Zarate AJ, Castro M, et al. Does obesity increase early postoperative complications after laparoscopic colorectal surgery? Results from a single center. Surg Endosc 2014;28(7):2090–6.
35. Hotouras A, Ribas Y, Zakeri SA, et al. The influence of obesity and body-mass index on the outcome of laparoscopic colorectal surgery: a systematic literature review. Colorectal Dis 2016;18(10):O337–66.
36. Offodile AC 2nd, Lee SW, Yoo J, et al. Does prior abdominal surgery influence conversion rates and outcomes of laparoscopic right colectomy in patients with neoplasia? Dis Colon Rectum 2008;51(11):1669–74.
37. Vignali A, De Nardi P, Ghirardelli L, et al. Short and long-term outcomes of laparoscopic colectomy in obese patients. World J Gastroenterol 2013;19(42): 7405–11.
38. Jadlowiec CC, Mannion EM, Thielman MJ, et al. Evolution of technique in performance of minimally invasive colectomies. Dis Colon Rectum 2014;57(9):1090–7.
39. Velchuru VR, Domajnko B, deSouza A, et al. Obesity increases the risk of postoperative peripheral neuropathy after minimally invasive colon and rectal surgery. Dis Colon Rectum 2014;57(2):187–93.
40. Yamamoto M, Okuda J, Tanaka K, et al. Effect of previous abdominal surgery on outcomes following laparoscopic colorectal surgery. Dis Colon Rectum 2013; 56(3):336–42.
41. Vignali A, Di Palo S, De Nardi P, et al. Impact of previous abdominal surgery on the outcome of laparoscopic colectomy: a case-matched control study. Tech Coloproctol 2007;11(3):241–6.
42. Aytac E, Stocchi L, De Long J, et al. Impact of previous midline laparotomy on the outcomes of laparoscopic intestinal resections: a case-matched study. Surg Endosc 2015;29(3):537–42.
43. Figueiredo MN, Campos FG, D'Albuquerque LA, et al. Short-term outcomes after laparoscopic colorectal surgery in patients with previous abdominal surgery: A systematic review. World J Gastrointest Surg 2016;8(7):533–40.
44. Kim IY, Kim BR, Kim YW. Impact of prior abdominal surgery on rates of conversion to open surgery and short-term outcomes after laparoscopic surgery for colorectal cancer. PLoS One 2015;10(7):e0134058.
45. Hasegawa H, Watanabe M, Nishibori H, et al. Laparoscopic surgery for recurrent Crohn's disease. Br J Surg 2003;90(8):970–3.
46. Lowney JK, Dietz DW, Birnbaum EH, et al. Is there any difference in recurrence rates in laparoscopic ileocolic resection for Crohn's disease compared with conventional surgery? A long-term, follow-up study. Dis Colon Rectum 2006;49(1): 58–63.
47. Vennix S, Abegg R, Bakker OJ, et al. Surgical re-interventions following colorectal surgery: open versus laparoscopic management of anastomotic leakage. J Laparoendosc Adv Surg Tech A 2013;23(9):739–44.
48. Franca A, Ramalho FS, Ramalho LN, et al. Effects of preoperative pelvic irradiation on colonic anastomosis healing. An experimental study in rats. Acta Cir Bras 2008;23(Suppl 1):24–30 [discussion: 30].
49. Geisler D, Marks J, Marks G. Laparoscopic colorectal surgery in the irradiated pelvis. Am J Surg 2004;188(3):267–70.

50. Buscail E, Blondeau V, Adam JP, et al. Surgery for rectal cancer after high-dose radiotherapy for prostate cancer: is sphincter preservation relevant? Colorectal Dis 2015;17(11):973–9.
51. Maschuw K, Kress R, Ramaswamy A, et al. Short-term preoperative radiotherapy in rectal cancer patients leads to a reduction of the detectable number of lymph nodes in resection specimens. Langenbecks Arch Surg 2006;391(4):364–8.
52. Tekkis PP, Senagore AJ, Delaney CP, et al. Evaluation of the learning curve in laparoscopic colorectal surgery: comparison of right-sided and left-sided resections. Ann Surg 2005;242(1):83–91.
53. Maeso S, Reza M, Mayol JA, et al. Efficacy of the Da Vinci surgical system in abdominal surgery compared with that of laparoscopy: a systematic review and meta-analysis. Ann Surg 2010;252(2):254–62.
54. Damle RN, Macomber CW, Flahive JM, et al. Surgeon volume and elective resection for colon cancer: an analysis of outcomes and use of laparoscopy. J Am Coll Surg 2014;218(6):1223–30.
55. Hopping JR, Bardakcioglu O. Single-port laparoscopic right hemicolectomy: the learning curve. JSLS 2013;17(2):194–7.
56. Kiran RP, Kirat HT, Ozturk E, et al. Does the learning curve during laparoscopic colectomy adversely affect costs? Surg Endosc 2010;24(11):2718–22.
57. Ozturk E, da Luz Moreira A, Vogel JD. Hand-assisted laparoscopic colectomy: the learning curve is for operative speed, not for quality. Colorectal Dis 2010; 12(10 Online):e304–9.
58. Pendlimari R, Holubar SD, Dozois EJ, et al. Technical proficiency in hand-assisted laparoscopic colon and rectal surgery determining how many cases are required to achieve mastery. Arch Surg 2012;147(4):317–22.
59. Stein S, Stulberg J, Champagne B. Learning laparoscopic colectomy during colorectal residency: what does it take and how are we doing? Surg Endosc 2012;26(2):488–92.
60. Langenfeld SJ, Thompson JS, Oleynikov D. Laparoscopic colon resection: is it being utilized? Adv Surg 2013;47:29–43.
61. Etzioni DA, Cannom RR, Madoff RD, et al. Colorectal procedures: what proportion is performed by American board of colon and rectal surgery-certified surgeons? Dis Colon Rectum 2010;53(5):713–20.
62. Steele SR, Stein SL, Bordeianou LG, et al. The impact of practice environment on laparoscopic colectomy utilization following colorectal residency: a survey of the ASCRS young surgeons. Colorectal Dis 2012;14(3):374–81.

Robotic Colorectal Surgery for Neoplasia

Ajit Pai, MD[a], Slawomir Marecik, MD[b],*, John Park, MD[c], Leela Prasad, MD[b]

KEYWORDS

- Robotic • Colorectal • Colon • Rectal • Cancer • Neoplasia
- Total mesorectal excision

KEY POINTS

- Robotic colorectal surgery has several advantages to surgeons, including improved visualization, enhanced control, and improved ergonomics.
- Robotic total mesorectal excision (RTME) is currently the main application for colorectal surgeons, and it is associated with a lower rate of conversion to open surgery than its laparoscopic counterpart.
- Outcomes after robotic colorectal surgery are similar to conventional laparoscopy.
- The learning curve for robotic colorectal surgery is short, but surgeons are often already experts in laparoscopy, which makes the number difficult to interpret.

INTRODUCTION

Minimally invasive surgery (MIS) for colon and rectal cancer is now universally accepted as providing equivalent oncologic outcomes to open surgery and offers added benefits, including earlier return of bowel function, shortened length of stay, and better cosmesis. The evidence for laparoscopy comes from multiple well-designed randomized controlled studies, meta-analyses, and case-matched and prospective cohort studies.[1-8] Laparoscopy, however, has several well-known limitations, including limited range of movement, 2-D vision, requirement of a highly trained assistant, and a long learning curve.[9]

Robotic surgery is in essence laparoscopy with sophisticated equipment designed to overcome these limitations. The key elements of the robotic platform include high-definition 3-D vision, EndoWrist (Intuitive Surgical, Sunnyvale, CA, USA) instruments

Disclosures and Conflicts of Interest: The authors have nothing to disclose.
[a] Department of Surgical Oncology, Apollo Hospitals, Apollo Cancer Institute, 21, Greams Lane, Off Greams Road, Chennai, Tamil Nadu 600006, India; [b] Division of Colorectal Surgery, Advocate Lutheran General Hospital, University of Illinois at Chicago College of Medicine, 1775 West Dempster Avenue, Park Ridge, IL 60068, USA; [c] Division of Colorectal Surgery, Advocate Lutheran General Hospital, Chicago Medical School, 1775 West Dempster Avenue, Park Ridge, IL 60068, USA
* Corresponding author.
E-mail address: smarecik@uic.edu

with greater degrees of freedom, and absence of tremors of the human hand to the instrument tips.[10]

Colon and rectal surgery was one of the earliest specialties to adopt robotic surgery, with Weber[11] and Hashizume[12] reporting the first operations for benign and malignant colorectal disease, respectively in 2002. D'Annibale[13] and Giulianotti[14] from Europe and Delaney and colleagues[15] from the United States were the early pioneers of this technology, publishing some of the seminal papers in this field.[11–17]

For the purpose of this article, the term *robot* refers to the da Vinci Si 4-arm system (Intuitive Surgical, Sunnyvale, California). The latest system is known as the Xi and is discussed in detail later. With the dual console system, it is possible to walk a trainee through the operation, with graded responsibility to complete more complex tasks as training progresses. The system also allows a more objective validation of surgical skill and competence using the skill simulator and external animate and inanimate models.

BENEFITS OF ROBOTIC SURGERY
Benefits to the Surgeon

The major advantage of robotic surgery for the surgeon is improved visualization, because robotic imaging includes depth perception akin to open surgery due to the stereoscopic 3-D image, a consequence of a dual telescope system. This allows a more precise dissection and preservation of critical structures, for example, the pelvic autonomic nerves during mesorectal excision.[18] Additionally, the heat generated at the tip of the dual lens system makes fogging and loss of clarity infrequent.

The second benefit is the instrumentation. The double-jointed EndoWrist has improved versatility compared with conventional nonarticulating laparoscopic instruments, and it maneuvers well in tight spaces, such as the pelvis. There is less dependence on a skilled assistant, because the surgeon controls the camera as well as a third operating arm, which can be used for retraction. Robot instruments also eliminate surgeon tremor, allowing for a more controlled dissection. When working in the deep pelvis, especially in obese men, the advantages of robotic instrumentation become the most apparent.

Another important advantage to robotics is improved ergonomics for the operating surgeon. The surgery is performed while sitting down, and the controls can be adjusted to reduce the pain and fatigue of a long, complex operation.[19] Conventional laparoscopy, on the other hand, is known to be associated with a high incidence of neck, back, and shoulder pain, muscle stiffness, headache, visual discomfort, and fatigue.[20,21]

Limitations

The major issue in robotic surgery is the significant increase in cost compared with laparoscopic and open surgery. The cost increase has 3 components[10]: (1) fixed costs of purchase and subsequent machine maintenance, (2) consumables (drapes and instruments with limited lifespan), and (3) increased operative time. Another limitation to robotics is the absence of haptics or tactile feedback. The surgeon understands tissue grip by visual cues, such as tissue blanching or shearing. Therefore, there is potential for suture fray and tissue injury if the surgeon is inexperienced. This is a component of the robotic learning curve, and practice in the dry, porcine, or cadaveric laboratory significantly improves understanding of tissue and suture tensile strength.

Benefits to the Patient

The MIS approach to colorectal surgery has several well-known benefits compared with open colectomy, including smaller incisions, less pain, and a quicker overall recovery. Additionally, some smaller studies report less pain with robotics compared with laparoscopy, presumably due to reduced movement at trocar sites and less torque on the abdominal wall. These same studies show a slightly quicker return of bowel function.[22]

Another benefit to the patient is a lower rate of conversion to open surgery for robotics (0%–4.9%) compared with laparoscopy (7.3%–34%), although these data are from heterogeneous studies.[2,23–30] Additionally, patient subgroups previously categorized as unsuitable for a minimally invasive approach, including the morbidly obese and those with locally advanced rectal cancers requiring exenteration have been operated successfully with the robotic platform, thereby extending the spectrum of MIS.[27,31]

TECHNIQUE
Robotic Total Mesorectal Excision

RTME is widely believed to be the area of greatest benefit compared with laparoscopic total mesorectal excision (TME). TME is a technically demanding operation whether performed open or by minimally invasive methods. It involves identification and separation of the rectum in the embryologic interface between the visceral and parietal fascia—along the holy plane, as described by Heald.[32] This plane can and often is obfuscated by edema after pelvic radiation, and the penalty for violating the mesorectal fascia is grave—a positive circumferential margin (CRM), tumor perforation, or an incomplete mesorectum are strongly associated with increased local recurrence, distant metastases, and decreased survival.[33,34] In the deep pelvis, especially in men, there is a paucity of space, and the need to preserve an intact mesorectal envelope often leads to damage to the autonomic nerves, which leads to inadequate bladder emptying, retention, and impotence in men.[18]

Technical Aspects

There are 2 main approaches to RTME (**Table 1**): a fully robotic dissection and a hybrid approach. In the latter, conventional laparoscopy is used to mobilize the left colon and control the major vessels, with the robot docked solely for the pelvic portion of the operation.[35]

The fully robotic approach is typically more challenging because the robotic system has limited range of external instrument arm movement and changes in cart position (redocking) are often required to accomplish mobilization of the splenic flexure, left colon, and rectum. Single docking has been described for select patients,[36,37] but a dual-docking approach allows for adequate mobilization of the splenic flexure.[26,38,39] Regardless of docking, the fully robotic approach is difficult in larger patients, and it is associated with more minor complications compared to a hybrid approach,[40] so it should be used selectively. The Xi system (discussed later) is better suited to the fully robotic approach with minimized arm collision.

The hybrid approach uses 2 minimally invasive techniques. Standard laparoscopy is used to mobilize the left colon and splenic flexure, and the robot is then docked for the

Table 1		
Main approaches to robotic total mesorectal excision		
Approach	**Colon Mobilization**	**Rectal Dissection**
Fully robotic	Robot	Robot
Hybrid	Laparoscopy	Robot

TME.[41] The inherent benefits of the robotic system, including the camera and 3 working arms that are controlled by a single surgeon, the stability of the platform, and the precision of movement due to motion scaling and wrist articulation, all make it well suited for the difficult work required in the pelvis. A reverse hybrid technique has also been described and involves completion of the RTME first robotically, followed by rectal transection and completion of the left colon mobilization, lymphadenectomy, and anastomosis laparoscopically.[42]

Principles of robotic cart positioning

For RTME, the robot is either placed between a patient's legs or at a patient's left hip. Positioning the cart between the legs allows for an ergonomic, fast, and forgiving setup, with the lowest risk for robotic arm collision, both inside and outside. It does, however, make it difficult to access the perineum for intraoperative finger examination, flexible sigmoidoscopy, or transanal stapler application.

    Conversely, positioning the cart at the left hip allows for easy access to the perineum, but it requires a clear understanding of spatial arm distribution and careful port placement. Even a small misplacement of the ports can lead to arm collisions. Positioning the cart at the left hip also gives the bedside assistant more room. The anatomic structures that can be accessed using the robotic device in either of these setup approaches are detailed in **Table 2**.

Robotic instruments: macroretraction and microretraction

Macroretraction refers to retraction of the necessary macrostructures during TME, for example, the rectosigmoid during the initial phase of dissection (opening of posterior plane) or the anterior pelvic structures during dissection along the Denonvilliers fascia. Microretraction refers to the application of tissue tension needed to perform cautery dissection in a desired tissue plane (**Table 3**).

    During RTME, the bedside assistant is actively working to allow tension and exposure. Additionally, each robotic arm has an assigned role as follows: right arm (#1) – cautery dissection; middle arm (#2) – microretraction and bipolar cautery; and left arm (#3) – macroretraction. The physical right hand of the operator controls the right arm (#1) of the robot, while the physical left hand of the operator controls the middle (#2) and the left (#3) robotic arms, switching in-between with the use of the clutch mechanism. The most common robotic instrument used by the right robotic arm (#1) is the cautery hook or monopolar scissors. The middle arm (#2) is often supplied with a bipolar fenestrated grasper and the left arm (#3) holds the Cadiere (Intuitive

Table 2
Anatomic structures that can be accessed using the robotic device

Anatomic Structure	Setup	
	Between the Legs	Right Hip
Splenic flexure	−	+ (Low splenic flexure/short patients)
Descending colon	−/+	+
Inferior mesenteric vein	−	+ (Potential reach/collision problem)
Inferior mesenteric artery	+	+
Rectosigmoid	+	+
Rectum		
Upper/mid	+	+
Low/levators	+	+ (Potential reach/collision problem in tall patients)

Table 3 Definitions of macroretraction and microretraction	
Macroretraction	Retraction of necessary macrostructures by freezing a retracting arm (rectosigmoid during posterior dissection, anterior pelvic structures during anterior dissection)
Microretraction	Application of necessary tissue tension by an active arm to perform dissection in desired tissue plane

Surgical, Sunnyvale, CA, USA) forceps. The summary of each instrument function is presented in **Table 4**.

Robotic rectal dissection

Dissection commences posteriorly, entering the avascular holy plane and avoiding injury to the hypogastric nerves,[43] and working down to the pelvic floor and coccyx. Dissection then continues laterally, and then finally the rectovesical/rectovaginal fold of the peritoneum is incised to expose Denonvilliers fascia, and the rectum is mobilized from the prostate/vagina. Maintaining the plane of dissection posterior to Denonvilliers fascia avoids troublesome bleeding from the vascular plexus that surrounds the seminal vesicles and prevents sexual dysfunction from occurring. Dissection anterior to this fascia is required only in anteriorly placed tumors. The fixed third-arm retraction on the bladder/vagina, provided by the retracting robotic arm #3, significantly facilitates surgical access and visualization during the anterior rectal dissection.

Distal rectal transection can be accomplished through several techniques. The robot can be undocked, and either the left lower quadrant or suprapubic ports upsized to facilitate a laparoscopic stapler. There is also a robotic stapler available, which can be used for arm #1. The specimen can then be removed through a small extraction site (Pfannenstiel incision, reversed McBurney incision, or lower midline incision) through the ileostomy site or through the anus. In obese patients, the authors' preferred method is the Pfannenstiel incision because it has the lowest incidence of incisional hernia.[44]

In patients who undergo abdominoperineal resection, TME can be combined with robotic intra-abdominal transection of levators. This allows the surgeon to obtain the cylindrical-shaped specimen while minimizing the perineal wound.[45] It also allows for controlled division of the levators under direct visualization and a narrowing transection perimeter of the levators on the side not affected by tumor.

Retraction and handling of the mesorectal specimen is important, especially with large tumors. A break in the mesorectal and colonic envelope can increase the risk

Table 4 Robotic instrument functions		
Arm	**Instrument**	**Function**
Robotic arm #1 (right)	Cautery hook/scissors	Dissection
Robotic arm #2 (middle)	Bipolar fenestrated grasper (ProGrasp)	Microretraction/dissection/ bipolar cautery
Robotic arm #3 (left)	Cadiere forceps, Graptor, double fenestrated grasper	Macroretraction/dissection
Assistant left arm (right upper quadrant)	Bowel grasper	Macroretraction and microretraction
Assistant right arm (suprapubic)	Suction-irrigator	Suction-irrigation, macroretraction, and microretraction

of tumor cell seeding. In the authors' experience, a majority of breaks in the mesorectal envelope happened during macroretraction that was applied during dissection in the presacral space. Rarely should the third robotic arm grasp the fascia propria of the rectum (mesorectal envelope).

OUTCOMES
Perioperative Outcomes

Robotic surgery is associated with comparable perioperative outcomes, such as length of stay and return of bowel function, as with laparoscopic surgery. Operative time and blood loss are similar to laparoscopy, whereas conversion rates are lower than with laparoscopy, varying from 0% to 4.9%, respectively, compared with 7.3% to 34%, respectively, in large laparoscopic series.[2,23–26,28–30,40,46] A 2012 meta-analysis also reported lower rates of conversion to open surgery (2% vs 7.5%, $P = .0007$).[47] Short-term complication rates are similar to laparoscopy, with an anastomotic leak rate of 1.8% to 12.1%.[24–26,28,35,40,46]

Oncologic Outcomes

Rates of CRM positivity are 0% to 7.1% for RTME, with a distal margin positivity of 0% to 1.9% and a lymph node yield of 13 to 20 nodes.[24–26,28,35,40,46] The number of studies with long-term outcomes data is limited, but emerging data indicate disease-free survival (DFS) and overall survival (OS) rates comparable to open and laparoscopic TME. Reported 3-year DFS rates are between 73.7% and 79.2% and OS rates between 90.1% and 97.0%.[24,35,40,46] There are only a few studies reporting 5-year survival data. Park and colleagues,[48] with a median follow-up of 58 months, found no significant differences in 5-year OS, DFS, or local recurrence rates between patients treated with robotic and laparoscopic surgery for rectal cancer. The 5-year OS rate was 92.8% in robotic and 93.5% in laparoscopic surgical procedures ($P = .829$). The 5-year DFS rates were 81.9% and 78.7%, respectively ($P = .547$). Local recurrence was similar: 2.3% and 1.2% ($P = .649$). In one of the largest series of 200 consecutive resections for rectal cancer, Hara and colleagues[49] reported local pelvic control and OS and DFS rates of stage III patients at 5 years as 93.0%, 88.6%, and 76.6%, respectively.

Functional Outcomes

Genitourinary function can be disturbed after TME due to injury to the superior hypogastric plexus around the root of the inferior mesenteric vein, hypogastric nerves, pelvic plexus, or splanchnic nerves (sacral and pelvic). Damage to the superior hypogastric plexus can lead to disturbances in ejaculation in men and to decreased lubrication in women, whereas a lesion in the pelvic splanchnic nerves or the pelvic plexus causes erectile dysfunction in men and cause diminished labial engorgement response in women. Both laparoscopy and robotic surgery lead to diminished libido and sexual dysfunction, but there is earlier recovery in the robotic arm (6 months) compared with laparoscopy (1 year). Bladder parameters, including filling and voiding function, deteriorate when measured at 1 month but recover within 3 months in robotic versus 6 months in laparoscopy.[50] Luca and colleagues[18] found no change in bladder function in the robotic arm and postulate that this is due to better visualization of the nerves and early catheter removal.

Robotic Versus Laparoscopic Resection for Rectal Cancer Trial

The Robotic versus Laaroscopic Resection for Rectal Cancer (ROLARR) trial is an ongoing international, multicenter, prospective randomized controlled trial of robotic-assisted versus laparoscopic surgery for the curative treatment of rectal cancer. The preliminary results were presented at the American Society of Colon and Rectal Surgeons 2015 meeting in Boston. The short-term postoperative and pathologic outcomes analysis showed that robotic systems had a nonsignificant reduction in conversion rates (8.1% vs 12.2%, $P = .158$).

No differences were observed in the short-term postoperative complication rate (33.1% in the robotic group vs 31.7% in the laparoscopic group) and oncological outcomes (CRM positivity 5.1% in the robotic group vs 6.3% in the laparoscopic group). The lack of a statistically significant difference could be explained by the limited number of patients enrolled in the study and by the bias related to differences in the surgeons' expertise in the robotic and laparoscopic approach.

Cost Data

Cost data were not evaluated in the ROLARR trial. A Korean study, however, reported total charges of $14,647 for RTME versus $9978 for laparoscopic TME.[51] Similarly, in the United States, the mean cost of robotic surgery was $22,640 versus $18,330 for the hand-assisted laparoscopic approach ($P = .005$).[35]

Robotic Colon Resections: Is There a Role?

Since the first reported robotic colon resections in 2002, robotic assistance has been used to perform all manner of colon resections: right, left, transverse, sigmoid, and total colectomy. The sigmoid robotic colectomy essentially represents the colonic mobilization and lymphadenectomy as for rectal cancer resections and is an important learning tool, although there was no oncologic superiority or clinical benefit found compared with laparoscopy.

Robotic right colectomy has been extensively studied in comparison to laparoscopy and provides no measurable benefit, either in terms of perioperative outcomes, including blood loss and conversion rates, or complications, including anastomotic leaks.[52] There is a significant increase in operative time and an increased cost of approximately $3000. An interest in robotic assistance in right colectomy has resurfaced due to its ability to facilitate complete mesocolic excision.[53] Complete mesocolic excision with central vascular ligation, as proposed by Hohenberger and colleagues,[54] is a technique to remove the right colon along its defined embryologic planes with dissection of all vessels up to the superior mesenteric axis with a complete lymphadenectomy.

At present, robotic colectomy (with the Si system) can only be recommended as a learning tool to develop the skills necessary to eventually perform a high-quality TME.[52] The advent of the Xi, however, may change this practice.

LEARNING CURVE FOR ROBOTIC SURGERY

The learning curve for performing robotic colorectal operations is shorter than for laparoscopy and is achieved after 15 to 30 cases.[26,36] There are 3 phases identified in the learning curve for robotic colorectal operations[47–49]:

Phase 1 – initial learning (1–15 cases)
Phase 2 – increased competence (15–25 cases)
Phase 3 – period of highest skill (>25 cases)

Systematic reviews of learning curves in laparoscopic and robotic colorectal surgery show that defining proficiency is difficult and subjective, depending on the parameters studied.[55] Operative time is commonly used as a surrogate for efficiency but is imperfect, and shorter operative time and conversion rates do not always translate into better patient outcomes.[56] A 2016 systematic review determined that the mean number of cases was 29.7 for phase 1 and 37.4 for phase 2, with 39 cases necessary to be considered an expert.[57]

Melich and colleagues[58] looked at perioperative outcomes and learning curves for a single surgeon trained in open colorectal surgery who simultaneously adopted laparoscopic and robotic surgery at the beginning of his minimally invasive career. This series provided a unique insight on MIS learning curves and allowed for direct comparisons.[58] Although initially slower than laparoscopy, operative times for robotic surgery improved rapidly and after 41 cases became faster than laparoscopy.

EVOLUTION OF ROBOTIC TECHNIQUE
The da Vinci Xi System

The da Vinci Xi surgical robotic system represents a natural, evolutionary progress of the da Vinci technology. It is the fourth generation of the robotic line and currently the most sophisticated surgical robotic system available. Released in 2015, the Xi has a completely new system of robotic arm support involving an overhead boom from which 4 independent robotic arms are suspended. This simplified the docking process for the bedside assistant and allowed all arms to rotate as a group in a coordinated, computer-controlled fashion. This approach, combined with smaller ports for the robot arms, extended range of motion and increased the reach of the instruments. The optical system was also significantly enhanced and simplified while the scope can be positioned in any robotic arm. The Xi system allows for work in multiple quadrants without redocking and may extend the indications for robotic colectomy.

da Vinci Sp Single-Port Flexible System

Since the advent of natural orifice transluminal endoscopic surgery and more recently transanal TME, high hopes were placed on robotics to mitigate the challenging aspects of single-port surgery. A highly anticipated da Vinci SP flexible system device is currently awaiting Food and Drug Administration (FDA) clearance and is thought to be a new promising avenue for MIS. The computer-enhanced and coordinated control of the flexible robotic arms, including the optical system, is expected to improve precision and efficacy especially during the transanal approach.

Reduced Port and Single-Incision/Single-Port Robotic Colorectal Surgery

There is no FDA-approved single-port device for robotic colorectal surgery as yet. A modified port using an Alexis wound retractor placed through a transumbilical incision, with a surgical glove to form the cover of the port has been used by Lim and colleagues to perform single- port sigmoid colectomy successfully.[59] Trocars are placed through the cut fingers of the glove and a 3-arm robot configuration is used. Short-term oncologic outcomes and perioperative parameters are acceptable with this technique.

Reduced port surgery, using the FDA-approved single port through a transumbilical incision, with an additional robotic port in the right lower quadrant, has been reported by Bae and colleagues[60] for left colon, sigmoid, and rectosigmoid cancers with no conversions and adequate node yield and negative margins. The da Vinci single-port system has 4 ports, 1 for an 8.5-mm robotic camera, 1 for the assistant, and 2 curved trocars that allow instruments to cross each other. The major advantage over SILS is that the computer is able to allocate each instrument to the hand on the side of the ipsilateral visual field, meaning the left instrument is controlled seamlessly with the right hand and vice versa.

SUMMARY

Robotic surgery is a natural evolution of the minimally invasive technique and should be considered one of the tools currently available for practicing surgeons. It is not likely to replace the traditional laparoscopy; however, it should be treated as its complement in selected cases. Surgery in the deep pelvis is particularly amenable to a robotic approach. New robotic technology is emerging that addresses some of the weaknesses of the earlier systems, which may lead to increased utilization in the near future. In general, the surgeon benefits more than the patient from the use of robotic technology, because it allows for improved ergonomics, visualization, versatility, and control of the case.

REFERENCES

1. Baik SH, Gincherman M, Mutch MG, et al. Laparoscopic vs open resection for patients with rectal cancer: comparison of perioperative outcomes and long-term survival. Dis Colon Rectum 2011;54(1):6–14.
2. Guillou PJ, Quirke P, Thorpe H, et al. Short-term endpoints of conventional versus laparoscopic-assisted surgery in patients with colorectal cancer (MRC CLASICC trial): multicentre, randomised controlled trial. Lancet 2005;365(9472):1718–26.
3. Jayne DG, Thorpe HC, Copeland J, et al. Five-year follow-up of the Medical Research Council CLASICC trial of laparoscopically assisted versus open surgery for colorectal cancer. Br J Surg 2010;97(11):1638–45.
4. Kang SB, Park JW, Jeong SY, et al. Open versus laparoscopic surgery for mid or low rectal cancer after neoadjuvant chemoradiotherapy (COREAN trial): short-term outcomes of an open-label randomised controlled trial. Lancet Oncol 2010;11(7):637–45.
5. Laurent C, Leblanc F, Wütrich P, et al. Laparoscopic versus open surgery for rectal cancer: long-term oncologic results. Ann Surg 2009;250(1):54–61.
6. Strohlein MA, Grützner KU, Jauch KW, et al. Comparison of laparoscopic vs. open access surgery in patients with rectal cancer: a prospective analysis. Dis Colon Rectum 2008;51(4):385–91.
7. Tsang WW, Chung CC, Kwok SY, et al. Laparoscopic sphincter-preserving total mesorectal excision with colonic J-pouch reconstruction: five-year results. Ann Surg 2006;243(3):353–8.
8. van der Pas MH, Haglind E, Cuesta MA, et al. Laparoscopic versus open surgery for rectal cancer (COLOR II): short-term outcomes of a randomised, phase 3 trial. Lancet Oncol 2013;14(3):210–8.
9. Kayano H, Okuda J, Tanaka K, et al. Evaluation of the learning curve in laparoscopic low anterior resection for rectal cancer. Surg Endosc 2011;25(9):2972–9.
10. Herron DM, MM. A Consensus Document on Robotic Surgery: Prepared by the SAGES-MIRA Robotic Surgery Consensus Group. 2007. Available at: http://www.sages.org/publication/id/ROBOT/. Accessed October 16, 2016.
11. Weber PA, Merola S, Wasielewski A, et al. Telerobotic-assisted laparoscopic right and sigmoid colectomies for benign disease. Dis Colon Rectum 2002;45(12):1689–94 [discussion: 1695–6].
12. Hashizume M, Shimada M, Tomikawa M, et al. Early experiences of endoscopic procedures in general surgery assisted by a computer-enhanced surgical system. Surg Endosc 2002;16(8):1187–91.

13. D'Annibale A, Morpurgo E, Fiscon V, et al. Robotic and laparoscopic surgery for treatment of colorectal diseases. Dis Colon Rectum 2004;47(12):2162–8.

14. Giulianotti PC, Coratti A, Angelini M, et al. Robotics in general surgery: personal experience in a large community hospital. Arch Surg 2003;138(7):777–84.

15. Delaney CP, Lynch AC, Senagore AJ, et al. Comparison of robotically performed and traditional laparoscopic colorectal surgery. Dis Colon Rectum 2003;46(12): 1633–9.

16. Pigazzi A, Ellenhorn JD, Ballantyne GH, et al. Robotic-assisted laparoscopic low anterior resection with total mesorectal excision for rectal cancer. Surg Endosc 2006;20(10):1521–5.

17. Rawlings AL, Woodland JH, Crawford DL. Telerobotic surgery for right and sigmoid colectomies: 30 consecutive cases. Surg Endosc 2006;20(11):1713–8.

18. Luca F, Valvo M, Ghezzi TL, et al. Impact of robotic surgery on sexual and urinary functions after fully robotic nerve-sparing total mesorectal excision for rectal cancer. Ann Surg 2013;257(4):672–8.

19. Plerhoples TA, Hernandez-Boussard T, Wren SM. The aching surgeon: a survey of physical discomfort and symptoms following open, laparoscopic, and robotic surgery. J Robot Surg 2012;6(1):65–72.

20. Stomberg MW, Tronstad SE, Hedberg K, et al. Work-related musculoskeletal disorders when performing laparoscopic surgery. Surg Laparosc Endosc Percutan Tech 2010;20(1):49–53.

21. Esposito C, Najmaldin A, Schier F, et al. Work-related upper limb musculoskeletal disorders in pediatric minimally invasive surgery: a multicentric survey comparing laparoscopic and sils ergonomy. Pediatr Surg Int 2014;30(4):395–9.

22. Casillas MA Jr, Leichtle SW, Wahl WL, et al. Improved perioperative and short-term outcomes of robotic versus conventional laparoscopic colorectal operations. Am J Surg 2014;208(1):33–40.

23. Agha A, Fürst A, Iesalnieks I, et al. Conversion rate in 300 laparoscopic rectal resections and its influence on morbidity and oncological outcome. Int J Colorectal Dis 2008;23(4):409–17.

24. Baek JH, McKenzie S, Garcia-Aguilar J, et al. Oncologic outcomes of robotic-assisted total mesorectal excision for the treatment of rectal cancer. Ann Surg 2010;251(5):882–6.

25. Baik SH, Kwon HY, Kim JS, et al. Robotic versus laparoscopic low anterior resection of rectal cancer: short-term outcome of a prospective comparative study. Ann Surg Oncol 2009;16(6):1480–7.

26. Choi DJ, Kim SH, Lee PJ, et al. Single-stage totally robotic dissection for rectal cancer surgery: technique and short-term outcome in 50 consecutive patients. Dis Colon Rectum 2009;52(11):1824–30.

27. deSouza AL, Prasad LM, Marecik SJ, et al. Total mesorectal excision for rectal cancer: the potential advantage of robotic assistance. Dis Colon Rectum 2010; 53(12):1611–7.

28. Hellan M, Anderson C, Ellenhorn JD, et al. Short-term outcomes after robotic-assisted total mesorectal excision for rectal cancer. Ann Surg Oncol 2007; 14(11):3168–73.

29. Rottoli M, Bona S, Rosati R, et al. Laparoscopic rectal resection for cancer: effects of conversion on short-term outcome and survival. Ann Surg Oncol 2009; 16(5):1279–86.

30. Yamamoto S, Fukunaga M, Miyajima N, et al. Impact of conversion on surgical outcomes after laparoscopic operation for rectal carcinoma: a retrospective study of 1,073 patients. J Am Coll Surg 2009;208(3):383–9.

31. Shin JW, Kim J, Kwak JM, et al. First report: Robotic pelvic exenteration for locally advanced rectal cancer. Colorectal Dis 2014;16(1):O9–14.
32. MacFarlane JK, Ryall RD, Heald RJ. Mesorectal excision for rectal cancer. Lancet 1993;341(8843):457–60.
33. Nagtegaal ID, Marijnen CA, Kranenbarg EK, et al. Circumferential margin involvement is still an important predictor of local recurrence in rectal carcinoma: not one millimeter but two millimeters is the limit. Am J Surg Pathol 2002;26(3):350–7.
34. Nagtegaal ID, van de Velde CJ, van der Worp E, et al. Macroscopic evaluation of rectal cancer resection specimen: clinical significance of the pathologist in quality control. J Clin Oncol 2002;20(7):1729–34.
35. Pai A, Marecik SJ, Park JJ, et al. Oncologic and clinicopathologic outcomes of robot-assisted total mesorectal excision for rectal cancer. Dis Colon Rectum 2015;58(7):659–67.
36. Ramos JR, Parra-Davila E. Four-arm single docking full robotic surgery for low rectal cancer: technique standardization. Rev Col Bras Cir 2014;41(3):216–23.
37. Kwak JM, Kim SH. The technique of single-stage totally robotic low anterior resection. J Robot Surg 2011;5(1):25–8.
38. Park YA, Kim JM, Kim SA, et al. Totally robotic surgery for rectal cancer: from splenic flexure to pelvic floor in one setup. Surg Endosc 2010;24(3):715–20.
39. Hellan M, Stein H, Pigazzi A. Totally robotic low anterior resection with total mesorectal excision and splenic flexure mobilization. Surg Endosc 2009;23(2): 447–51.
40. Baik SH, Kim NK, Lim DR, et al. Oncologic outcomes and perioperative clinicopathologic results after robot-assisted tumor-specific mesorectal excision for rectal cancer. Ann Surg Oncol 2013;20(8):2625–32.
41. Fleshman J, Branda M, Sargent DJ, et al. Effect of laparoscopic-assisted resection vs open resection of stage II or III rectal cancer on pathologic outcomes: the ACOSOG Z6051 randomized clinical trial. JAMA 2015;314(13):1346–55.
42. Park IJ, You YN, Schlette E, et al. Reverse-hybrid robotic mesorectal excision for rectal cancer. Dis Colon Rectum 2012;55(2):228–33.
43. Kinugasa Y, Murakami G, Suzuki D, et al. Histological identification of fascial structures posterolateral to the rectum. Br J Surg 2007;94(5):620–6.
44. DeSouza A, Domajnko B, Park J, et al. Incisional hernia, midline versus low transverse incision: what is the ideal incision for specimen extraction and hand-assisted laparoscopy? Surg Endosc 2011;25(4):1031–6.
45. Marecik SJ, Zawadzki M, Desouza AL, et al. Robotic cylindrical abdominoperineal resection with transabdominal levator transection. Dis Colon Rectum 2011; 54(10):1320–5.
46. Pigazzi A, Luca F, Patriti A, et al. Multicentric study on robotic tumor-specific mesorectal excision for the treatment of rectal cancer. Ann Surg Oncol 2010;17(6): 1614–20.
47. Trastulli S, Farinella E, Cirocchi R, et al. Robotic resection compared with laparoscopic rectal resection for cancer: systematic review and meta-analysis of short-term outcome. Colorectal Dis 2012;14(4):e134–56.
48. Park EJ, Cho MS, Baek SJ, et al. Long-term oncologic outcomes of robotic low anterior resection for rectal cancer: a comparative study with laparoscopic surgery. Ann Surg 2015;261(1):129–37.
49. Hara M, Sng K, Yoo BE, et al. Robotic-assisted surgery for rectal adenocarcinoma: short-term and midterm outcomes from 200 consecutive cases at a single institution. Dis Colon Rectum 2014;57(5):570–7.

50. Kim JY, Kim NK, Lee KY, et al. A comparative study of voiding and sexual function after total mesorectal excision with autonomic nerve preservation for rectal cancer: laparoscopic versus robotic surgery. Ann Surg Oncol 2012;19(8):2485–93.

51. Baek SJ, Kim SH, Cho JS, et al. Robotic versus conventional laparoscopic surgery for rectal cancer: a cost analysis from a single institute in Korea. World J Surg 2012;36(11):2722–9.

52. deSouza AL, Prasad LM, Park JJ, et al. Robotic assistance in right hemicolectomy: is there a role? Dis Colon Rectum 2010;53(7):1000–6.

53. Spinoglio G, Marano A, Bianchi PP, et al. Robotic right colectomy with modified complete mesocolic excision: long-term oncologic outcomes. Ann Surg Oncol 2016;23(Suppl 5):684–91.

54. Hohenberger W, Weber K, Matzel K, et al. Standardized surgery for colonic cancer: complete mesocolic excision and central ligation–technical notes and outcome. Colorectal Dis 2009;11(4):354–64 [discussion: 364–5].

55. Barrie J, Jayne DG, Wright J, et al. Attaining surgical competency and its implications in surgical clinical trial design: a systematic review of the learning curve in laparoscopic and robot-assisted laparoscopic colorectal cancer surgery. Ann Surg Oncol 2014;21(3):829–40.

56. Chen G, Liu Z, Han P, et al. The learning curve for the laparoscopic approach for colorectal cancer: a single institution's experience. J Laparoendosc Adv Surg Tech A 2013;23(1):17–21.

57. Jimenez-Rodriguez RM, Rubio-Dorado-Manzanares M, Díaz-Pavón JM, et al. Learning curve in robotic rectal cancer surgery: current state of affairs. Int J Colorectal Dis 2016;31(12):1807–15.

58. Melich G, Hong YK, Kim J, et al. Simultaneous development of laparoscopy and robotics provides acceptable perioperative outcomes and shows robotics to have a faster learning curve and to be overall faster in rectal cancer surgery: analysis of novice MIS surgeon learning curves. Surg Endosc 2015;29(3):558–68.

59. Lim MS, Melich G, Min BS. Robotic single-incision anterior resection for sigmoid colon cancer: access port creation and operative technique. Surg Endosc 2013; 27(3):1021.

60. Bae SU, Jeong WK, Baek SK. Robotic anterior resection for sigmoid colon cancer using reduced port access. Dis Colon Rectum 2016;59(3):245–6.

Local Excision of Rectal Cancer

Daniel Owen Young, MD, Anjali S. Kumar, MD, MPH*

KEYWORDS

- Rectal cancer • Local excision • TEM • TAMIS

KEY POINTS

- Several techniques are commonly used for local excision of early-stage rectal cancer, including conventional local excision, transanal endoscopic microsurgery (TEM), and transanal minimally invasive surgery (TAMIS).
- There are strict criteria for selecting patients for local excision of rectal cancer, all of which are calculated to minimize the likelihood of lymph node involvement.
- Local excision avoids the morbidity of radical surgery for rectal cancer, but for advanced tumors it is associated with a higher risk of local and distant tumor recurrence.
- Newer techniques, such as TEM and TAMIS, improve visualization and versatility, and may have superior oncologic outcomes to conventional local excision.
- The use of neoadjuvant and adjuvant therapy in conjunction with local excision is an active area of research and there is no current consensus regarding these multimodality treatments.

INTRODUCTION

The ideal surgical treatment for rectal cancer would have negligible morbidity, and would be curative while maintaining intestinal continuity and excellent function. In most cases, this is an unrealized standard. In terms of oncologic outcome, total mesorectal excision (TME) provides the best long-term prognosis for rectal cancer, with low rates of local recurrence and excellent long-term survival. Depending on tumor location and morphology, TME can be performed with restoration of intestinal continuity (low anterior resection) or with removal of the anus and creation of a permanent colostomy (abdominoperineal resection). This type of radical surgery removes the tumor and its organ of origin en bloc with associated perirectal lymph nodes.

Although it does provide the best oncologic outcomes, TME is associated with a panoply of complications, including urinary tract infections, nonhealing perineal

Disclosures: The authors have nothing to disclose.
Colorectal Surgery Program, Section of General, Thoracic, and Vascular Surgery, Virginia Mason Medical Center, 1100 9th Avenue Seattle, WA 98101, USA
* Corresponding author.
E-mail address: askumarmd@gmail.com

wounds, functional disorders, anastomotic leaks, strictures, and perioperative death.[1–3] Moreover, the 5-year local recurrence rates for radical surgery, even in cases of early-stage rectal cancers, still range from 2% to 8%.[4,5] Therefore, physicians have often used less-invasive techniques when possible that could mitigate the morbidity of rectal resection while providing the patient with acceptable oncologic results, particularly for early-stage rectal cancer.

Local excision (LE) of rectal cancer involves removal of the tumor itself without proctectomy. Interest in LE for early distal rectal cancers began in earnest after Morson and colleagues[6] published their experience at St. Mark's Hospital in London in 1977 demonstrating a low rate of local recurrence after excision with negative margins. This suggested that early rectal cancer could be definitively treated with LE, thereby sparing patients many of the morbidities of radical surgery. As enthusiasm for LE has grown, so has its use in the United States for early-stage rectal cancer.[7]

LE involves full-thickness resection of the tumor and a margin of rectum, down to the perirectal fat, but not necessarily including any draining lymphatics. Several different approaches to local excision have been used, including older transsphincteric and transcoccygeal techniques. Currently, the most widely used technique for LE is transanal excision (TAE). Conventional techniques are somewhat limited due to poor visualization and confinement to the distal rectum. Transanal endoscopic microsurgery (TEM) and transanal minimally invasive surgery (TAMIS) are more recent additions to the surgeon's armamentarium, and allow for improved visualization and access to the more proximal rectum.

PATIENT SELECTION
Premalignant Polyps

Adenomatous polyps often develop within the rectum, but size and morphology may prevent them from being amenable to complete endoscopic removal. Full-thickness or partial-thickness excision of these lesions can be done successfully via LE, and can avoid the morbidity of major pelvic surgery in a patient without an invasive cancer.

Rectal Adenocarcinoma

In general, LE should be reserved for favorable T1 lesions without irregular or enlarged lymph nodes. Patients under consideration for LE of rectal cancer should undergo routine staging, including computed tomography (CT) imaging of the chest, abdomen, and pelvis and serum carcinoembryonic antigen (CEA) level, as well as digital rectal examination, proctoscopy, and dedicated rectal imaging with MRI or endorectal ultrasound[8] to assess the depth of local invasion. Because lymphatics are not reliably removed with LE, the goal is to select patients with early-stage tumors that have a low risk for lymphatic involvement at the time of operation. A combination of physical examination findings, preoperative imaging, and histopathologic characteristics are taken into account (**Table 1**).

On digital examination, the tumor should be freely mobile, as fixed tumors are predictive of advanced disease.[9,10] Proctoscopic examination should determine tumor size, extent of rectal circumference involvement, and distance from the anal verge. Tumors larger than 4 cm or involving more than 50% of the rectal circumference are often excluded from local excision for technical reasons,[11] although large tumors still can be removed via LE with a selective approach, and circumferential or near-circumferential resections have been described in models.[12] Conventional local excision is limited to distal tumors (usually within 6–8 cm of the anal verge), whereas TEM and TAMIS have allowed for successful resection of more proximal lesions (8–20 cm from the anal verge).

Table 1
Criteria for local excision of rectal cancer

Anatomic	Histologic	Staging
• <50% circumference of bowel • <4 cm in size • Mobile and nonfixed • Within 8 cm of the anal verge for conventional local excision and 20 cm for transanal endoscopic microsurgery or transanal minimally invasive surgery	• T1 • sm1 or sm2 • Absence of tumor budding • Absence of lymphovascular invasion • Well to moderate differentiation	• No evidence of T2 disease or lymphadenopathy on MRI or endorectal ultrasound

Histologic features of the endoscopic biopsy also impact the appropriateness for LE. Features including poor differentiation and lymphovascular invasion predict unacceptably high rates of lymph node metastasis and local recurrence, and these lesions should not be considered for LE.[13] Tumor budding or sprouting, in which groups of a few tumor cells are seen invading ahead of the main front of tumor, is another risk factor for lymph node metastasis and should exclude patients from LE.[14–16]

Depth of tumor invasion into the bowel wall (T-stage) not only impacts the feasibility of a complete resection with negative margins, but it is also correlated with the likelihood of lymph node metastasis.[17,18] Preoperative imaging provides an essential but imperfect estimate for depth of invasion. MRI can be used to assess depth of rectal wall invasion, but in select patients, transrectal ultrasound may better discriminate between T1 and T2 lesions.[19,20]

Some evidence suggests that further subclassification of T1 lesions based on depth of invasion of the submucosa allows for even better stratification of risk for lymph node metastasis (LNM). By dividing the submucosal layer into thirds, tumors can be classified by depth of infiltration, as tumors with deeper invasion correlate with increased risk for metastasis (SM1 = superficial 1/3, 3% risk LNM; SM2 = middle 1/3, 8% risk LNM; SM3 = deep 1/3, 23% risk LNM).[14,17,21]

Any patient with clinical evidence of LNM should not be considered for LE. Transrectal ultrasound is used to evaluate mesorectal lymph nodes, but has limited accuracy and relies mostly on size.[18] MRI, although also imperfect, may be the most sensitive and specific preoperative test for lymph node involvement, as it can appreciate irregularities in subcentimeter nodes.[19]

Other indications

Patients with more advanced tumors also may be appropriate for LE if their comorbidities prohibit them from being candidates for major pelvic surgery. LE also may be used for these tumors when curative resection is not the goal, and the focus is instead on palliation. There are also some patients who simply refuse radical surgery for personal reasons. For example, if patients are adamantly against having a permanent colostomy, they demonstrate understanding, and they are willing to accept a higher risk of cancer recurrence to maintain intestinal continuity, it is appropriate to respect their wishes and perform LE despite the potential for an inferior oncologic outcome.

As alluded to previously, LE of rectal lesions also may be considered in patients without a definitive diagnosis of rectal cancer, such as in cases of high-grade dysplasia, large polyps not amenable to endoscopic resection, or submucosal tumors, including carcinoid or gastrointestinal stromal tumors.[22]

Some surgeons also have advocated for LE for those with a complete clinical response to neoadjuvant chemotherapy and radiation. They use LE as a biopsy to confirm or deny a pathologic complete response. Currently, however, there is no role for this approach outside of a clinical trial.[23]

TECHNIQUE

Conventional LE of rectal tumors can be done via transanal, transcoccygeal, or transsphincteric approach. Among these, the transanal approach is the most common; our technique is described in the following section. Transcoccygeal and transsphincteric excision are reviewed elsewhere.[24] Regardless of the approach, the principles of LE are the same: full-thickness resection of an intact tumor with 1 cm margin of benign tissue circumferentially, and the absence of tissue fragmentation.

Transanal Excision

In selecting the bowel preparation for these procedures, the patient's description of his or her bowel habits can be used to determine if cleansing enemas will be adequate, or if a full mechanical bowel preparation will be necessary. For patients with a history of constipation and straining, a mechanical bowel preparation can reduce the likelihood that a patient will strain immediately after resection. For those with regular bowel habits, an enema the night before surgery and another on the morning of the resection is enough to allow for proper visualization. Preoperative intravenous antibiotics are often given within 1 hour of the procedure, although there is no evidence that this decreases the risk for surgical site infection in anorectal surgery. These procedures usually take less than an hour to perform. They can be done with a combination of intravenous sedation (monitored anesthesia care) and a local anesthetic, or alternatively with the use of general anesthesia, with the approaches being equally effective. A pudendal nerve and perianal block relaxes the anal sphincter and has the additional benefit of improving postoperative pain control.

Lithotomy positioning is usually adequate, even for anterior tumors. However, it is typically easier to operate with the lesion oriented toward the floor, and certain anterior tumors may be accessed more readily in the prone jackknife position. Using a headlamp maximizes visualization.

When the patient is positioned, the rectum is further irrigated with a bulb syringe. Irrigation with betadine is unnecessary and may stain the specimen, obscuring the borders of the lesion. The authors typically use Ferguson plastic anoscopes (CS Surgical, Inc, Slidell, LA) for retraction. These anoscopes are reusable and come in myriad diameters and lengths (**Fig. 1**). Other retractors, such as the Lone Star (Lone Star Medical Products, Inc, Stafford, TX), Sawyer, Hill-Ferguson retractors, or Parks retractors are preferred by others.

The anus is gently dilated until good visualization is obtained. Next, the lesion is marked by scoring the mucosa circumferentially with electrocautery. This preserves the intended 1-cm margin, as the tissue often becomes distorted during the resection. Cautery is then used to incise the full thickness of the rectum along the scored outline around the lesion. The needle-tip cautery is often used with a combination of cut and coagulation settings, as this distorts and shrinks the benign tissue less than the spatulated cautery tip on the coagulation setting alone. The perirectal fat should be visible in the wound once the specimen is removed. For all LE procedures (TAE, TEM, and TAMIS), the specimen should be pinned out and oriented on a cork board immediately after removal while fresh (**Fig. 2**). This prevents retraction of the benign tissue margin once placed in formalin.

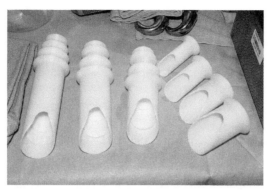

Fig. 1. Ferguson anoscope set provides varying lengths and diameters for access. The soft bevel allows for the lesion to fall into view for resection. (CS Surgical, Inc, Slidell, LA.)

We thoroughly irrigate the wound bed and typically close the defect transversely with interrupted 3-0 Vicryl sutures, although smaller, distal defects can be left open to heal secondarily. A rigid or flexible proctoscope then can be used to assess for rectal patency after closure of the defect. Patients are typically discharged home from the recovery area.

Transanal Endoscopic Microsurgery and Transanal Minimally Invasive Surgery

Use of TEM and TAMIS instrumentation has become more prevalent in recent years, relying on laparoscopic technology to assist with lesion removal. Although the technique was initially aimed at more proximal tumors, many surgeons use these techniques for distal tumors as well because of the improved visualization and versatility. Selection of TEM versus TAMIS is usually based on surgeon preference and the relative availability of the 2 platforms. In general, the 2 techniques have very similar goals and capabilities, although TAMIS is newer and lacks long-term data.

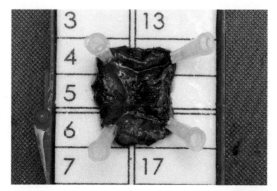

Fig. 2. After excision, the full-thickness specimen is pinned to a cork board and oriented to the patient's anatomy and laterality on the pathology slip by using the numbers on the board (ie, 4 = right proximal, 14 = left proximal, 6 = right distal, 16 = left distal). Seen here is an adenocarcinoma arising in a polyp that was incompletely excised by snare polypectomy for which we performed conventional transanal excision.

Because more proximal tumors are approached with TEM and TAMIS, a full mechanical and antibiotic bowel preparation is usually used to minimize intraoperative contamination should peritoneal violation occur. This also lessens the bacterial load of stool passing by the excision site in the first few postoperative days. It is imperative that a complete mechanical preparation is achieved, as the propensity of liquid stool to obscure the view or seep out into the wound bed is a legitimate concern.

Transanal endoscopic microsurgery

TEM was first introduced in Germany in 1984 by Dr Gerhard Buess, and it has slowly gained momentum globally over the past 30 years as more outcomes data became available.[25] It uses a rigid, beveled proctoscope that is 4 cm in diameter and 12 to 20 cm in length, a laparoscopic camera, and modified laparoscopic instruments. Specialized equipment is necessary for TEM, including disposable tubing, a dedicated machine for pneumorectum, and equipment to position the patient and secure the proctoscope to the bed.[25] The cost of that equipment, along with TEM's steep learning curve, has prevented the technique from being widespread.

The procedure works best when the patients are positioned with the lesion in a dependent orientation, and the bevel of the proctoscope holds up the opposite bowel wall (**Fig. 3**). In this way, visualization is optimized. We have found that even in morbidly obese patients, the rigid proctoscope provides excellent retraction for safe excision.[26]

Transanal minimally invasive surgery

TAMIS was introduced in 2009 as an alternative to TEM, offering similar visibility and versatility without the need for certain expensive and specialized pieces of equipment.[25] TAMIS also allows for dissection in multiple quadrants, and so has fewer limitations on patient positioning. It uses a flexible and disposable single-port laparoscopic entry device through which trocars are inserted or are pre-embedded. Pneumorectum is achieved with a regular laparoscopic CO_2 insufflator, and conventional laparoscopic cameras and graspers are inserted. Because bellowing and fogging of the lens is more common with TAMIS than with TEM, use of insufflators designed to constantly recirculate and warm the gases can be helpful.

Techniques for dissection are similar for TEM and TAMIS; 1-cm margins are scored circumferentially with hook electrocautery. The full-thickness resection can then be performed using electrocautery, with great care taken to

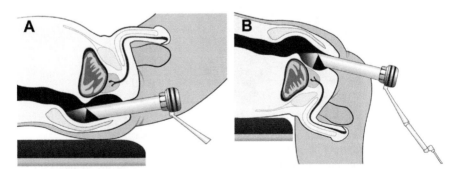

Fig. 3. Illustration of the beveled end of the TEM proctoscope, which holds up the opposite wall of the rectum. The lesion is placed in the dependent position; thus, the patient is placed (A) supine for a posterior tumor, or (B) prone for an anterior tumor.

avoid coning in on the specimen. For TAMIS, ultrasonic shears can counteract the previously described smoke and fog. Some advocate for dissecting the proximal margin first, whereas others work in the more traditional distal-to-proximal manner. Although both techniques are effective, the surgeon must remain focused and remove the tissue in a way that minimizes errors in orientation. After the specimen has been extracted and properly oriented for pathology, a suction irrigation device is used to wash the wound bed and ensure hemostasis.

Defects in the rectal wall can be very large after TEM and TAMIS, and it is best to achieve a watertight closure. Suturing is typically done using laparoscopic sutures and needle drivers, closing the defect in the rectal wall transversely. Both running and interrupted techniques can be used, typically using an absorbable suture. If the peritoneal cavity was entered during dissection, either intentionally or unintentionally depending on the intended depth of resection, this typically can be repaired primarily with sutures without any significant consequences.

Of note, laparoscopic suturing in this very small field can be technically challenging. To assist in closure, silver beads can be fastened like clips to the ends of the suture to allow knotless closure. Another approach is to use barbed suture, and even specialized suturing devices such as the Endostitch (TM, Covidien, Mansfield, MA, USA).[25] Once closure is completed, it is crucial to ensure that the lumen of the bowel was not compromised. Adequate tension placed on the edges of the wound closure helps mitigate this, as does a combination of linear and transverse closure approaches. At the conclusion of the case, flexible or rigid proctoscopy is used to ensure bowel patency and the absence of luminal narrowing.

COMPLICATIONS
Conventional Local Excision

Overall, morbidity and complication rates for LE of rectal tumors are much lower than for radical surgery.[7] Common complications include urinary tract infection and bleeding, as well as gastrointestinal complaints, such as diarrhea. Other uncommon complications include wound infections or abscesses, thromboembolic events, and, rarely, rectal strictures or rectovaginal fistulas.[7]

Transanal Endoscopic Microsurgery and Transanal Minimally Invasive Surgery

Like conventional LE, TEM and TAMIS have a low rate of complications. The most common complications are urinary retention, perioperative bleeding, and peritoneal violation.[27] In TEM, both urinary retention and peritoneal violation are associated with anterior and lateral locations of the excised tumor. Entry into the peritoneum has not been shown to have any increased morbidity,[27] and this risk is further reduced if full mechanical and antibiotic bowel preparation is used and patients are observed overnight with 24 hours of intravenous antibiotics.

Increased rates of intraoperative bleeding (more than 50 mL) are associated with larger tumor size. Rectovaginal fistula is reported in fewer than 1.5% of patients in large series.[28–30] Anal dysfunction and fecal incontinence due to anal stretch during the procedure have been hypothetical concerns due to the size of the operating proctoscope, but several studies have demonstrated that fecal incontinence scores do not change significantly after TEM or TAMIS, and long-term fecal incontinence is rare.[31–33]

OUTCOMES
Conventional Local Excision

The 3 most important outcome measures with regard to LE for rectal cancer are local recurrence, disease-free survival, and overall survival. There are no prospective randomized trials comparing conventional LE with radical surgery, and most studies are small single-institution reviews. There is great variability in reported outcomes for both locally excised T1 and T2 tumors in these studies, reflecting the varied nature of the studies themselves. Local recurrence, for instance, varies from 5% to 28% with LE of T1 lesions and 13% to 37% for T2 lesions.[34] Disease-free survival at 5 years is also a range: 64% to 93% for T1 lesions and 63% to 90% for T2 lesions.[34] These findings compare unfavorably with radical surgery for similar lesions. Nevertheless, despite the increased local recurrence seen with LE of T1 tumors, most studies do not show any statistical difference in 5-year overall survival as compared with radical surgery, although the trend favors radical surgery.[7,35–38] Conventional LE for T2 lesions, however, is clearly inferior to radical surgery.[7,35–38]

Transanal Endoscopic Microsurgery and Transanal Minimally Invasive Surgery

The benefit of endoscopic and minimally invasive resection of rectal tumors is an extended anatomic range, allowing access to more proximal tumors than conventional excision. Moreover, visualization of the tumor is enhanced, leading to a theoretic oncologic advantage with improved margins and less specimen fragmentation when compared with conventional LE. There are no randomized studies that directly compare TEM or TAMIS to conventional LE. A recent meta-analysis concluded that local recurrence rates are lower with TEM than with conventional LE.[39] Several studies directly compare TEM with radical surgery. A single small randomized trial for T1 tumors found no significant difference in local recurrence or overall survival between TEM and radical surgery.[40] This is consistent with other retrospective studies for TEM in T1 tumors.[41,42]

INDICATIONS TO PROCEED WITH RADICAL SURGERY

Because of the uncertainty that surrounds clinical staging of a rectal tumor, LE may be thought of as a full-thickness biopsy. For patients with clinically staged T1 tumors who want to pursue LE as a definitive resection, the final treatment plan should nevertheless be based on the final pathologic tumor stage. If there are high-risk features (see **Table 1**) after LE or if the tumor is T2 or greater, radical surgery should be recommended in patients physiologically fit for such an operation.

Other indications for radical surgery include inadequate circumferential margins or piecemeal extraction of the specimen.[43] Outcomes for patients who undergo delayed radical resection of an early-stage rectal cancer within 30 days of initial LE are similar to those who undergo immediate radical resection.[44] Some patients may refuse radical surgery despite high-risk features or more advanced tumor penetration (T2 or T3); under those circumstances, it is crucial to convey the inferior oncologic outcomes for LE as compared with radical surgery, but ultimately respect the patients' wishes.

Posttreatment Surveillance

Standard posttreatment surveillance of rectal adenocarcinoma includes clinical abdominal and digital rectal examination; CT imaging of the chest, abdomen, and pelvis; serial serum CEA levels; and endoscopic evaluation.[8] For patients who have undergone LE alone, the optimal surveillance protocol has not been determined,[45] but a more aggressive surveillance regimen may be appropriate to allow early identification of recurrence. Some studies have suggested routine use of transrectal ultrasound and pelvic MRI.[46,47] The authors' favored approach adheres to protocols designed for nonoperative management of rectal cancer in patients with a complete response to chemoradiation therapy,[48] using annual endoscopic surveillance of the wound bed by flexible sigmoidoscopy for the first 5 years and assessing the lymph node basin by alternating endoscopic ultrasounds and pelvic MRI (rectal cancer staging protocols) spaced at 3-month intervals during the year after resection. The imaging interval is lengthened to 6 months and then annually with continued negative findings.

ADDITIONAL THERAPY
Neoadjuvant Therapy

Neoadjuvant chemoradiation therapy combined with radical surgery has become the standard of care for locally advanced rectal cancer because of evidence for decreased local recurrence.[49,50] This has kindled interested in applying this approach to LE, especially in T2 or T3 rectal cancers, with the hope of decreasing local recurrence and avoiding radical surgery.

Several small studies[51–54] have suggested improved local tumor control with neoadjuvant chemoradiotherapy plus LE. A multicenter phase II clinical trial using LE (TEM or conventional LE) after neoadjuvant therapy for T2N0 rectal cancer recently reported 4% local recurrence and 3-year disease-free survival of 88%, although it did not meet its predetermined statistical threshold for efficacy.[55] This result is nevertheless promising, although such efforts remain within the realm of clinical study and outside the scope of standard practice.

Adjuvant Therapy

The role for adjuvant chemoradiation after LE is not well defined. In contrast to the increase over recent years in rates of LE for early-stage rectal cancer, there has been a decrease in the number of patients who undergo adjuvant therapy after LE.[56] There is retrospective evidence suggesting that LE plus adjuvant radiation therapy may be equivalent to radical surgery alone for overall survival in T1 and T2 tumors.[56] It is not clear that LE plus adjuvant radiation maintains the benefits of LE alone in terms of quality of life versus radical surgery. At least 1 randomized trial comparing radical surgery to LE plus chemoradiation therapy for T1-2 rectal cancers is planned.[57]

Salvage

The prognosis for local recurrence after TAE of T1 adenocarcinoma is poor compared with those initially resected with radical surgery. Five-year disease-free survival ranges from 53% to 79% despite salvage therapy.[34,58,59] A recent single-institution retrospective review found that most patients (87%) with recurrence after LE for T1 rectal cancer were able to undergo a salvage operation, although 5-year overall survival was only 69%.[59] In addition to the dramatic decrease in overall survival, sphincter-sparing approaches that were possible at first presentation may not be possible with salvage surgery. This underscores the importance of patient selection; it is especially critical to discuss these findings with patients who fall outside the strict criteria for LE but are averse to radical surgery.

SUMMARY

LE for rectal cancer is enticing because of the decreased morbidity and mortality as compared with radical surgery, but it is best used in highly selected patients who have early-stage cancers with favorable histology. It is also appropriate for those who otherwise would be unfit or unwilling to undergo a more aggressive surgical approach. Oncologic outcomes of LE are inferior to radical surgery, but newer literature suggests that TEM and TAMIS may partially bridge the outcomes gap due to improved visibility and lower margin positivity. Any locally excised tumor, regardless of approach, merits meticulous follow-up and surveillance for local and distant recurrence.

ACKNOWLEDGMENTS

The authors gratefully acknowledge the efforts of Alexandria J. Kent, BA, for editorial and administrative assistance in preparation and submission of this article. The authors also thank the ASCRS CREST project for use of the figures in this article.

REFERENCES

1. Pollard CW, Nivatvongs S, Rojanasakul A, et al. Carcinoma of the rectum. Dis Colon Rectum 1994;37(9):866–74.
2. Stewart DB, Hollenbeak C, Boltz M. Laparoscopic and open abdominoperineal resection for cancer: how patient selection and complications differ by approach. J Gastrointest Surg 2011;15(11):1928–38.
3. Luna-Pérez P, Rodríguez-Ramírez S, Vega J, et al. Morbidity and mortality following abdominoperineal resection for low rectal adenocarcinoma. Rev Invest Clin 2001;53(5):388–95.
4. Mccall JL, Cox MR, Wattchow DA. Analysis of local recurrence rates after surgery alone for rectal cancer. Int J Colorectal Dis 1995;10(3):126–32.
5. Enríquez-Navascués JM, Borda N, Lizerazu A, et al. Patterns of local recurrence in rectal cancer after a multidisciplinary approach. World J Gastroenterol 2011; 17(13):1674.
6. Morson BC, Bussey HJ, Samoorian S. Policy of local excision for early cancer of the colorectum. Gut 1977;18(12):1045–50.
7. You YN, Baxter NN, Stewart A, et al. Is the increasing rate of local excision for stage I rectal cancer in the United States justified? Ann Surg 2007;245(5):726–33.
8. National Comprehensive Cancer Network. Rectal cancer. Available at: https://www. nccn.org/professionals/physician_gls/pdf/rectal_blocks.pdf. Accessed September 5, 2016.
9. Rafaelsen SR, Kronborg O, Fenger C. Digital rectal examination and transrectal ultrasonography in staging of rectal cancer: a prospective, blind study. Acta Radiol 1994;35(3):300–4.
10. Nicholls RJ, Mason AY, Morson BC, et al. The clinical staging of rectal cancer. Br J Surg 1982;69:404–9.
11. Brunner W, Widmann B, Marti L, et al. Predictors for regional lymph node metastasis in T1 rectal cancer: a population-based SEER analysis. Surg Endosc 2016; 30(10):4405–15.
12. Denk PM, Swanström LL, Whiteford MH. Transanal endoscopic microsurgical platform for natural orifice surgery. Gastrointest Endosc 2008;68(5):954–9.
13. Blumberg D, Paty PB, Guillem JG, et al. All patients with small intramural rectal cancers are at risk for lymph node metastasis. Dis Colon Rectum 1999;42:881–5.
14. Kitajima K, Fujimori T, Fujii S, et al. Correlations between lymph node metastasis and depth of submucosal invasion in submucosal invasive colorectal carcinoma: a Japanese collaborative study. J Gastroenterol 2004;39:534–43.
15. Hase K, Shatney C, Johnson D, et al. Prognostic value of tumor "budding" in patients with colorectal cancer. Dis Colon Rectum 1993;36(7):627–35.

16. Ueno H, Mochizuki H, Hashiguchi Y, et al. Risk factors for an adverse outcome in early invasive colorectal carcinoma. Gastroenterology 2004;127(2):385–94.

17. Nascimbeni R, Burgart LJ, Nivatvongs S, et al. Risk of lymph node metastasis in T1 carcinoma of the colon and rectum. Dis Colon Rectum 2002;45(2):200–6.

18. Landmann RG, Wong DW, Hoepfl J, et al. Limitations of early rectal cancer nodal staging may explain failure after local excision. Dis Colon Rectum 2007;50(10): 1520–5.

19. Kwok H, Bissett IP, Hill GL. Preoperative staging of rectal cancer. Int J Colorectal Dis 2000;15(1):9–20.

20. Kennedy E, Vella E, Macdonald DB, et al. Optimisation of preoperative assessment in patients diagnosed with rectal cancer. Clin Oncol 2015;27(4):225–45.

21. Kudo S. Endoscopic mucosal resection of flat and depressed types of early colorectal cancer. Endoscopy 1993;25:455–61.

22. Kumar AS, Sidani SM, Kolli K, et al. Transanal endoscopic microsurgery for rectal carcinoids: the largest reported United States experience. Colorectal Dis 2012; 14(5):562–6.

23. Hallam S, Messenger DE, Thomas MG. A systematic review of local excision after neoadjuvant therapy for rectal cancer. Dis Colon Rectum 2016;59(10):984–97.

24. Irani JL, Bleday R. Local excision of rectal cancer. Shackelford's Surgery of the Alimentary Tract. 7th edition. Philadelphia: Elsevier/Saunders; 2013. p. 2077–8.

25. Rai V, Mishra N. Transanal approach to rectal polyps and cancer. Clin Colon Rectal Surg 2016;29(1):65–70.

26. Kumar AS, Chhitwal N, Coralic J, et al. Transanal endoscopic microsurgery: safe for midrectal lesions in morbidly obese patients. Am J Surg 2012;204(3):402–5.

27. Keller DS, Tahilramani RN, Flores-Gonzalez JR, et al. Transanal minimally invasive surgery: review of indications and outcomes from 75 consecutive patients. J Am Coll Surg 2016;222(5):814–22.

28. Allaix ME, Arezzo A, Caldart M, et al. Transanal endoscopic microsurgery for rectal neoplasms: experience of 300 consecutive cases. Dis Colon Rectum 2009;52:1831–6.

29. Tsai BM, Finne CO, Nordenstam JF, et al. Transanal endoscopic microsurgery resection of rectal tumors: outcomes and recommendations. Dis Colon Rectum 2010;53:16–23.

30. Kumar AS, Coralic J, Kelleher DC, et al. Complications of transanal endoscopic microsurgery are rare and minor: a single institution's analysis and comparison to existing data. Dis Colon Rectum 2013;56:295–300.

31. Cataldo PA, O'Brien S, Osler T. Transanal endoscopic microsurgery: a prospective evaluation of functional results. Dis Colon Rectum 2005;48:1366–71.

32. Kreis ME, Jehle EC, Haug V, et al. Functional results after transanal endoscopic microsurgery. Dis Colon Rectum 1996;39:1116–21.

33. Planting A, Phang PT, Raval MJ, et al. Transanal endoscopic microsurgery: impact on fecal incontinence and quality of life. Can J Surg 2013;56:243–8.

34. Kim E, Hwang JM, Garcia-Aguilar J. Local excision for rectal carcinoma. Clin Colorectal Cancer 2008;7(6):376–85.

35. Nascimbeni R, Nivatvongs S, Larson DR, et al. Long-term survival after local excision for T1 carcinoma of the rectum. Dis Colon Rectum 2004;47(11):1773–9.

36. Endreseth BH, Myrvold HE, Romundstad P, et al. Transanal excision vs. major surgery for T1 rectal cancer. Dis Colon Rectum 2005;48(7):1380–8.

37. Mellgren A, Sirivongs P, Rothenberger DA, et al. Is local excision adequate therapy for early rectal cancer? Dis Colon Rectum 2000;43(8):1064–71.

38. Bentrem DJ, Okabe S, Wong WD, et al. T1 adenocarcinoma of the rectum: transanal excision or radical surgery? Ann Surg 2005;242:472–7.
39. Clancy C, Burke JP, Albert MR, et al. Transanal endoscopic microsurgery versus standard transanal excision for the removal of rectal neoplasms: a systematic review and meta-analysis. Dis Colon Rectum 2015;58(2):254–61.
40. Winde G, Nottberg H, Keller R, et al. Surgical cure for early rectal carcinomas (T1). Transanal endoscopic microsurgery vs. anterior resection. Dis Colon Rectum 1996;39:969–76.
41. Heintz A, Mörschel M, Junginger T. Comparison of results after transanal endoscopic microsurgery and radical resection for T1 carcinoma of the rectum. Surg Endosc 1998;12:1145–8.
42. Lee W, Lee D, Choi S, et al. Transanal endoscopic microsurgery and radical surgery for T1 and T2 rectal cancer. Surg Endosc 2003;17:1283–7.
43. Baron PL, Enker WE, Zakowski MF, et al. Immediate vs. salvage resection after local treatment for early rectal cancer. Dis Colon Rectum 1995;38:177–81.
44. Hahnloser D, Wolff BG, Larson DW, et al. Immediate radical resection after local excision of rectal cancer: an oncologic compromise? Dis Colon Rectum 2005;48: 429–37.
45. Im YC, Kim CW, Park S, et al. Oncologic outcomes and proper surveillance after local excision of rectal cancer. J Korean Surg Soc 2013;84(2):94.
46. de Anda EH, Lee SH, Finne CO, et al. Endorectal ultrasound in the follow-up of rectal cancer patients treated by local excision or radical surgery. Dis Colon Rectum 2004;47:818–24.
47. Doornebosch PG, Ferenschild FT, de Wilt JH, et al. Treatment of recurrence after transanal endoscopic microsurgery (TEM) for T1 rectal cancer. Dis Colon Rectum 2010;53:1234–9.
48. Smith JJ, Chow OS, Gollub MJ, et al. Organ preservation in rectal adenocarcinoma: a phase II randomized controlled trial evaluating 3-year disease-free survival in patients with locally advanced rectal cancer treated with chemoradiation plus induction or consolidation chemotherapy, and total mesorectal excision or nonoperative management. BMC Cancer 2015;15(1):767.
49. van Gijn W, Marijnen CA, Nagtegaal ID, et al. Preoperative radiotherapy combined with total mesorectal excision for resectable rectal cancer: 12-year follow-up of the multicentre, randomised controlled TME trial. Lancet Oncol 2011;12:575–82.
50. Sauer R, Liersch T, Merkel S, et al. Preoperative versus postoperative chemoradiotherapy for locally advanced rectal cancer: results of the German CAO/ARO/AIO-94 randomized phase III trial after a median follow-up of 11 years. J Clin Oncol 2012;30:1926–33.
51. Borschitz T, Wachtlin D, Mohler M, et al. Neoadjuvant chemoradiation and local excision for T2–3 rectal cancer. Ann Surg Oncol 2008;15:712–20.
52. Nair RM, Siegel EM, Chen DT, et al. Long-term results of transanal excision after neoadjuvant chemoradiation for T2 and T3 adenocarcinomas of the rectum. J Gastrointest Surg 2008;12:1797–806.
53. Kim CJ, Yeatman TJ, Coppola D, et al. Local excision of T2 and T3 rectal cancers after downstaging chemoradiation. Ann Surg 2001;234:352–9.
54. Lezoche E, Baldarelli M, Lezoche G, et al. Randomized clinical trial of endoluminal locoregional resection versus laparoscopic total mesorectal excision for T2 rectal cancer after neoadjuvant therapy. Br J Surg 2012;99:1211–8.
55. Garcia-Aguilar J, Renfro LA, Chow OS, et al. Organ preservation for clinical T2N0 distal rectal cancer using neoadjuvant chemoradiotherapy and local excision

(ACOSOG Z6041): results of an open-label, single-arm, multi-institutional, phase 2 trial. Lancet Oncol 2015;16(15):1537–46.

56. Stitzenberg KB, Sanoff HK, Penn DC, et al. Practice patterns and long-term survival for early-stage rectal cancer. J Clin Oncol 2013;31(34):4276–82.

57. Borstlap WAA, Tanis PJ, Koedam TWA, et al. A multi-centred randomised trial of radical surgery versus adjuvant chemoradiotherapy after local excision for early rectal cancer. BMC Cancer 2016;16:513.

58. Bikhchandani J, Ong GK, Dozois EJ, et al. Outcomes of salvage surgery for cure in patients with locally recurrent disease after local excision of rectal cancer. Dis Colon Rectum 2015;58(3):283–7.

59. Vaid S, Park JS, Sinnott RJ. Outcomes of recurrent rectal cancer after transanal excision. Am Surg 2016;82:152–5.

New Strategies in Rectal Cancer

Guilherme Pagin São Julião, MD[a], Angelita Habr-Gama, MD, PhD[a],
Bruna Borba Vailati, MD[a], Sergio Eduardo Alonso Araujo, MD, PhD[b],
Laura Melina Fernandez, MD[a], Rodrigo Oliva Perez, MD, PhD[a,*]

KEYWORDS

- Transanal TME • Organ-preserving strategies • Local excision • Watch and wait

KEY POINTS

- Neoadjuvant chemoradiation may lead to significant tumor regression and to complete pathologic response in rectal cancer.
- Assessment of tumor response may identify patients who could be managed with organ-preserving strategies, including the Watch and Wait strategy and local excision.
- When organ-preserving strategies are used for rectal cancer, close surveillance may allow early detection of local recurrences and salvage alternatives.
- In case of incomplete response to chemoradiation, the best alternative for most patients will still be proper total mesorectal excision: minimally invasive or conventional open surgery.

INTRODUCTION

The development and implementation of newer treatment modalities have significantly increased the complexity in the management of rectal cancer,[1] with surgical treatment remaining as the main pillar. Interest into the different approaches for total mesorectal excision (TME), including standard laparoscopy, robotic surgery, and transanal TME are increasing rapidly. This interest is not only based on the advantages of smaller incisions, but also on the desire to obtain a better specimen quality, which may translate into a better oncological outcome.

Several recent trials have focused on the oncological outcomes of laparoscopic rectal cancer surgery compared with the standard open approach, and results have been mixed,[2–5] with some showing laparoscopy to be either equivalent or even favorable to open surgery, whereas others were unable to establish noninferiority for

Disclosures: The authors have nothing to disclose.
[a] Department of Colorectal Surgery, Angelita & Joaquim Gama Institute, Rua Manoel da Nóbrega 1564, São Paulo 04001, Brazil; [b] Department of Colorectal Surgery, Hospital Israelita Albert Einstein, Avenida Albert Einstein 627, Suite 219, São Paulo 05652, Brazil
* Corresponding author.
E-mail address: rodrigo.operez@gmail.com

Surg Clin N Am 97 (2017) 587–604
http://dx.doi.org/10.1016/j.suc.2017.01.008
0039-6109/17/© 2017 Elsevier Inc. All rights reserved.

surgical.theclinics.com

laparoscopy.[4,5] Most experts agree that laparoscopic rectal cancer surgery is very complex and technically demanding, and it cannot be universally applied to all patients. To overcome specific technical complexities associated with laparoscopic TME, transanal total mesorectal excision (TaTME) has emerged as a technique that enables meticulous endoscopic dissection from the bottom up, which reduces the technical constraints of the narrow pelvis.

In addition to changes in the surgical approach to rectal cancer, there have also been many advances in neoadjuvant therapy with subsequent management tailored to the tumor response. Neoadjuvant chemoradiation (nCRT) may lead to significant tumor regression, ultimately leading to complete pathologic response in up to 42% of patients.[6] Assessment of tumor response after nCRT and before radical surgery may identify patients with complete clinical response that could be managed nonoperatively with strict follow-up (watch and wait [WW] strategy) and thus avoiding unnecessary postoperative morbidity with good long-term oncological outcomes and excellent functional results.[7–11] In addition, close surveillance may allow for early detection of local recurrences and subsequent salvage surgery without a significant compromise in the oncological outcome.[12]

This article discusses these new strategies for the management of rectal cancer.

ORGAN PRESERVATION IN RECTAL CANCER

Different organ-preserving strategies for the treatment of rectal cancer have gained popularity in recent years. Regardless of approach, proctectomy is associated with significant postoperative morbidity, including long-term urinary, sexual, and fecal continence dysfunction in addition to the requirement for temporary or definitive stomas associated with the procedure. Also, depending on age and comorbidities, postoperative mortality also may be quite significant.[13] Therefore, in selected patients, surgical and even nonsurgical approaches that spare the rectum have been suggested.[14]

The observation that rectal cancers could develop significant tumor regression with reduction in primary tumor size (downsizing), depth of tumor penetration, and even potential nodal sterilization (downstaging) after nCRT could set the ideal stage for organ-preserving alternatives, including local excision of small and superficial residual tumors.[15] In addition, regression of the primary tumor could result in complete disappearance of the tumor in the resected specimen (complete pathologic response [pCR]) in some patients. In a subset of these patients, complete regression of the primary tumor is clinically detected before surgical resection, referred to as a complete clinical response (cCR).[16] It is in these patients with a cCR after nCRT that we have considered a WW strategy without immediate surgical resection.[9] To consider these approaches, surgeons must take into consideration several aspects of the disease, patients, and treatment modalities that may be quite relevant during their clinical decision-making process.

Assessment of Tumor Response

When considering patients for the WW strategy, assessment of tumor response is crucial. However, this assessment can be challenging due to uncertainties regarding the optimal timing of the assessment, and the most accurate clinical and radiological tools for this purpose.

Of note, assessment of tumor response is also recommended for patients with a partial clinical response in which organ-preserving strategies are not being considered. Even if the plan after nCRT is a radical resection, one needs to consider that after nCRT, the surgeon may be facing a considerably different tumor. Knowing this potentially new "anatomy" ahead of time may allow the surgeon to optimize intraoperative surgical strategy and to know in advance what challenges could be anticipated during the procedure.[17] Therefore, reassessment of tumor response should be performed in all patients.

Timing for the Assessment of Tumor Response

The grade of tumor regression after nCRT appears to be a time-dependent phenomenon. The first randomized trial to consider the effect of different time intervals in the response to CRT was a French study comparing 2 versus 6 weeks from nCRT. In this study, all patients underwent radical surgery after these 2 time intervals and patients with 6-week intervals presented significantly more tumor regression after nCRT.[18] Due to this study, a 6-week time interval between nCRT completion and performance of radical surgery has been considered the standard of care for many years. However, retrospective studies consistently reported that patients undergoing radical surgery after longer than 6 to 8 weeks from nCRT were more likely to develop pCR.[19–22] One of these studies suggested that the rates of pCR after nCRT may keep rising after nCRT for as long as 12 weeks from treatment completion.[20] However, there was a question of whether these prolonged intervals from nCRT would result in excessive tissue fibrosis in the area included in the radiation therapy field that could lead to increased technical difficulty and postoperative morbidity after radical surgery.

In 2015, Garcia-Aguilar and colleagues[23] performed a prospective, nonrandomized study evaluating patients in nCRT regimens with progressively longer interval periods before surgery. Although one group received surgery 6 weeks after cCRT completion, the other 3 groups had extended intervals of 12, 16, and 20 weeks, with supplemental chemotherapy during the extended intervals. Even though this was not a randomized study, patients in different groups had similar baseline demographics and tumor stages. The investigators found that extended intervals were associated with significantly higher rates of pCR (6 weeks = 18%, 12 weeks = 25%, 16 weeks = 30%, and 20 weeks = 38%). In addition, the investigators found that the extended intervals did not have a deleterious impact on overall morbidity, blood loss, or the technical difficulty of the case.[23]

Another recently published randomized study came to different conclusions. In the GRECCAR-6 trial, patients were randomized to post-CRT intervals of 7 or 11 weeks. The investigators found that pCR rates were similar with the 2 intervals, but the morbidity rates were higher in the 11-week group (higher for Clavien Dindo classes 1 and 2, similar for classes 3–5), and the quality of mesorectal excision was worse in the 11-week group, suggesting the detrimental effects of prolonged time after nCRT on fibrotic changes in the surgical and previously irradiated fields.[24] Of note, there were several limitations to this trial, including issues with adherence to the prescribed time interval, resulting in several patients from the 7-week group having longer intervals before surgery.

The optimal interval after nCRT remains undetermined, and additional ongoing trials will definitely provide more data to allow us to understand the benefits and risks of using prolonged intervals after treatment. In fact, it may be the case that a single and fixed interval may not be appropriate for all patients. Instead, patients/tumors may respond differently as a function of time to nCRT. Ultimately, responsive tumors may require and actually benefit from prolonged intervals from nCRT, whereas unresponsive tumors may not. It is likely that responsive tumors that are being considered for organ-preserving strategies should have their assessment of response and ultimately surgical strategy decision deferred to longer than 12 weeks. On the other hand, tumors with little response that still require radical TME may benefit from 6-week to 8-week intervals between nCRT completion and radical surgery.[25]

Tools in Assessment of Tumor Response

Clinical and endoscopic assessment

Clinical assessment is one of the most important tools to evaluate tumor response. Commonly, patients with tumor regression would have relief of their symptoms. Digital rectal examination (DRE) is an irreplaceable tool for the evaluation of response. The stringent criteria to consider a complete clinical response (cCR) includes the absence of any irregularity, mass, ulceration, or stenosis during the DRE. The surface has to be regular and smooth.[16]

Endoscopic evaluation of the area harboring the original tumor is the remaining key component of clinical assessment. It is important to look for any irregularity or superficial ulcers missed during DRE. A flat white scar and telangiectasia are common endoscopic findings among patients with a cCR (**Fig. 1**). Even though flexible scopes provide photographic documentation of endoscopic response, rigid proctoscopy may suffice for most patients.[16]

In the presence of a cCR by DRE and proctoscopy, endoscopic biopsies are not recommended. Even in the setting of incomplete clinical response, endoscopic biopsy results should be interpreted with caution. Among patients with significant response, negative predictive values of these endoscopic biopsies have been reported to be consistently low.[26] Residual mucosal disease can be missed due to adjacent scarring, and residual disease within the bowel wall or mesorectum may be accompanied by a normal mucosal surface. Therefore, a negative biopsy in the setting of incomplete clinical response does not rule out microscopic residual cancer.

Radiological assessment

Even though historically the definition of a cCR has been based on clinical and endoscopic findings by direct assessment of the rectal wall, radiological studies have always attempted to provide additional information unavailable to the finger or the proctoscope, particularly regarding nodal or mesorectal status of the disease. Currently, however, significant developments in imaging definition and interpretation have resulted in significant increases in accuracy for the assessment of response not only within the mesorectum compartment, but also within the rectal wall.

High-resolution magnetic resonance (MR) is now routinely used for the assessment of response. The ability to discriminate between fibrosis and residual disease has

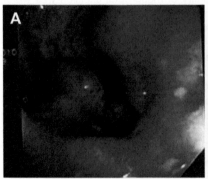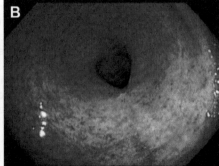

Fig. 1. Endoscopic view of rectal cancer before (A) and after 10 weeks from nCRT completion (B) showing a complete clinical response (cCR).

improved with advances in technology, placing the resonance as an essential tool to confirm clinical and endoscopic findings of a cCR.[27] MR may provide an accurate radiological (mrTRG) estimate of the pathologic tumor regression grade (TRG). The utilization of this mrTRG score may identify good and poor responders with significant impact in disease-free and overall survival[28,29] (**Fig. 2**).

Even though clinical and endoscopic assessment using stringent criteria will result in high specificity rates for the detection of a pCR, a significant number of patients with incomplete clinical response will still harbor complete pathologic response.[30,31] In fact, it seems that most patients with pCR after nCRT have incomplete clinical response after 8 to 12 weeks from nCRT.[30] Therefore, there is a potential role for MR studies to identify patients with incomplete clinical response who may ultimately harbor pCR. Currently, these patients would be referred for immediate radical surgery; however, radiological tools may be able to accurately identify these patients and avoid potentially unnecessary surgery.[32]

Recently, a study that compared mrTRG and residual mucosal abnormalities following nCRT suggested that the mrTRG system may identify nearly 10 times more complete pathologic responses compared with clinical endoscopic findings. These findings may improve the selection of patients with pCR despite initial incomplete clinical response and that may be appropriate candidates for deferral of surgery.[32]

Diffusion-weighted magnetic resonance imaging (DWI-MR) may add significant functional information to standard MRI. The fact that diffusion properties of water molecules may vary in areas of tissue necrosis, high cellularity (frequently observed within tumor tissues), or fibrosis may be used to help assess tumor response to nCRT (**Fig. 3**). Absence of restriction to diffusion of water molecules has been associated with the absence of residual cancer (complete response). On the other hand, restriction to diffusion of water molecules (seen as high signal intensity in the area of the previous tumor) may indicate the presence of residual cancer cells (incomplete response). Initial reports with DWI-MR for the assessment of response to nCRT have shown promising results with high accuracy rates and may constitute a useful tool during assessment of response.[33,34]

PET/computed tomography (CT) imaging has been studied for the prediction of response to CRT. The use of molecular imaging may provide additional information

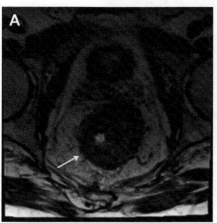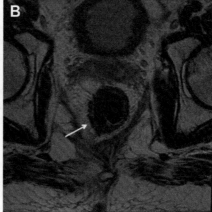

Fig. 2. Image showing baseline mrT2/3a cancer (*A, yellow arrow*) and post-CRT images showing mrTRG1 (low signal intensity, *yellow arrow*) (*B*) consistent with complete response to nCRT.

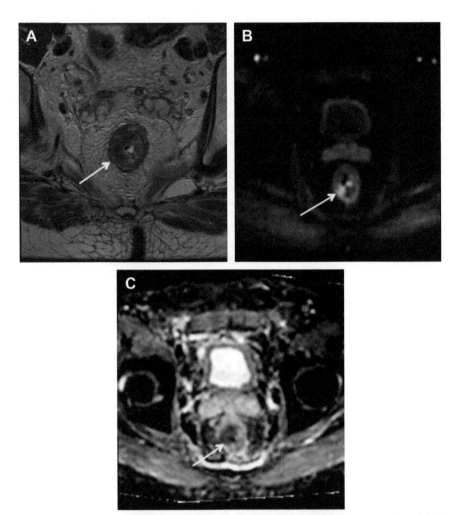

Fig. 3. Image showing a residual ymrT2 cancer following nCRT (*A, yellow arrow*) and diffusion restriction (high signal intensity, *yellow arrow*) (*B*) with correspondent low signal intensity in the apparent diffusion coefficient map (*C, yellow arrow*) (suggestive of residual cancer by DWI-MR).

to standard structural/anatomic features to help distinguish between fibrosis or residual tumor. The use of fludeoxyglucose (FDG) allows for the estimate of tissue metabolism (standard uptake values [SUV]) within areas of interest and fused images of PET and CT may indicate precise anatomic areas of residual cancer cells, even among mucinous histologic subtypes.[35]

Most of the available studies have focused on SUV variation for the identification of complete responders to nCRT using variable interval periods and sequential PET/CT imaging.[36–38] Accuracies, however, have been insufficient for its routine recommendation into clinical practice. A recently reported study suggested that the combination of SUV variation and volumetric reduction in tumors could predict complete response to nCRT. Using individual technical calibration for determining metabolic tumor volumes estimates, variation in total lesion glycolysis (determined by metabolic tumor volume and mean SUV values) was found to be the best predictor of response to nCRT using sequential PET/CT imaging at baseline and 12 weeks from nCRT completion[39] (**Fig. 4**).

Complete Response: Watch and Wait Strategy

Watch and wait strategy: follow-up

When a nonoperative strategy for cCR in rectal cancer is considered, a relatively intensive follow-up is certainly required. Patients should be encouraged to adhere to this strict follow-up program to allow early recognition of any local or systemic recurrence and, therefore, increasing the chance of a successful salvage treatment. After initial assessment of response confirming a cCR, visits should be performed every 1 to 2 months during the first year, every 3 months during the second year, and every 6 months thereafter. DRE, proctoscopy, and carcinoembryonic antigen level determination are recommended for all visits. Timing for radiological assessment during follow-up has not yet been standardized. Routine MR for the assessment of the rectal wall, mesorectum, and pelvic nodes every 6 months for the first 2 years and yearly thereafter has been our practice.[14]

Outcomes

Patients managed nonoperatively under the WW strategy after a cCR following neoadjuvant chemoradiation were originally reported to have similar long-term oncological outcomes to patients with complete pathologic response after radical surgery.[9] Additional retrospective studies reported by others have consistently shown similar oncological outcomes between these subgroups of patients.[10,11,40–44] These findings further support the idea that patients with a cCR may be spared from the morbidity and mortality of radical surgery with no oncological compromise.[13] In addition, functional outcomes of patients managed nonoperatively not only appear to be better than with radical surgery, but also better than other organ-preserving strategies (transanal local excision).[7,11]

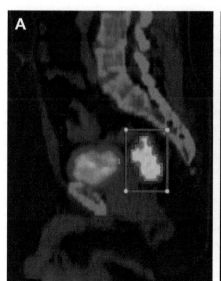 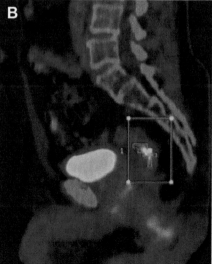

Fig. 4. PET/CT showing a baseline tumor with significant FDG uptake and precise metabolic tumor volume (*green lines*) delineation (*A*) and post-CRT images showing significant metabolic volume reduction (*B*) within the region of interest (green squares - ROI). (*From* Dos Anjos DA, Perez RO, Habr-Gama A, et al. Semiquantitative volumetry by sequential PET/CT may improve prediction of complete response to neoadjuvant chemoradiation in patients with distal rectal cancer. Dis Colon Rectum 2016;59:805–12; with permission.)

Local recurrences after this treatment strategy are still a concern and may develop at any time during follow-up. Most local recurrences appear to develop within the first 12 months of follow-up and may represent limitations in the precise identification of microscopic residual disease among "apparent" complete clinical responders. For these reasons, these "early recurrences" developing within the initial 12 months of follow-up have been called "early regrowths" instead.[12,44,45] Still, close and strict follow-up may allow early detection of regrowths, leading to oncological outcomes equivalent to those who have an incomplete clinical response and underwent surgery 8 to 12 weeks after CRT completion.[46] In addition, local recurrences (late and early regrowths) are usually amenable to salvage therapies, often allowing sphincter preservation, and associated with excellent long-term local disease control.[12]

Considering that the rate of cCR or pCR was historically fewer than 30% of patients across most of the studies, one could assume that this treatment strategy could benefit a rather limited proportion of patients with rectal cancer. However, the observation of increased rates of complete response (clinical or pathologic) using regimens with consolidation chemotherapy and with the inclusion of earlier stages of disease (cT2N0 otherwise candidates for ultra-low resections or abdominoperineal resections) may result in nearly 50% who ultimately avoid surgical resection.[8,23] This has been further confirmed in a prospective trial including patients with T2 and T3 rectal cancers managed by CRT and an additional endorectal high-dose brachytherapy boost (total 65 Gy) that showed a 58% cCR rate at 2 years of follow-up without surgical resection.[10]

Finally, in the era of evidence-based medicine, a randomized prospective trial is still lacking to definitively demonstrate the oncological equivalence of WW and radical surgery in the setting of a cCR following nCRT.[47] Even though such a trial is not likely to be performed, a recent study using a propensity-score matched cohort analysis comparing WW and radical surgery has been designed to demonstrate noninferiority of the WW approach. Curiously however, the comparison between groups demonstrated a slight superiority of the nonoperative management of these patients in terms of survival and a clear benefit in colostomy-free survival even when accounting for the development of local recurrences.[44]

Organ Preservation After Incomplete Response

As previously mentioned, transanal local excision with or without the use of endoscopic microsurgical platforms has been suggested to provide insufficient oncological outcomes for most patients with T1 or T2 rectal cancer. A very small subset of patients fulfilling strict favorable criteria are considered to be appropriate candidates for this organ-preserving strategy.[48] Local recurrence rates have mirrored the risk of mesorectal nodal metastases for T1 and T2 cancer, respectively. Of note, advanced techniques, such as transanal endoscopic microsurgery (TEMS) and transanal minimally invasive surgery (TAMIS), have allowed the surgeon to selectively perform larger resections that include mesorectal tissue. However, conventional local excision is a procedure that typically removes the primary cancer with no associated mesorectal tissue, and thus oncological failures after this treatment strategy have been associated with the risk of unsuspected and unremoved metastatic mesorectal nodes. In this setting, the potential effects of nCRT on primary tumor size, depth of tumor penetration, and mesorectal nodal sterilization could result in a residual tumor amenable to local excision even in the setting of an incomplete response to nCRT.

Indeed this organ-preserving strategy may be a valid alternative in the treatment of select patients with rectal cancer after nCRT. The only randomized study comparing TEMS to laparoscopic TME in the management of cT2N0 rectal cancer after nCRT has suggested similar local recurrence-free survival and postoperative morbidity favoring the TEMS group.[49] However, a later update of this trial suggested that patients undergoing TEMS were more likely to develop any disease recurrence.[50] Another prospective single-arm study reported on long-term outcomes with local excision after nCRT for the management of cT2N0 rectal adenocarcinomas. This study reported considerably low local recurrence rates (<5%), suggesting that this organ-preserving strategy could be safe for the management of these patients after nCRT.[51]

Certain issues must be considered when evaluating the 2 previously mentioned studies. First, in both studies, only select (small) cT2N0 rectal cancers were included. Particularly for the ACOSOG Z6041 study, it becomes difficult to understand whether there is a chance that "unfavorable" cT2N0 never entered the study.[51] Second, local recurrences in both studies were exclusively observed among poor responders to nCRT. This means that none of the recurrences observed were among patients with complete pathologic response of the primary tumor (ypT0)

Ultimately, local excision of primary tumors that respond poorly to nCRT may prove to be insufficient. Data from 2 prospective European studies revealed that patients with residual ypT2 cancers that refused subsequent TME, and instead underwent local excision, developed considerably high rates of local recurrence.[50,52] Despite an appropriate R0 resection of these residual ypT1 or ypT2 cancers, the presence of remote islands of cancer cells away from the primary residual visible ulcer/tumor can develop during the partial response to nCRT (also known as the "fragmented" pattern of tumor regression or tumor scatter). These fragments may contribute to local failures after local excision.[53–55] Fragmented patterns of tumor regression are possible regardless of baseline staging features among these unresponsive tumors.[53] Therefore, one could argue that the patients who can be safely managed by local excision after nCRT are those who experience complete tumor regression (ypT0). In this subset of patients with a favorable response, the oncological outcome is usually excellent after local excision.[56]

To further complicate the decision process in selecting this organ-preserving strategy, one has to consider the consequences of local excision in the setting of a previously irradiated field. Suturing of 2 radiated borders of the rectum together may lead to significant difficulties in tissue healing and seems to justify the considerable rates of associated morbidity after this procedure.[57,58] Wound complications, including partial separation and even complete dehiscence occur in 25% to 70% of patients after nCRT, which has several clinical consequences, including significant anal pain, requiring readmission in up to 30% of patients, and even occasional diverting stomas. Such complications have been clearly observed in a prospective trial using short-course radiation therapy followed by delayed TEMS. The observation of severe postoperative complications (including rectal-sacral fistulas) among patients led the investigators to interrupt the trial.[59]

In addition, significant scarring of these separated wounds may have other clinically relevant consequences. Even though TEMS has been associated with minimal long-term detrimental functional consequences, in the setting of nCRT and frequent wound dehiscences, local resection may lead to significant anorectal dysfunction. Patients managed by nCRT followed by TEMS compared with patients with cCR managed by WW showed consistently worse functional outcomes for the former group of patients.

There is also concern that oncological outcomes may be compromised in the event that salvage TME is required after nCRT and local excision, and some studies have shown a negative impact on the quality of the mesorectal excision.[60] The risk that salvage TME will require an abdominal perineal excision instead of a restorative proctectomy is quite significant.[61,62] A recently reported study on the outcomes for salvage TME for local recurrences after nCRT and TEMS suggested considerably high local re-recurrence rates, frequent need for abdominoperineal resections (APRs) and frequent risk for achieving an R1 resection with circumferential resection margin positivity (CRM+).[63]

Altogether, these data may suggest that local excision should be offered with extreme caution after nCRT to patients with selected rectal cancers. Patients with suspected pCR are probably the best indication for this strategy. However, these patients will probably do better if no surgical resection is undertaken, provided that they have developed complete clinical response. A few patients with incomplete clinical response harboring ypT0 lesion or even residual adenomas (**Fig. 5**) within the area or border of previously invasive cancers may be a specific subset of patients for whom a WW strategy is inappropriate.[64] In these patients, local excision with TEMS may be both diagnostic and therapeutic. Small and early baseline cancers (cT2N0) are preferred even though poor responders (ypT1-2) may still harbor a significant risk for local recurrences.[65] Fragmented patterns of regression to nCRT may constitute a significant source for local recurrences, even in small residual ypT1-2 cancers (**Fig. 6**). Postoperative morbidity in the event that salvage TME is required may be quite significant. Even though good (complete) responders are preferred, worse functional and similar oncological outcomes compared with nonoperative management of such patients may further limit the use and indication of such procedure.

Ultimately, in the setting of an incomplete response to nCRT the best alternative for most patients will still be proper total mesorectal excision, regardless of the surgical access (minimally invasive or conventional TME).

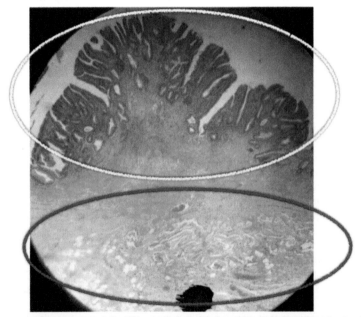

Fig. 5. Microscopic view of a full-thickness fragment locally excised by TEMS harboring a residual adenoma within the area of the original invasive cancer (*yellow*) and the presence of acellular mucin deposits (*red*).

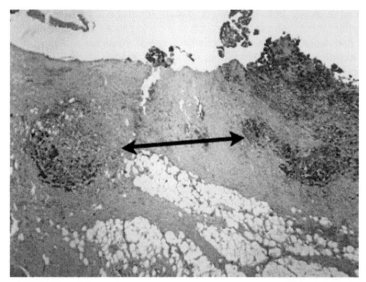

Fig. 6. Microscopic view of "fragmented" pattern of regression after nCRT with isolated foci of cancer cells separated by areas (*double arrow*) of fibrotic non-neoplastic tissue.

TOTAL MESORECTAL EXCISION: OPEN, LAPAROSCOPIC, AND ROBOTIC

Despite considerable postoperative morbidity, functional consequences, and even mortality, TME with an intact mesorectum, and proper radial margins (>1 mm) and distal margins (≥1 cm) provides excellent local disease control.[66] Oncological outcomes (particularly in terms of local disease control) seem to be directly related to achieving a proper TME specimen regardless of the exact surgical approach. Historically, open TME has been considered the standard approach for this operation; however, the development of minimally invasive approaches with laparoscopic colorectal procedures led to significant improvements in short-term outcomes for colon cancer surgery with similar long-term oncological outcomes.

In theory, optimal visualization of the pelvis and standardization of key technical steps were expected to result in at least similar oncological outcomes and potentially maintaining the short-term outcomes benefits observed for colon cancer surgery. However, regarding laparoscopic TME (lap TME), the issues of nCRT, the need for autonomic nerve preservation, and the technical demands of a TME and a well-constructed low colorectal or coloanal anastomosis challenge even the most specialized surgeon. Therefore, it was only recently that randomized trials specifically addressed these issues for the management of rectal cancer.[2–5] A premise to most if not all of these studies was the use of pathologic findings (quality of the mesorectum and CRM+) as a surrogate for oncological outcomes.

The COREAN trial, demonstrating similar oncological outcomes between open and laparoscopic TME, was promising in supporting routine use of the minimally invasive approach.[3] The COLOR II trial performed in Europe also suggested similar oncological outcomes between laparoscopic and open surgery for rectal cancer.[2] Two interesting aspects of this particular trial are worth noting. First, there was a significant difference in the CRM+ rate between the 2 arms favoring the open approach among mid-rectal cancers. On the other hand, among distal rectal cancers, the opposite was observed, with rate of CRM+ favoring the laparoscopic approach. Even though oncological outcomes were similar between groups (except for stage III disease, in which it was actually better for the laparoscopic group), one could argue that worse pathologic outcomes for mid-rectal cancers could possibly suggest worse surgical performance with the laparoscopic approach. The worse results observed in the open group for distal cancers could be possibly related to the APR technique rather than TME surgery itself, as APRs have been historically associated with worse pathologic outcomes.[67]

These controversial findings were further complicated by 2 well-designed and highly publicized randomized controlled trials (RCTs) comparing open and laparoscopic surgery for TME, both of which were published in the October 2015 issue of the *Journal of the American Medical Association*. In the ACOSOG Z6051 trial, surgeons underwent previous credentialing to ensure proper surgical expertise before entering the trial.[4] In this study, investigators decided to use as the primary endpoint a composite of pathologic variables including quality of the mesorectum specimen, CRM status, and distal resection margin. Originally designed to demonstrate noninferiority of laparoscopic to open TME, the study failed to demonstrate that laparoscopy was not inferior to open surgery. Possible reasons for these unexpected findings include the use of an endpoint (composite pathologic endpoint) not previously validated. In addition, the power calculations were based on a higher-than-observed composite success rate for open ("standard") TME.

Another important and similarly designed RCT was performed in Australia and Asia (ALaCaRT trial), and reported similar outcomes failing to demonstrate noninferiority of laparoscopic surgery to open surgery for the performance of TME.[5] These 2 recent studies, both of which involved master surgeons with extensive experience performing laparoscopic TME, resulted in a proper amount of concern in the colorectal community that laparoscopic TME is not appropriate for all patients with locally advanced rectal cancer, and patients must be selected carefully for this technique.

Another promising improvement in minimally invasive TME involves the surgical robot. Robotic technology reports improved visualization using a stable high-definition camera and a more precise rectal dissection using articulated instruments with motion scaling. Surgeon ergonomics also may be improved, which reduces the physical demands of an already-difficult pelvic dissection. However, although these advantages were presumed to translate into improved surgical outcomes, systematic reviews and meta-analyses have failed to show significant benefits to robot TME when compared with laparoscopic TME, with the exception of a decreased rate of conversion to open surgery.[68]

Moreover, it has been demonstrated in the same reviews that robotic TME is associated with a prolonged operating time when compared with laparoscopic TME, with several contributing factors, including surgeon and assistant familiarity, learning curves, and extra time taken to dock the robot. Results from the single randomized study comparing robotic to laparoscopic TME surgery (ROLARR trial) remain unpublished, and the current role of robotic surgery for rectal cancer remains controversial.

TRANSANAL TOTAL MESORECTAL EXCISION

Regardless of the exact reasons for the unexpected negative findings for laparoscopic and robotic TME surgery, it is clear that minimally invasive TME is a challenging procedure for even the best endoscopic surgeons. Pelvic exposure during TME is especially difficult in obese men with low tumors, as the visualization is poor, and the narrow pelvis and fatty mesorectum leave little space for dissection. Perhaps the most challenging cases involve these difficult patients in combination with an anterior distal tumor, in whom there is high risk for a positive circumferential resection margin regardless of the chosen technique. From this challenge, arose a new technique to battle the anatomic constraints of the narrow pelvis.

Previous experience with transanal surgery for local excision and developments in microsurgical endoscopic platforms led surgeons to consider performing TME via a transanal approach (taTME).[69] The mesorectal dissection is performed transanally from bottom to up using a variety of flexible or rigid transanal platforms. The first key step of the procedure includes closure and transection of the rectum distal to the tumor, thus ensuring a proper distal margin (one of the key surrogate markers for long-term oncological outcomes). This replaces one of the most challenging elements of the abdominal approach, in which the distal rectum is transected with linear staples, which often requires multiple staple loads, and can be associated with poor visualization and unintentional incorporation of adjacent organs, such as the vagina.

Once the rectum is fully incised in a circumferential manner, CO_2 insufflation and laparoscopic instrumentation (including a high-definition camera) are used to perform TME under direct vision. Dissection proceeds cranially through the same surgical planes that are used for the abdominal approach. TaTME enthusiasts report improved identification of the proper planes using this technique in the narrow pelvis.

Although the taTME surgeon works from below, a separate surgeon typically works from above, completing the abdominal portions of the operation, including proximal vessel ligation and splenic flexure mobilization. The 2 dissections then meet, typically at the peritoneal reflection, which completes the dissection. There is still controversy about whether a single or 2-team approach results in different outcomes during the procedure.[70]

Initial experience with case-control studies suggest that taTME allows similar (if not superior) pathologic outcomes compared with the abdominal approach, including distal margins, CRM status, and the quality of the mesorectum.[71] In fact, some surgeons prefer taTME for difficult pelvic dissections even when an open abdominal approach is used.

Despite this promising initial experience, caution must be taken before definitive implementation of taTME into surgical practice. TaTME requires proper training, and, as in any other surgical procedure, there is a learning curve for the procedure. Previous experience with TME and transanal surgery with endoscopic microsurgical platforms may be useful to accelerate overcoming the learning curve and preventing complications.[72] In fact, considering the change in anatomic landmarks during taTME when compared with abdominal TME, certain intraoperative complications may be more likely to develop when compared with abdominal TME, including injuries to the prostate or urethra, as well as damage to the iliac/obturator vessels and presacral veins.[73] In addition, long-term functional outcomes after taTME are not yet available. In the meantime, registries provide an opportunity to compare and scrutinize individual results with the technique, and ultimately a randomized trial comparing taTME with conventional and minimally invasive TME is necessary before widespread adoption of the technique.

SUMMARY

Organ preservation in the management of rectal cancer has become a valid option for select patients after significant response to neoadjuvant CRT. Patients who develop complete tumor regression with no clinical, endoscopic, or radiological evidence of residual cancer may be offered no immediate surgery and enrolled in a strict surveillance program (WW) with excellent functional and acceptable oncological outcomes. Good responders to nCRT (ypT0 or ypTis), despite incomplete clinical response, may warrant local excision as a diagnostic and therapeutic tool also with good oncological outcomes but at the cost of a slightly worse functional outcome and significant post-operative morbidity. Poor responders to nCRT (ypT1-2) are still at risk of significant local recurrence rates after local excision of the visible residual disease. Proper selection of these patients for organ-preserving strategies remains a challenge, and TME may provide considerably better oncological outcomes. Obtaining a proper TME specimen with adequate distal and radial margins may be challenging by minimally invasive techniques. In this setting, the transanal approach (taTME) is promising alternative to be investigated in future prospective trials.

REFERENCES

1. Kosinski L, Habr-Gama A, Ludwig K, et al. Shifting concepts in rectal cancer management: a review of contemporary primary rectal cancer treatment strategies. CA Cancer J Clin 2012;62:173–202.
2. Bonjer HJ, Deijen CL, Abis GA, et al. A randomized trial of laparoscopic versus open surgery for rectal cancer. N Engl J Med 2015;372:1324–32.
3. Jeong SY, Park JW, Nam BH, et al. Open versus laparoscopic surgery for mid-rectal or low-rectal cancer after neoadjuvant chemoradiotherapy (COREAN trial): survival outcomes of an open-label, non-inferiority, randomised controlled trial. Lancet Oncol 2014;15:767–74.
4. Fleshman J, Branda M, Sargent DJ, et al. Effect of laparoscopic-assisted resection vs open resection of stage II or III rectal cancer on pathologic outcomes: the ACOSOG Z6051 randomized clinical trial. JAMA 2015;314:1346–55.
5. Stevenson AR, Solomon MJ, Lumley JW, et al. Effect of laparoscopic-assisted resection vs open resection on pathological outcomes in rectal cancer: the ALaCaRT randomized clinical trial. JAMA 2015;314:1356–63.
6. Sanghera P, Wong DW, McConkey CC, et al. Chemoradiotherapy for rectal cancer: an updated analysis of factors affecting pathological response. Clin Oncol (R Coll Radiol) 2008;20:176–83.
7. Habr-Gama A, Lynn PB, Jorge JMN, et al. Impact of organ-preserving strategies on anorectal function in patients with distal rectal cancer following neoadjuvant chemoradiation. Dis Colon Rectum 2016;59:264–9.
8. Habr-Gama A, Sabbaga J, Gama-Rodrigues J, et al. Watch and wait approach following extended neoadjuvant chemoradiation for distal rectal cancer: are we getting closer to anal cancer management? Dis Colon Rectum 2013;56:1109–17.
9. Habr-Gama A, Perez RO, Nadalin W, et al. Operative versus nonoperative treatment for stage 0 distal rectal cancer following chemoradiation therapy: long-term results. Ann Surg 2004;240:711–7 [discussion: 717–8].
10. Appelt AL, Ploen J, Harling H, et al. High-dose chemoradiotherapy and watchful waiting for distal rectal cancer: a prospective observational study. Lancet Oncol 2015;16:919–27.
11. Maas M, Beets-Tan RG, Lambregts DM, et al. Wait-and-see policy for clinical complete responders after chemoradiation for rectal cancer. J Clin Oncol 2011; 29:4633–40.
12. Habr-Gama A, Gama-Rodrigues J, Sao Juliao GP, et al. Local recurrence after complete clinical response and watch and wait in rectal cancer after neoadjuvant chemoradiation: impact of salvage therapy on local disease control. Int J Radiat Oncol Biol Phys 2014;88:822–8.
13. Smith FM, Rao C, Oliva Perez R, et al. Avoiding radical surgery improves early survival in elderly patients with rectal cancer, demonstrating complete clinical

response after neoadjuvant therapy: results of a decision-analytic model. Dis Colon Rectum 2015;58:159–71.

14. Habr-Gama A, Sao Juliao GP, Perez RO. Nonoperative management of rectal cancer: identifying the ideal patients. Hematol Oncol Clin North Am 2015;29: 135–51.

15. Smith FM, Waldron D, Winter DC. Rectum-conserving surgery in the era of chemoradiotherapy. Br J Surg 2010;97:1752–64.

16. Habr-Gama A, Perez RO, Wynn G, et al. Complete clinical response after neoadjuvant chemoradiation therapy for distal rectal cancer: characterization of clinical and endoscopic findings for standardization. Dis Colon Rectum 2010;53:1692–8.

17. Brown G. Thin section MRI in multidisciplinary pre-operative decision making for patients with rectal cancer. Br J Radiol 2005;78(Spec No 2):S117–27.

18. Francois Y, Nemoz CJ, Baulieux J, et al. Influence of the interval between preoperative radiation therapy and surgery on downstaging and on the rate of sphincter-sparing surgery for rectal cancer: the Lyon R90-01 randomized trial. J Clin Oncol 1999;17:2396.

19. Tulchinsky H, Shmueli E, Figer A, et al. An interval >7 weeks between neoadjuvant therapy and surgery improves pathologic complete response and disease-free survival in patients with locally advanced rectal cancer. Ann Surg Oncol 2008;15:2661–7.

20. Kalady MF, de Campos-Lobato LF, Stocchi L, et al. Predictive factors of pathologic complete response after neoadjuvant chemoradiation for rectal cancer. Ann Surg 2009;250:582–9.

21. Evans J, Tait D, Swift I, et al. Timing of surgery following preoperative therapy in rectal cancer: the need for a prospective randomized trial? Dis Colon Rectum 2011;54:1251–9.

22. Wolthuis AM, Penninckx F, Haustermans K, et al. Impact of interval between neoadjuvant chemoradiotherapy and TME for locally advanced rectal cancer on pathologic response and oncologic outcome. Ann Surg Oncol 2012;19:2833–41.

23. Garcia-Aguilar J, Chow OS, Smith DD, et al. Effect of adding mFOLFOX6 after neoadjuvant chemoradiation in locally advanced rectal cancer: a multicentre, phase 2 trial. Lancet Oncol 2015;16:957–66.

24. Lefevre JH, Mineur L, Kotti S, et al. Effect of interval (7 or 11 weeks) between neoadjuvant radiochemotherapy and surgery on complete pathologic response in rectal cancer: a multicenter, randomized, controlled trial (GRECCAR-6). J Clin Oncol 2016. [Epub ahead of print].

25. Perez RO, Habr-Gama A, Sao Juliao GP, et al. Optimal timing for assessment of tumor response to neoadjuvant chemoradiation in patients with rectal cancer: do all patients benefit from waiting longer than 6 weeks? Int J Radiat Oncol Biol Phys 2012;84:1159–65.

26. Perez RO, Habr-Gama A, Pereira GV, et al. Role of biopsies in patients with residual rectal cancer following neoadjuvant chemoradiation after downsizing: can they rule out persisting cancer? Colorectal Dis 2012;14:714–20.

27. Lambregts DM, Maas M, Bakers FC, et al. Long-term follow-up features on rectal MRI during a wait-and-see approach after a clinical complete response in patients with rectal cancer treated with chemoradiotherapy. Dis Colon Rectum 2011;54:1521–8.

28. Patel UB, Brown G, Rutten H, et al. Comparison of magnetic resonance imaging and histopathological response to chemoradiotherapy in locally advanced rectal cancer. Ann Surg Oncol 2012;19:2842–52.

29. Patel UB, Taylor F, Blomqvist L, et al. Magnetic resonance imaging-detected tumor response for locally advanced rectal cancer predicts survival outcomes: MERCURY experience. J Clin Oncol 2011;29:3753–60.

30. Smith FM, Wiland H, Mace A, et al. Clinical criteria underestimate complete pathological response in rectal cancer treated with neoadjuvant chemoradiotherapy. Dis Colon Rectum 2014;57:311–5.

31. Nahas SC, Rizkallah Nahas CS, Sparapan Marques CF, et al. Pathologic complete response in rectal cancer: can we detect it? Lessons learned from a proposed randomized trial of watch-and-wait treatment of rectal cancer. Dis Colon Rectum 2016;59:255–63.

32. Bhoday J, Smith F, Siddiqui MR, et al. Magnetic resonance tumor regression grade and residual mucosal abnormality as predictors for pathological complete response in rectal cancer postneoadjuvant chemoradiotherapy. Dis Colon Rectum 2016;59:925–33.

33. Lambregts DM, Vandecaveye V, Barbaro B, et al. Diffusion-weighted MRI for selection of complete responders after chemoradiation for locally advanced rectal cancer: a multicenter study. Ann Surg Oncol 2011;18:2224–31.

34. Curvo-Semedo L, Lambregts DM, Maas M, et al. Rectal cancer: assessment of complete response to preoperative combined radiation therapy with chemotherapy–conventional MR volumetry versus diffusion-weighted MR imaging. Radiology 2011;260:734–43.

35. Dos Anjos DA, Habr-Gama A, Vailati BB, et al. 18F-FDG uptake by rectal cancer is similar in mucinous and nonmucinous histological subtypes. Ann Nucl Med 2016;30:513–7.

36. Cascini GL, Avallone A, Delrio P, et al. 18F-FDG PET is an early predictor of pathologic tumor response to preoperative radiochemotherapy in locally advanced rectal cancer. J Nucl Med 2006;47:1241–8.

37. Kristiansen C, Loft A, Berthelsen AK, et al. PET/CT and histopathologic response to preoperative chemoradiation therapy in locally advanced rectal cancer. Dis Colon Rectum 2008;51:21–5.

38. Perez RO, Habr-Gama A, Gama-Rodrigues J, et al. Accuracy of positron emission tomography/computed tomography and clinical assessment in the detection of complete rectal tumor regression after neoadjuvant chemoradiation: long-term results of a prospective trial (National Clinical Trial 00254683). Cancer 2012;118:3501–11.

39. Dos Anjos DA, Perez RO, Habr-Gama A, et al. Semiquantitative volumetry by sequential PET/CT may improve prediction of complete response to neoadjuvant chemoradiation in patients with distal rectal cancer. Dis Colon Rectum 2016;59:805–12.

40. Vaccaro CA, Yazyi FJ, Ojra Quintana G, et al. Locally advanced rectal cancer: preliminary results of rectal preservation after neoadjuvant chemoradiotherapy. Cir Esp 2016;94:274–9.

41. Smith RK, Fry RD, Mahmoud NN, et al. Surveillance after neoadjuvant therapy in advanced rectal cancer with complete clinical response can have comparable outcomes to total mesorectal excision. Int J Colorectal Dis 2015;30:769–74.

42. Dalton RS, Velineni R, Osborne ME, et al. A single-centre experience of chemoradiotherapy for rectal cancer: is there potential for nonoperative management? Colorectal Dis 2012;14:567–71.

43. Araujo RO, Valadao M, Borges D, et al. Nonoperative management of rectal cancer after chemoradiation opposed to resection after complete clinical response. A comparative study. Eur J Surg Oncol 2015;41:1456–63.

44. Renehan AG, Malcomson L, Emsley R, et al. Watch-and-wait approach versus surgical resection after chemoradiotherapy for patients with rectal cancer (the OnCoRe project): a propensity-score matched cohort analysis. Lancet Oncol 2015;17:174–83.

45. Martens MH, Maas M, Heijnen LA, et al. Long-term outcome of an organ preservation program after neoadjuvant treatment for rectal cancer. J Natl Cancer Inst 2016;108(12).

46. Habr-Gama A, Perez RO, Proscurshim I, et al. Interval between surgery and neoadjuvant chemoradiation therapy for distal rectal cancer: does delayed surgery have an impact on outcome? Int J Radiat Oncol Biol Phys 2008;71:1181–8.

47. Perez RO. Complete clinical response in rectal cancer: a turning tide. Lancet Oncol 2016;17:125–6.

48. Bach SP, Hill J, Monson JR, et al. A predictive model for local recurrence after transanal endoscopic microsurgery for rectal cancer. Br J Surg 2009;96:280–90.

49. Lezoche G, Baldarelli M, Guerrieri M, et al. A prospective randomized study with a 5-year minimum follow-up evaluation of transanal endoscopic microsurgery versus laparoscopic total mesorectal excision after neoadjuvant therapy. Surg Endosc 2008;22:352–8.

50. Lezoche E, Baldarelli M, Lezoche G, et al. Randomized clinical trial of endoluminal locoregional resection versus laparoscopic total mesorectal excision for T2 rectal cancer after neoadjuvant therapy. Br J Surg 2012;99:1211–8.

51. Garcia-Aguilar J, Renfro LA, Chow OS, et al. Organ preservation for clinical T2N0 distal rectal cancer using neoadjuvant chemoradiotherapy and local excision (ACOSOG Z6041): results of an open-label, single-arm, multi-institutional, phase 2 trial. Lancet Oncol 2015;16:1537–46.

52. Verseveld M, de Graaf EJ, Verhoef C, et al. Chemoradiation therapy for rectal cancer in the distal rectum followed by organ-sparing transanal endoscopic microsurgery (CARTS study). Br J Surg 2015;102:853–60.

53. Perez RO, Habr-Gama A, Smith FM, et al. Fragmented pattern of tumor regression and lateral intramural spread may influence margin appropriateness after TEM for rectal cancer following neoadjuvant CRT. J Surg Oncol 2014;109:853–8.

54. Hayden DM, Jakate S, Pinzon MC, et al. Tumor scatter after neoadjuvant therapy for rectal cancer: are we dealing with an invisible margin? Dis Colon Rectum 2012;55:1206–12.

55. Smith FM, Wiland H, Mace A, et al. Depth and lateral spread of microscopic residual rectal cancer after neoadjuvant chemoradiation: implications for treatment decisions. Colorectal Dis 2014;16:610–5.

56. Hallam S, Messenger DE, Thomas MG. A systematic review of local excision after neoadjuvant therapy for rectal cancer: are ypT0 tumors the limit? Dis Colon Rectum 2016;59:984–97.

57. Perez RO, Habr-Gama A, Sao Juliao GP, et al. Transanal endoscopic microsurgery for residual rectal cancer after neoadjuvant chemoradiation therapy is associated with significant immediate pain and hospital readmission rates. Dis Colon Rectum 2011;54:545–51.

58. Marks JH, Valsdottir EB, DeNittis A, et al. Transanal endoscopic microsurgery for the treatment of rectal cancer: comparison of wound complication rates with and without neoadjuvant radiation therapy. Surg Endosc 2009;23:1081–7.

59. Arezzo A, Arolfo S, Allaix ME, et al. Results of neoadjuvant short-course radiation therapy followed by transanal endoscopic microsurgery for t1-t2 n0 extraperitoneal rectal cancer. Int J Radiat Oncol Biol Phys 2015;92:299–306.

60. Hompes R, McDonald R, Buskens C, et al. Completion surgery following transanal endoscopic microsurgery: assessment of quality and short- and long-term outcome. Colorectal Dis 2013;15:e576–81.

61. Morino M, Allaix ME, Arolfo S, et al. Previous transanal endoscopic microsurgery for rectal cancer represents a risk factor for an increased abdominoperineal resection rate. Surg Endosc 2013;27:3315–21.

62. Bujko K, Richter P, Smith FM, et al. Preoperative radiotherapy and local excision of rectal cancer with immediate radical re-operation for poor responders: a prospective multicentre study. Radiother Oncol 2013;106:198–205.

63. Perez RO, Habr-Gama A, Sao Juliao GP, et al. Transanal endoscopic microsurgery (TEM) following neoadjuvant chemoradiation for rectal cancer: outcomes of salvage resection for local recurrence. Ann Surg Oncol 2016;23:1143–8.

64. Habr-Gama A, Vianna MR, Sao Juliao GP, et al. Management of adenomas within the area of rectal cancer that develop complete pathological response. Int J Colorectal Dis 2015;30:1285–7.

65. Perez RO, Habr-Gama A, Lynn PB, et al. Transanal endoscopic microsurgery for residual rectal cancer (ypT0-2) following neoadjuvant chemoradiation therapy: another word of caution. Dis Colon Rectum 2013;56:6–13.

66. Heald RJ, Ryall RD. Recurrence and survival after total mesorectal excision for rectal cancer. Lancet 1986;1:1479–82.

67. Nagtegaal ID, van de Velde CJ, Marijnen CA, et al. Low rectal cancer: a call for a change of approach in abdominoperineal resection. J Clin Oncol 2005;23: 9257–64.

68. Lorenzon L, Bini F, Balducci G, et al. Laparoscopic versus robotic-assisted colectomy and rectal resection: a systematic review and meta-analysis. Int J Colorectal Dis 2016;31:161–73.

69. Sylla P, Rattner DW, Delgado S, et al. NOTES transanal rectal cancer resection using transanal endoscopic microsurgery and laparoscopic assistance. Surg Endosc 2010;24:1205–10.

70. Knol J, Chadi SA. Transanal total mesorectal excision: technical aspects of approaching the mesorectal plane from below. Minim Invasive Ther Allied Technol 2016;25:257–70.

71. Araujo SE, Perez RO, Seid VE, et al. Laparo-endoscopic transanal total mesorectal excision (TATME): evidence of a novel technique. Minim Invasive Ther Allied Technol 2016;25:278–87.

72. Atallah S, Albert M, Monson JR. Critical concepts and important anatomic landmarks encountered during transanal total mesorectal excision (taTME): toward the mastery of a new operation for rectal cancer surgery. Tech Coloproctol 2016;20:483–94.

73. Atallah S, Martin-Perez B, Drake J, et al. The use of a lighted stent as a method for identifying the urethra in male patients undergoing transanal total mesorectal excision: a video demonstration. Tech Coloproctol 2015;19:375.

Hereditary Colorectal Cancer Syndromes

Katerina Wells, MD, MPH[a], Paul E. Wise, MD[b],*

KEYWORDS

- Inherited colon cancer • Hereditary nonpolyposis colorectal cancer
- Lynch syndrome • Familial adenomatous polyposis • MUTYH-associated polyposis
- Serrated polyposis syndrome

KEY POINTS

- Hereditary colorectal cancer syndromes are rare and affected patients are at increased risk for early onset, synchronous and metachronous colorectal malignancies, and extracolonic malignancies.

- Understanding the genetic basis of cancer syndromes and unique genotype-phenotype profiles allows clinicians to tailor surveillance and treatment strategies based on individual risk.

- Lynch syndrome follows an autosomal-dominant inheritance pattern characterized by early onset, aggressive colorectal cancer, and extracolonic malignancies. The genetic basis is a defect in mismatch repair genes.

- Familial adenomatous polyposis (FAP) follows an autosomal-dominant inheritance pattern characterized by intestinal polyposis and extracolonic malignancies. Patients exhibit a spectrum of disease severity from attenuated to extensive disease with clinical overlap with MUTYH-associated polyposis.

- Serrated polyposis syndrome is characterized by multiple, sometimes large, serrated polyps and associated with increased colorectal cancer risk. The morphology of the precursor polyps makes endoscopic management challenging, underscoring the need for short interval surveillance.

INTRODUCTION

It is estimated that 20% to 30% of colorectal cancers (CRCs) are familial with 5% to 10% related to a known genetic syndrome.[1,2] The hereditary CRCs are broadly divided into nonpolyposis and polyposis syndromes. Individuals with hereditary CRC syndromes are at risk for earlier development of cancer, increased risk of

Disclosure Statement: The authors have nothing to disclose.
[a] Department of Surgery, Division of Colon and Rectal Surgery, Baylor University Medical Center, 3409 Worth Street, Suite 640, Dallas, TX 75246, USA; [b] Division of General Surgery, Section of Colon and Rectal Surgery, Washington University Inherited Colorectal Cancer and Polyposis Registry, Washington University General Surgery Residency, Washington University in St Louis School of Medicine, 660 South Euclid Avenue, Campus Box 8109, St Louis, MO 63110, USA
* Corresponding author.
E-mail address: wisep@wustl.edu

metachronous cancers, and extracolonic manifestations. As such, identification of these individuals is critical for prevention and early detection and treatment of associated malignancies to reduce associated morbidity and mortality. Although there are a multitude of hereditary syndromes associated with increased risk of CRC, this article focuses on the most common nonpolyposis and polyposis syndromes.

HEREDITARY NONPOLYPOSIS COLORECTAL CANCER/LYNCH SYNDROME

Hereditary nonpolyposis CRC (HNPCC), also often used synonymously with the term Lynch syndrome, is the most common hereditary CRC syndrome, accounting for at least 2% to 3% of all CRCs. Lynch syndrome and HNPCC are associated with a predisposition to CRC and other cancers following an autosomal-dominant inheritance pattern, although rare sporadic mutations are described.[3] HNPCC defines a patient who meets particular clinical criteria (**Box 1**), regardless of the results of genetic assessment. Lynch syndrome is reserved for patients with a known mismatch repair (MMR) gene mutation regardless of whether they fulfill the clinical criteria for HNPCC (**Fig. 1**).

Both syndromes are associated with onset of CRC earlier than the general population with a mean age at CRC diagnosis of 45 years. Cancers are typically proximal to the splenic flexure; have a high degree of microsatellite instability (MSI-high); and have histologic features including poor differentiation, Crohn's-like host-lymphocytic infiltration, lymphoid aggregation at the tumor margins, and mucinous features.[4,5] They are associated with synchronous cancers,[6,7] and metachronous cancers are common with an annual incidence rate of 2.1%.[8,9] Despite the apparent high-risk histologic features, HNPCC-related CRC demonstrates less nodal and distant metastatic spread compared with sporadic CRC.[5,10] The "nonpolyposis" label of HNPCC can be misleading to less experienced physicians, because colorectal adenomatous polyps are the precursor lesions in these syndromes, with adenomas typically demonstrating a villous growth pattern and having a high degree of dysplasia.[4,11] Degeneration through the adenoma-carcinoma sequence is accelerated with CRC developing within a 5-year interval compared with 10 or more years in the case of sporadic CRC.[12,13]

Risk of Cancer

Regardless of the patient populations studied, the risk of CRC extracolonic malignancy is clearly elevated in HNPCC. Most studies present these risks reported in

---

Box 1
Revised HNPCC criteria (Amsterdam criteria II)

Criterion

1. There should be at least three relatives with an HNPCC-associated cancer (CRC, cancer of the endometrium, small bowel, ureter, or renal pelvis)

2. One should be a first-degree relative of the other two

3. At least two successive generations should be affected

4. At least one should be diagnosed before age 50

5. Familial adenomatous polyposis should be excluded in the CRC cases if any

6. Tumors should be verified by pathologic examination

From Vasen HF, Watson P, Mecklin JP, et al. New clinical criteria for hereditary nonpolyposis colorectal cancer (HNPCC, Lynch syndrome) proposed by the International Collaborative group on HNPCC. Gastroenterology 1999;116(6):1455; with permission.

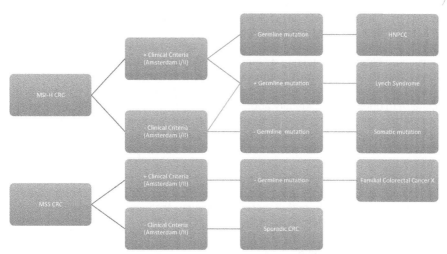

Fig. 1. Relationship between HNPCC and Lynch syndrome. MSI-H, microsatellite instability, high; MSS, microsatellite stable.

aggregate of all potentially associated gene mutations; however, each MMR mutation confers a unique genotype-phenotype cancer-risk profile.[14,15] Prior literature reports higher lifetime risk of CRC, up to 69% in men and 52% in women by the age of 70 years,[16,17] emphasizing the variable penetrance among individuals. Dowty and colleagues reports an average CRC cumulative risk by age 70 years for patients with *MLH1* and *MSH2* mutations of 34% and 47% for male carriers and 36% and 37% for female carriers, respectively; however, there is significant heterogeneity within these groups with some proportion of carriers having CRC risk similar to that of the general population and some having near absolute likelihood of developing CRC.[18,19]

Patients are also at increased risk of extracolonic malignancies, in particular endometrial, ovarian, gastric and small bowel, pancreatic, hepatobiliary, brain, and upper urothelial tract.[7,18] The average endometrial cancer risk is 18% to 60% with a mean age of diagnosis at 50 years.[19–21] *MSH6* is associated with a higher risk of endometrial cancer and a one-third lower risk of CRC compared with *MLH1* and *MSH2* carriers.[22,23] The estimated risk for gastric cancer is 6% to 13%[3]; however, this varies by the endemicity of gastric cancer in the population. For example, in Korea the lifetime risk of Lynch-related gastric cancer approaches 30% and surpasses endometrial cancer risk.[24] There are also subtypes of HNPCC/Lynch syndrome including Muir-Torre syndrome, associated with sebaceous carcinomas and keratocanthomas, and Turcot syndrome, which is associated with brain malignancies and colonic adenomas.[25]

Diagnosis of Hereditary Nonpolyposis Colorectal Cancer

The Amsterdam I clinical criteria for HNPCC were created in 1990 to standardize inclusion criteria for clinical research studies.[4] For kindred of families meeting Amsterdam criteria, the chance of identifying a germline mutation is 45% to 50%.[26] However, 40% of patients with an identified genetic mutation fail to meet Amsterdam criteria.[17] Concern of the Amsterdam I criteria missing clear familial clustering of extracolonic malignancies led to establishment of the Amsterdam II criteria (see **Box 1**), which broadens the HNPCC definition to include associated cancers (eg, endometrial, small bowel).[4] The revised Bethesda guidelines were then published in 2004 to identify CRC patients who should undergo pathologic examination for HNPCC/Lynch syndrome (**Box 2**).[27] For patients meeting these criteria, further pathologic analysis of the CRC specimen includes MSI testing or immunohistochemistry (IHC) assessment for the presence of the MMR proteins. Jerusalem guidelines further broaden the indications for MSI or IHC testing to CRC in individuals younger than 70 years.[28] Regardless, Amsterdam criteria fail to identify approximately 50% of cases, and Bethesda guidelines fail to identify at least 30% of cases,[29] which has led to increased support for the universal application of polymerase chain reaction (for detection of MSI-high tumors) and/or IHC testing (for MMR protein deficiency) to all CRC specimens.[30] This justification also supports universal testing of endometrial cancer.[31] Universal testing followed by germline testing offers the highest sensitivity (and somewhat lower specificity) than alternative screening strategies, although the increase in the diagnostic yield is modest compared with criteria-based screening techniques (**Table 1**).[32] Cost-effectiveness analyses demonstrate varying results.[33,34]

Etiology of Lynch Syndrome

Lynch syndrome is caused by a germline mutation in DNA MMR genes (most common being *MLH1*, *MSH2*, *MSH6*, and *PMS2*). As cellular division occurs, errors in replicated DNA are identified and corrected by the MMR protein complexes. Loss-of-function mutations in the MMR genes may result in DNA replication errors, which can occur in tumor suppressor genes or proto-oncogenes leading to carcinogenesis. DNA replication errors are propagated through daughter cells, leading to repetitive DNA sequences called microsatellites, making them unstable (MSI-high). MSI testing via polymerase chain reaction is an effective and highly reproducible method for identifying tumors with an underlying germline MMR defect (93% sensitivity).[35] Using a panel of microsatellite markers, tissue is classified as being MSI-high if two or more of five core markers show instability.[36] If more expansive panels are used, a greater than 30% rate of instability is considered MSI-high.[37] Sporadic CRC MSI

Box 2
Revised Bethesda guidelines

Criterion

1. CRC in a patient <50 years of age

2. Synchronous or metachronous CRC or the presence of other HNPCC-associated tumors,[a] regardless of age

3. Pathologic features of a microsatellite instability–high cancer (tumor infiltrating lymphocytes, Crohn's-like lymphocytic reaction, mucinous/signet-ring differentiation, or medullary growth pattern) in a patient <60 years

4. CRC in one or more first-degree relatives with an HNPCC-related tumor[a] with one of the cancers diagnosed by the age of 50 years (including adenoma by the age of 40 years)

5. CRC in two or more first- or second-degree relatives with HNPCC-related tumors, regardless of age

[a] Endometrial, stomach, ovarian, pancreas, small bowel, biliary tract, ureter or renal pelvis, brain, sebaceous gland adenoma, or keratoacanthoma.

From Umar A, Boland CR, Terdiman JP, et al. Revised Bethesda guidelines for hereditary non-polyposis colorectal cancer (Lynch syndrome) and microsatellite instability. J Natl Cancer Inst 2004;96(4):266; with permission.

Table 1 Sensitivity, specificity, and diagnostic yield of screening techniques for HNPCC			
Screening Approach	**Sensitivity (%)**	**Specificity (%)**	**Diagnostic Yield (%)**
Universal screening	100 (95% CI, 99.3–100)	93 (95% CI, 92–93.7)	2.2 (95% CI, 1.7–2.7)
Bethesda guidelines	87.8 (95% CI, 78.9–93.2)	97.5 (95% CI, 96.9–98.0)	2.0 (95% CI, 1.5–2.4)
Jerusalem recommendations	85.4 (95% CI, 77.1–93.6)	96.7 (95% CI, 96–97.2)	1.9 (95% CI, 1.4–2.3)
Selective MMR testing CRC in patients <70 y meeting Bethesda guidelines	95.1 (95% CI, 89.8–99)	95.5 (95% CI, 94.7–96.1)	2.1 (95% CI, 1.6–2.6)

Abbreviation: CI, confidence interval.

From Moreira L, Balaguer F, Lindor N, et al. Identification of Lynch syndrome among patients with colorectal cancer. JAMA 2012;308(15):1555; with permission.

testing typically reveals no instability and are considered microsatellite stable (MSS)[36]; however, 15% of sporadic CRCs are identified as being MSI-high and likely occur through the epigenetic pathway of hypermethylation of the *MLH1* promoter region and also harbor *BRAF* mutations, distinguishing them from germline-related pathways, which are typically BRAF wild-type.[15] Of note, a small percentage of CRCs that fulfill HNPCC clinical criteria are found to be MSS. Patients meeting these criteria have been designated "familial colorectal cancer type X" and have a moderately increased risk of CRC but no increased risk for extracolonic cancers (see **Fig. 1**).[38,39]

Genetic Testing for Hereditary Nonpolyposis Colorectal Cancer/Lynch Syndrome

Genetic testing should always be done in a thoughtful, stepwise fashion in the setting of effective counseling to ensure that the patient and kindred understand the implications of any test results, whether they confirm the presence of a mutation or not. When an MSI-high CRC is identified through tumor testing, IHC for the MMR proteins is performed to identify the likely mutated gene. Alternatively, IHC can replace MSI as the initial tumor test because IHC is technically easy to perform and has demonstrated 92% sensitivity in identifying mutations.[3] Although identification of a particular MMR protein loss on IHC guides germline testing, the finding of the loss of *MLH1* or *MLH1/PMS2* in the tumor is not sufficient for the diagnosis of Lynch because of the potential for sporadic loss from hypermethylation as described previously and requires additional testing for hypermethylation[40,41] or *BRAF* testing to identify somatic mutations. The presence of a *BRAF* mutation is thought to be rare in Lynch syndrome and usually excludes the diagnosis.[42]

When genetic testing is initiated after MMR IHC tumor testing, the implicated genes are tested for first with further gene testing performed only if the result is unrevealing. There are times when the clinical criteria for HNPCC are so impressive in a family (eg, significant phenotypes with multiple associated cancers in multiple individuals) that it is logical to proceed directly to germline testing of an affected individual without prior tumor testing. This is performed using a multigene panel to test for the MMR genes and any other CRC-related genes. Cost for these tests has decreased significantly in recent years because of more affordable testing methods; however, panels may vary greatly between laboratories. Regardless of method used, if a pathogenic mutation is found, the patient's at-risk kindred can be tested for that particular mutation.

Surveillance of Hereditary Nonpolyposis Colorectal Cancer/Lynch Syndrome

The recommendation for CRC surveillance of at-risk and affected individuals is colonoscopy every 1 to 2 years initiated at 20 to 25 years of age or 2 to 5 years before the age of the earliest diagnosed CRC, whichever comes first (**Table 2**).[6,43] Compliance with surveillance is paramount to reduce the incidence of CRC in affected individuals. In a prospective cohort study, 95% compliance rates of colonoscopic and gynecologic screening over a 10-year period found no difference in mortality in affected individuals compared with their nonaffected relatives.[44] Additional screening guidelines for extracolonic malignancies are outlined in **Table 2**.[6]

Surgical Approach to Hereditary Nonpolyposis Colorectal Cancer/Lynch Syndrome

Surgical options include segmental or extended resection, both requiring informed consent regarding implications on future cancer development balanced with the changes in bowel function and quality of life associated with each procedure. Extended colectomy is the recommended treatment of young to middle-aged patients with colon cancer, both for treatment of the primary lesion and risk reduction for metachronous CRC.[45] Subtotal colectomy or total abdominal colectomy with ileorectal anastomosis (TAC/IRA) decreases the risk of metachronous cancer by 31% for every 10 cm of bowel removed.[46] In the elderly, incontinent, and/or comorbid patient, the morbidity of and quality-of-life implications of an extended resection must be weighed heavily against the benefit of cancer risk reduction, and in some cases, a segmental colectomy may be more appropriate. In the case of rectal cancer, a total proctocolectomy with end ileostomy or restorative ileal pouch-anal anastomosis (IPAA) should be considered; however, when patients have a locally advanced rectal cancer with high risk for metastatic disease, prophylactic surgery becomes less of a concern, and low anterior resection or abdominoperineal resection may be more appropriate.[47] The decision to perform an extended versus segmental resection for CRC is also influenced by the patient's anticipated compliance with surveillance, which is paramount for early detection of recurrence and metachronous lesions.

There is not an established role for prophylactic colectomy in the asymptomatic Lynch syndrome patient. However, the role of prophylactic hysterectomy with bilateral salpingoophorectomy is well supported and recommended for women who have completed child bearing. In the setting of a planned CRC resection, concomitant prophylactic hysterectomy with bilateral salpingoophorectomy should be considered.[15]

FAMILIAL ADENOMATOUS POLYPOSIS

Familial adenomatous polyposis (FAP) has an incidence of 0.6 to 2.3 per million and accounts for approximately 0.5% to 1% of all CRCs.[48] FAP is characterized by the development of numerous (>100) colorectal adenomatous polyps (**Fig. 2**), often exceeding effective endoscopic management, and follows an autosomal-dominant inheritance pattern, although 20% to 30% of cases present as a result of a *de novo* mutation.[49] Onset of polyposis occurs in adolescence with progression to CRC by middle-age. The penetrance of FAP is 100%, with an incidence of CRC approaching 100% by the age of 50 years.[50] Enhanced awareness of this disease and more aggressive strategies for screening and surveillance have substantially decreased the incidence of CRC and associated mortality.[51,52]

Patients with FAP may present with extracolonic findings depending on the specific gene mutation involved. Duodenal adenomas are a significant contributor to FAP-related mortality with the risk of malignant progression guided by the Spigelman classification.[53] Desmoid tumors occur in approximately 15% to 20% of patients over the

Table 2
National Comprehensive Cancer Network surveillance recommendations for hereditary CRC syndromes

Syndrome	Site	Age to Begin Surveillance (y)	Surveillance Interval (y)	Procedures
HNPCC	Colon	20–25 or 2–5 y before earliest CRC diagnosis	1–2	Colonoscopy
	Endometrial and ovarian	No evidence to support	1	Consider annual endometrial sampling
				Consider prophylactic hysterectomy/BSO in women who have completed childbearing
				No evidence to support routine ovarian screening (transvaginal ultrasound or CA-125)
	Urinary tract	30–35	1	Consider annual urinalysis
	Small bowel	30–35	3–5	Consider EGD with extended duodenoscopy in at-risk individuals
	and gastric	No evidence to support		
Familial	Colon	10–15	1	Flexible sigmoidoscopy or colonoscopy
adenomatous	Upper GI	20–25	1–5	EGD with complete visualization of the papilla
polyposis		Earlier if colectomy at <20 y		Surveillance by Spigelman staging
				Consider CT or MRI for small bowel if duodenal polyposis is advanced
	Thyroid	Late teenage years	1	Annual thyroid examination
				Consider annual thyroid ultrasound
	Intra-abdominal desmoids	No evidence to support	1	Annual abdominal examination
				Consider CT or MRI 1–3 y after colectomy, then every 5–10 y or symptom-based

(continued on next page)

Table 2
(continued)

Syndrome	Site	Age to Begin Surveillance (y)	Surveillance Interval (y)	Procedures
Attenuated familial adenomatous polyposis	Colon	Late teenage years	2–3	Colonoscopy
	Upper GI	20–25 Earlier if colectomy at <20 y	1–5	EGD with complete visualization of the papilla
	Thyroid		1	Annual thyroid examination and thyroid ultrasound
MUTYH-associated polyposis	Colon	25–30	2–3	Colonoscopy
	Upper GI	30–35	1–5	EGD with complete visualization of the papilla
Serrated polyposis syndrome	Colon	40 10 y before earliest CRC diagnosis	1–3	Colonoscopy

Abbreviations: BSO, bilateral salpingoophorectomy; CT, computed tomography; EGD, esophagogastroduodenoscopy; GI, gastrointestinal.
Adapted from Provenzale D, Gupta S, Ahnen DJ, et al. Genetic/familial high-risk assessment: colorectal version 1.2016, NCCN Clinical Practice Guidelines in Oncology. J Natl Compr Canc Netw 2016;14(8):1010–30; with permission.

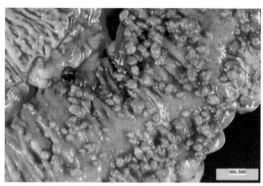

Fig. 2. Gross pathology of a colectomy specimen from a patient with FAP. (*From* Hawkins AT, Wise PE. Colon cancer in hereditary syndromes. Semin Colon Rectal Surg 2016. http://dx.doi. org/10.1053/j.scrs.2016.04.021; with permission.)

second and third decades of life (**Fig. 3**) with risk factors being prior abdominal surgery,[54,55] positive family history, and *APC* mutation 3′ to codon 1399.[56] Thyroid cancer risk is five times higher than that of the general population with a strong female preponderance.[57] Other benign findings include osteomas (~20%); lipomas; epidermoid cysts; fibromas; dental abnormalities; and congenital hypertrophy of the retinal pigment epithelium, which is pathognomonic for the diagnosis, albeit without known clinical import.[57] These unusual extracolonic manifestations often precede colonic symptoms and may aid in early diagnosis.[58]

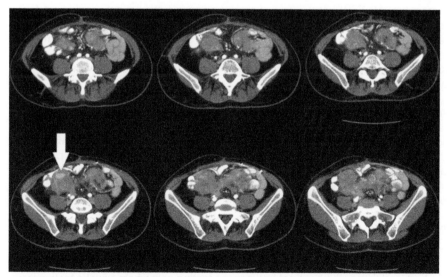

Fig. 3. Sections from a contrasted abdominal computed tomography scan of a patient with FAP with intra-abdominal desmoid originating from the mesentery and retroperitoneum, including areas with fistulization with oral contrast within the desmoid (*arrow*). (*From* Hawkins AT, Wise PE. Colon cancer in hereditary syndromes. Semin Colon Rectal Surg 2016. http://dx.doi.org/10.1053/j.scrs.2016.04.021; with permission.)

Etiology of Familial Adenomatous Polyposis

FAP is caused by a mutation in the adenomatous polyposis coli (*APC*) gene. The *APC* gene encodes a large multifunctional scaffolding protein that acts as a tumor suppressor within the *wnt*-signaling pathway to downregulate the activity of β-catenin. With loss of APC function, accumulation of β-catenin upregulates several genes that mediate cell proliferation, differentiation, and apoptosis. APC also mediates microtubule stabilization, with defects resulting in aberrant mitosis. More than 1100 mutations of the *APC* gene are identified, mostly resulting in a loss of function.[59]

Variations in the loci of *APC* mutations and other genetic modifiers result in genotype-phenotype variation in FAP. Three major phenotypes are described. The first is profuse polyposis exhibiting an aggressive phenotype with early onset of polyposis, symptoms, and CRC-related death at an average of 10 years earlier than typically described. Deletions at codon 1309 and truncating mutations at codons 1250 and 1464 are associated with this phenotype.[60] Second, intermediate polyposis, with most mutations located between codon 157 and codon 1595.[61] Third, attenuated polyposis (AFAP) characterized by a reduced polyp burden (10–100 polyps) with later age of onset and lower risk of CRC.[61] Diagnosis of AFAP is challenging because some features of AFAP are similar to those of *MUTYH*-associated polyposis (MAP), discussed later.[11]

Work-up of Familial Adenomatous Polyposis

It is important to emphasize that approximately 20% to 30% of patients with FAP present without a family history of CRC often via *de novo APC* mutations.[49,62] Historically, up to 40% to 50% of patients with FAP included in hereditary cancer registries are diagnosed based on symptomatic presentation (eg, rectal bleeding, changes in bowel habits) in the third or fourth decade and are significantly more likely to have an initial diagnosis of CRC compared with those diagnosed based on family history or other risk factors for FAP.[51,63,64] At the time of clinical diagnosis, the patient should be referred to a genetic counselor and testing performed to confirm the diagnosis. If a genetic mutation is identified, gene testing is extended to all at-risk kindred. If a genetic mutation is not identified for testing, surveillance must be extended to all at-risk kindred. In kindred born into an FAP family, genetic screening is recommended in midadolescence, before the initiation of cancer screening.

The gold standard and current method for genetic testing is direct sequencing of the *APC* gene. This method identifies greater than 85% of mutations with remaining mutations resulting from large gene rearrangements that are diagnosed on multiplex ligation-dependent probe amplification testing.[37] Approximately 20% of clinically diagnosed patients with FAP do not have an identified *APC* mutation. If the patient expresses a polyposis phenotype despite negative *APC* testing, genetic testing for MAP should be considered.[65] Occasionally, panel testing identifies other genotypes beyond those typically associated with FAP and MAP.

Surveillance for Familial Adenomatous Polyposis

In a study of 170 patients by Bussey,[66] rectal involvement with polyposis was identified in all cases. Based on this finding, it is reasonable for affected individuals, at-risk kindred, and those who have not had genetic testing or in whom genetic testing is uninformative to undergo annual flexible sigmoidoscopy beginning in the early teenage years. If polyps are detected, full colonoscopy is indicated. Annual surveillance should be life-long regardless of findings because of 100% penetrance of the disease.[67] In the case of AFAP, onset of CRC is later and there is a propensity for right-sided adenomas, so screening can be initiated in late teenage years, but colonoscopy should be used instead of flexible sigmoidoscopy. Further screening recommendations are outlined in **Table 2**.

Chemoprevention for Familial Adenomatous Polyposis

Various chemoprevention strategies have been considered to delay proctocolectomy in young patients and to manage upper and lower gastrointestinal polyps when surgical intervention is unfavorable. Sulindac and celecoxib are the most widely studied agents. The mechanism of nonsteroidal anti-inflammatory drug–mediated chemoprevention is not completely understood; however, cyclooxygenase-2 inhibition is known to inhibit angiogenesis and neovascularization, and restore normal apoptosis signaling in CRC cells.[68] These agents demonstrate significantly reduced colon polyp burden in placebo-controlled trials[69,70] and offer a moderate effect in the reduction in duodenal epithelial proliferation[71]; however, effects are incomplete and temporary with recurrence following cessation of therapy. It is also not clear that a reduced polyp burden translates into reduced CRC risk. Currently, chemoprophylaxis is not a suitable alternative to surgical therapy. Chemoprevention is considered if contraindications or unavoidable delay to surgery exist and also serves as an effective adjunct to endoscopic polypectomy in the management of ileal pouch polyposis.[72] Studies are underway examining other therapeutic agents and combination therapies for chemoprevention.[73]

Surgery for Familial Adenomatous Polyposis

Surgery is the mainstay of CRC risk reduction for FAP. Timing is not clearly defined by guidelines because multiple factors must play into the decision-making process shared by the surgeon and the patient. Ideally, surgical intervention is an elective procedure with the indication of prophylaxis in the asymptomatic patient. This can be delayed until adolescence, usually 15 to 20 years of age, considering the psychological impact to the young patient, because the incidence of CRC before that age is low.[67] Patients with large or dysplastic lesions, severe disease either clinically or by genotype, or with symptoms should proceed to colectomy as soon as possible because of the risk of underlying CRC. Patients with a family history or genotype predisposing to desmoid disease may opt to delay surgery provided CRC risk allows for this. It is reasonable for patients with AFAP or mild disease to delaying surgery into young adulthood (21–25 years of age) or later, especially if the disease can be endoscopically controlled.[74] Three main surgical options for FAP are described next (**Table 3**).

Total proctocolectomy with end ileostomy

Total proctocolectomy with end ileostomy is the gold standard treatment and offers complete extirpation of at-risk colorectal mucosa at the expense of permanent ileostomy. Although less commonly performed, this procedure should be included in the discussion of surgical options for patients with low rectal cancers that preclude IPAA, those with poor sphincter function, and desmoid disease or other anatomic constraints that prevent IPAA construction.

Total proctocolectomy with ileal pouch–anal anastomosis

Total proctocolectomy with IPAA is the most widely used procedure and is considered standard of care for the treatment of FAP other than for the previously noted contraindications. This is a near-complete extirpative procedure with the benefit of preserved continence. Historically, mucosectomy with handsewn IPAA was the recommended approach to remove remaining at-risk mucosa from the retained

Surgery	Indications	Contraindications
Table 3 **Surgical management options for FAP**		
Total proctocolectomy with end ileostomy	• Low rectal cancer precluding sphincter preservation • Mesenteric foreshortening (desmoids) • Poor sphincter function • Refusal of IPAA • Noncompliance to surveillance	• Refusal of permanent ileostomy
Total abdominal colectomy with ileorectal anastomosis	• AFAP/mild polyposis • <1000 colonic adenomas • <20 rectal adenomas • Desire for preserved fertility/potency	• Noncompliance to surveillance • Rectal polyposis (>20 rectal adenomas) • Rectal dysplasia/carcinoma • Rectal polyp >3 cm • Predisposition to desmoid disease • APC mutation predisposing to rectal cancer
Total proctocolectomy with ileal pouch–anal anastomosis	• Acceptable anticipated functional outcome	• Poor baseline sphincter function • Low rectal cancer precluding sphincter preservation • Noncompliance to surveillance

rectal cuff; however, the incidence of dysplasia is not statistically different in comparisons of either method.[75] The relative procedural ease and functional benefit afforded by stapled IPAA makes this the preferred method in most clinical scenarios.[76] The risk of cancer in the residual rectal cuff or anal transition zone or pouch approaches 1.2%.[77] Risk factors related to pouch cancer include preoperative diagnosis of dysplasia or carpeting polyposis of the rectum.[76] Endoscopic surveillance of the anal transition zone and pouch should be performed every 1 to 3 years depending on polyp burden. Surveillance should be increased to every 6 months in the case of large polyps, villous architecture, and/or dysplasia in the pouch or cuff.[6]

Total abdominal colectomy with ileorectal anastomosis

TAC/IRA is technically easier to perform with the benefit of improved fecal and urinary continence and sexual function compared with IPAA.[78–80] This option is considered in patients who have a limited rectal polyp burden (<20 polyps), a low-risk genotype, and are able to comply with surveillance. This is a good option for patients with AFAP and rectal sparing. Endoscopic surveillance of the residual rectum should be performed every 6 to 12 months depending on the extent of polyp burden.[6] Patients considering IRA must be counseled regarding the risk of metachronous lesions within the retained rectum and progression to polyposis that exceeds endoscopic management because both are indications for completion proctectomy. In a registry-based review of 427 patients undergoing IRA for FAP, 11% of patients developed rectal cancer with 50% of patients undergoing proctectomy by age 60. Risk factors for progression of rectal disease include rectal polyp burden greater than 20, colonic polyp burden greater than

500, and an *APC* mutation at codon 1250 to 1450 suggesting that IRA may not be appropriate for these patients.[8]

MUTYH-ASSOCIATED POLYPOSIS

MAP was first described in 2002 with a report of a biallelic germline mutation in the *MUTYH* gene in a family expressing a recessive inheritance pattern of colon adenomas and CRC.[10] As the body of knowledge regarding genotypic contributors to polyposis has grown, MAP shares clinical features with FAP/AFAP such that 10% to 20% of patients with suspected FAP/AFAP without an identified *APC* mutation exhibit a mutation in *MUTYH*.[11] Affected patients have a 50-fold increased lifetime risk of CRC with a mean age of diagnosis at 50 years. Heterozygote carriers exhibit a three-fold increased risk of CRC.[12] MAP polyposis includes conventional adenomas, serrated adenomas, and hyperplastic polyps.[14] A family history of polyposis is rarely evident because of an autosomal-recessive inheritance pattern. Affected individuals are also at risk for extracolonic neoplasm with duodenal adenomas found in 17% to 25%[18] of patients with a 4% lifetime risk of duodenal cancer.[16] MAP is also associated with late-onset gynecologic, urothelial, and skin cancers.[18]

Etiology of MUTYH-Associated Polyposis

The *MUTYH* gene encodes a glycosylase involved in base excision repair. *MUTYH* deficiency results in genetic instability of the *APC* gene and perhaps others, including *KRAS* and *p53*. The pathogenesis of MAP-related tumors is unique but has overlap with FAP, perhaps accounting for phenotypic similarities.[20]

Diagnosis of MUTYH-Associated Polyposis

Genetic testing for MAP should be considered in the case of clinically diagnosed polyposis without an identified *APC* mutation. Genetic testing is initially mutation-specific, because 80% of patients exhibit one of two major mutations. If a mutation is identified, then sequencing of the remaining allele is performed to confirm the presence of biallelic mutations. If a known mutation is not identified, primary sequencing is performed.[81]

Surveillance and Surgical Approach to MUTYH-Associated Polyposis

Colonoscopic surveillance is recommended to start at 25 years of age with surveillance every 1 to 2 years and extracolonic screening as outlined in **Table 2**. Screening for heterozygote carriers is similar to population screening guidelines for high-risk individuals. Indications for surgical intervention and considerations for type of resection are similar to those outlined for FAP/AFAP.[6]

SERRATED POLYPOSIS SYNDROME

Serrated polyposis syndrome (SPS) has an incidence of 1:100,00,0[82] and is characterized by the presence of multiple or large serrated polyps and a predisposition to CRC. SPS is associated with a lifetime risk of CRC approaching 70%. There is no known genetic basis for SPS, and identifying at-risk patients is limited because a positive family history is reported in 0% to 59% of patients without a consistent mode of inheritance.[83] Therefore, diagnosis is based on specific clinical criteria outlined by the World Health Organization (**Box 3**),[84] which underscore the considerable phenotypic variation of the condition (eg, patients may have multiple lesions throughout their colons or few, large, right-sided lesions on cumulative surveillance).

Box 3
World Health Organization criteria for diagnosis of SPS

Criterion

1. At least five serrated class polyps proximal to the sigmoid of which at least two are greater than 1 cm in size

2. Any serrated class polyp proximal to the sigmoid in a first-degree relative with SPS

3. ≥20 serrated class polyps distributed throughout the colon.

Satisfaction of any one of the three criteria establishes the diagnosis of SPS.

Data from Snover DC, Ahnen DJ, Burt RW, et al. Serrated polyps of the colon and rectum and serrated polyposis. In: Bosman FT, Carneiro F, Hruban RH, et al, editors. WHO Classification of Tumours of the Digestive System. 4th edition. Lyon: IARC; 2010. p. 160–65.

Sessile serrated polyps (SSPs) account for 25% of serrated lesions and seem to be the precursor lesions for SPS-associated CRC. SSPs are flat with an overlying mucus cap making identification and complete endoscopic clearing challenging. SSPs are generally located in the proximal colon but up to 30% are found distally.[85] SPS-associated CRCs can present with synchronous and/or metachronous lesions. Interval cancers most often occur in the proximal colon and are often MSI-high via an epigenetically mediated pathway involving CpG island hypermethylation. This pathway is described in greater detail next.

Etiology of Serrated Polyposis Syndrome

Although no gene mutation has clearly been linked to SPS, the serrated adenoma–carcinoma pathway is well described. This is an epigenetically mediated mechanism whereby hypermethylation of CpG islands occurs in the promoter region of tumor suppressor genes. Hypermethylation results in silencing of the tumor promoter region resulting in MSI. Tumors arising via this pathway are characterized by the CpG island mutation phenotype (CIMP-high). CIMP-high phenotypes are found in 15% to 20% of sporadic colon carcinomas.[86] The serrated adenoma–carcinoma pathway is also associated with methylation of *MLH1*, wherein gene dysfunction predisposes to dysplasia and rapid progression to carcinoma, much like MSI-high lesions seen in HNPCC/Lynch syndrome.[87] There is significant heterogeneity in the molecular profiles of SSPs suggesting that other pathways for carcinogenesis exist (**Fig. 4**).[88] *KRAS* mutations are associated with CIMP-low, SPS-associated CRC.[89] Germline mutations in genes that regulate cellular senescence pathways have also been identified in SSPs of patients with SPS.[90]

Screening and Surveillance for Serrated Polyposis Syndrome

Surveillance recommendations for patients with SPS include colonoscopy every 1 to 3 years depending on polyp burden (see **Table 2**).[43] In at-risk kindred, colonoscopy should begin at age 40 or 10 years earlier than the youngest relative diagnosed with SPS if complicated by CRC, whichever is earlier. Colonoscopy is repeated every 5 years in the absence of findings or every 1 to 3 years if polyps are identified.[6]

Although based on best available data, screening guidelines may underdiagnose patients resulting in prolonged screening intervals before a diagnosis is realized, placing patients at increased risk for interval carcinomas. Some argue that the finding of two or more serrated lesions on colonoscopy qualifies as screening criteria for close interval surveillance despite not meeting World Health Organization criteria. In a retrospective review of 500 patients with at least two or more serrated lesions, a median of

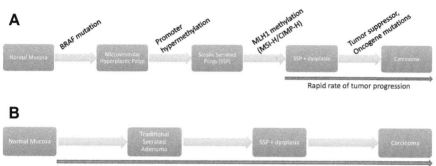

Fig. 4. Pathways for SPS-associated carcinogenesis. (*A*) Serrated adenoma-carcinoma pathway: hypermethylation of CpG islands results in MSI-H, CIMP-H carcinoma similar to Lynch-associated CRC. (*B*) KRAS serrated polyp pathway: resulting in MSI-L, CIMP-L carcinoma. (*Data from* Snover DC, Ahnen DJ, Burt RW, et al. Serrated polyps of the colon and rectum and serrated polyposis. In: Bosman FT, Carneiro F, Hruban RH, et al, editors. WHO Classification of Tumours of the Digestive System. 4th edition. Lyon: IARC; 2010. p. 160–65.)

four colonoscopies was performed before the diagnosis of SPS was made. Of the 40 patients (8%) with SPS, only one was diagnosed at initial colonoscopy and all 16 patients with CRC were diagnosed with SPS at the time of cancer diagnosis.[91]

Because of the subtle appearance of serrated polyps, chromoendoscopy or virtual chromoendoscopy with narrow band imaging is recommended to aid in detection of these lesions.[82] Increased withdrawal times of at least 9 minutes are associated with improved adenoma detection rates.[92] SSPs have indistinct borders and complete removal of these flat lesions is challenging. The rate of incomplete resection for SSPs is higher than conventional adenomas at 31% versus 7.2%.[93] This may contribute to the higher rate of interval carcinomas previously discussed and emphasizes the need for shorter screening intervals for lesions greater than 1 cm. In the case of numerous (>5), large (>2 cm), or dysplastic lesions, some authors support the use of serial endoscopic mucosal resection every 3 to 6 months until endoscopically cleared.[94]

Surgical Approach to Serrated Polyposis Syndrome

Surgical intervention is warranted when the polyp burden exceeds endoscopic management or when dysplasia/CRC is diagnosed. There is limited experience regarding the benefit of segmental versus TAC/IRA; however, the rate of synchronous and metachronous CRC approaches 26%, favoring extended colectomy.[88] In the case of segmental resection, annual colonoscopy of the remaining colon is recommended. If at least two successive colonoscopies reveal no lesions greater than 1 cm, no dysplastic lesions, or the mean number and size of the lesions is declining, this interval can be expanded to every 2 years.[94]

SUMMARY

Inherited CRC syndromes are a rare cause of CRC within the general population. Nevertheless, awareness of these unique syndromes leads to early diagnosis and prevention of cancer-related morbidity and mortality in affected individuals and families. Moreover, screening, counseling, and testing of at-risk kindred can translate into significant benefit across multiple generations, emphasizing the tremendous importance of understanding the heritable risks of each syndrome. Currently, surgery is the mainstay of CRC prevention and treatment of all of these syndromes. Operative decision-making must take into account the life-long cancer risk of each patient and balance this against long-term function. The pathogenesis of most heritable CRC syndromes remains poorly understood. The use of cancer registries, genetic counseling and testing, and ongoing academic pursuits are instrumental in defining the genetic basis of this heterogeneous group, broadening the understanding of unique genotype-phenotype profiles, and customizing treatment strategies based on individual risk.

REFERENCES

1. Lichtenstein P, Holm NV, Verkasalo PK, et al. Environmental and heritable factors in the causation of cancer: analyses of cohorts of twins from Sweden, Denmark, and Finland. N Engl J Med 2000;343(2):78–85.
2. Jasperson KW, Tuohy TM, Neklason DW, et al. Hereditary and familial colon cancer. Gastroenterology 2010;138(6):2044–58.
3. Kohlmann W, Gruber SB. Lynch syndrome [updated 2014 May 22]. In: Pagon RA, Adam MP, Ardinger HH, et al, editors. GeneReviews [Internet]. Seattle (WA): University of Washington; 2004. p. 1993–2016.
4. Vasen HF, Watson P, Mecklin JP, et al. New clinical criteria for hereditary nonpolyposis colorectal cancer (HNPCC, Lynch syndrome) proposed by the International Collaborative group on HNPCC. Gastroenterology 1999;116(6):1453–6.
5. Guillem JG, Calle JP-L, Cellini C, et al. Varying features of early age-of-onset "sporadic" and hereditary nonpolyposis colorectal cancer patients. Dis Colon Rectum 1999;42(1):36–42.
6. Provenzale D, Gupta S, Ahnen DJ, et al. Genetic/familial high-risk assessment: colorectal version 1.2016, NCCN clinical practice guidelines in oncology. J Natl Compr Canc Netw 2016;14(8):1010–30.
7. Lynch HT, la Chapelle de A. Hereditary colorectal cancer. N Engl J Med 2003; 348(10):919–32.
8. Sinha A, Tekkis PP, Rashid S, et al. Risk factors for secondary proctectomy in patients with familial adenomatous polyposis. Br J Surg 2010;97(11):1710–5.
9. Lin KM, Shashidharan M, Ternent CA, et al. Colorectal and extracolonic cancer variations in MLH1/MSH2 hereditary nonpolyposis colorectal cancer kindreds and the general population. Dis Colon Rectum 2016;41(4):428–33.
10. Al-Tassan N, Chmiel NH, Maynard J, et al. Inherited variants of MYH associated with somatic G: C→T: A mutations in colorectal tumors. Nat Genet 2002;30(2):227–32.
11. Burt RW, Leppert MF, Slattery ML, et al. Genetic testing and phenotype in a large kindred with attenuated familial adenomatous polyposis. Gastroenterology 2004; 127(2):444–51.
12. Jenkins MA. Risk of colorectal cancer in monoallelic and biallelic carriers of MYH mutations: a population-based case-family study. Cancer Epidemiol Biomarkers Prev 2006;15(2):312–4.
13. Edelstein DL, Axilbund J, Baxter M, et al. Rapid development of colorectal neoplasia in patients with Lynch syndrome. Clin Gastroenterol Hepatol 2011; 9(4):340–3.
14. Boparai KS, Dekker E, van Eeden S, et al. Hyperplastic polyps and sessile serrated adenomas as a phenotypic expression of MYH-associated polyposis. Gastroenterology 2008;135(6):2014–8.
15. Lindor NM, Petersen GM, Hadley DW, et al. Recommendations for the care of individuals with an inherited predisposition to Lynch syndrome: a systematic review. JAMA 2006;296(12):1507–17.

16. Nielsen M, Poley JW, Verhoef S, et al. Duodenal carcinoma in MUTYH-associated polyposis. J Clin Pathol 2006;59(11):1212–5.
17. Hampel H, Stephens JA, Pukkala E, et al. Cancer risk in hereditary nonpolyposis colorectal cancer syndrome: later age of onset. Gastroenterology 2005;129(2): 415–21.
18. Vogt S, Jones N, Christian D, et al. Expanded extracolonic tumor spectrum. Gastroenterology 2009;137(6):1976–85.e1-e10.
19. Dowty JG, Win AK, Buchanan DD, et al. Cancer risks for MLH1and MSH2 mutation carriers. Hum Mutat 2013;34(3):490–7.
20. Lipton L, Halford SE, Johnson V, et al. Carcinogenesis in MYH-associated polyposis follows a distinct genetic pathway. Cancer Res 2003;63(22):7595–9.
21. Win AK, Lindor NM, Young JP, et al. Risks of primary extracolonic cancers following colorectal cancer in Lynch syndrome. J Natl Cancer Inst 2012; 104(18):1363–72.
22. Plaschke J. Lower incidence of colorectal cancer and later age of disease onset in 27 families with pathogenic MSH6 germline mutations compared with families with MLH1 or MSH2 Mutations: the German Hereditary Nonpolyposis Colorectal Cancer Consortium. J Clin Oncol 2004;22(22):4486–94.
23. Hendriks YMC, Wagner A, Morreau H, et al. Cancer risk in hereditary nonpolyposis colorectal cancer due to MSH6 mutations: impact on counseling and surveillance. Gastroenterology 2004;127(1):17–25.
24. Park YJ, Shin KH, Park JG. Risk of gastric cancer in hereditary nonpolyposis colorectal cancer in Korea. Clin Cancer Res 2000;6(8):2994–8.
25. Felton K, Gilchrist DM, Andrew SE. Constitutive deficiency in DNA mismatch repair: is it time for Lynch III? Clin Genet 2007;71(6):499–500.
26. Wijnen J, Khan PM, Vasen H, et al. Hereditary nonpolyposis colorectal cancer families not complying with the Amsterdam criteria show extremely low frequency of mismatch-repair-gene mutations. Am J Hum Genet 1997;61:329–35.
27. Umar A, Boland CR, Terdiman JP, et al. Revised Bethesda guidelines for hereditary nonpolyposis colorectal cancer (Lynch Syndrome) and microsatellite instability. J Natl Cancer Inst 2004;96(4):261–8.
28. Boland CR, Shike M. Report from the Jerusalem workshop on Lynch syndrome-hereditary nonpolyposis colorectal cancer. Gastroenterology 2010;138(7): 2197.e1-7.
29. Sjursen W, Haukanes BI, Grindedal EM, et al. Current clinical criteria for Lynch syndrome are not sensitive enough to identify MSH6 mutation carriers. J Med Genet 2010;47(9):579–85.
30. Evaluation of Genomic Applications in Practice and Prevention (EGAPP) Working Group. Recommendations from the EGAPP Working Group: genetic testing strategies in newly diagnosed individuals with colorectal cancer aimed at reducing morbidity and mortality from Lynch syndrome in relatives. Genet Med 2009; 11(1):35–41.
31. Moline J, Mahdi H, Yang B, et al. Implementation of tumor testing for Lynch syndrome in endometrial cancers at a large academic medical center. Gynecol Oncol 2013;130(1):121–6.
32. Moreira L, Balaguer F, Lindor N, et al. Identification of Lynch syndrome among patients with colorectal cancer. JAMA 2012;308(15):1555.
33. Chen Y-E, Kao S-S, Chung R-H. Cost-effectiveness analysis of different genetic testing strategies for Lynch syndrome in Taiwan. PLoS One 2016;11(8):e0160599.
34. Severin F, Stollenwerk B, Holinski-Feder E, et al. Economic evaluation of genetic screening for Lynch syndrome in Germany. Genet Med 2015;17(10):765–73.

35. Shia J. Immunohistochemistry versus microsatellite instability testing for screening colorectal cancer patients at risk for hereditary nonpolyposis colorectal cancer syndrome. Part I. The utility of immunohistochemistry. J Mol Diagn 2008; 10(4):293–300.

36. Boland CR, Thibodeau SN, Hamilton SR, et al. A National Cancer Institute workshop on microsatellite instability for cancer detection and familial predisposition: development of international criteria for the determination of microsatellite instability in colorectal cancer. Cancer Res 1998;58(22):5248–57.

37. Hegde M, Ferber M, Mao R, et al. ACMG technical standards and guidelines for genetic testing for inherited colorectal cancer (Lynch syndrome, familial adenomatous polyposis, and MYH-associated polyposis). Genet Med 2014;16(1):101–16.

38. Lindor NM, Rabe K, Petersen GM, et al. Lower cancer incidence in Amsterdam-I criteria families without mismatch repair deficiency: familial colorectal cancer type X. JAMA 2005;293(16):1979–85.

39. Stoffel EM, Chittenden A. Genetic testing for hereditary colorectal cancer: challenges in identifying, counseling, and managing high-risk patients. Gastroenterology 2010;139(5):1436–41.e1.

40. Niessen RC, Hofstra RMW, Westers H, et al. Germline hypermethylation of MLH1 and EPCAM deletions are a frequent cause of Lynch syndrome. Genes Chromosomes Cancer 2009;48(8):737–44.

41. Nagasaka T, Rhees J, Kloor M, et al. Somatic hypermethylation of MSH2 is a frequent event in Lynch syndrome colorectal cancers. Cancer Res 2010;70(8): 3098–108.

42. Bouzourene H, Hutter P, Losi L, et al. Selection of patients with germline MLH1 mutated Lynch syndrome by determination of MLH1 methylation and BRAF mutation. Fam Cancer 2009;9(2):167–72.

43. Syngal S, Brand RE, Church JM, et al. ACG clinical guideline: genetic testing and management of hereditary gastrointestinal cancer syndromes. Am J Gastroenterol 2015;110(2):223–62.

44. Järvinen HJ, Renkonen-Sinisalo L, Aktan-Collan K, et al. Ten years after mutation testing for Lynch syndrome: cancer incidence and outcome in mutation-positive and mutation-negative family members. J Clin Oncol 2009;27(28):4793–7.

45. Natarajan N, Watson P, Silva-Lopez E, et al. Comparison of extended colectomy and limited resection in patients with Lynch syndrome. Dis Colon Rectum 2010; 53(1):77–82.

46. Parry S, Win AK, Parry B, et al. Metachronous colorectal cancer risk for mismatch repair gene mutation carriers: the advantage of more extensive colon surgery. Gut 2011;60(7):950–7.

47. Maeda T, Cannom RR, Beart RW, et al. Decision model of segmental compared with total abdominal colectomy for colon cancer in hereditary nonpolyposis colorectal cancer. J Clin Oncol 2010;28(7):1175–80.

48. Järvinen HJ. Epidemiology of familial adenomatous polyposis in Finland: impact of family screening on the colorectal cancer rate and survival. Gut 1992;33(3): 357–60.

49. Aretz S, Uhlhaas S, Caspari R, et al. Frequency and parental origin of de novo APC mutations in familial adenomatous polyposis. Eur J Hum Genet 2004; 12(1):52–8.

50. Bisgaard ML, Fenger K, Bülow S, et al. Familial adenomatous polyposis (FAP): frequency, penetrance, and mutation rate. Hum Mutat 1994;3:121–3.

51. Bülow S. Results of national registration of familial adenomatous polyposis. Gut 2003;52(5):742–6.

52. Mallinson EKL, Newton KF, Bowen J, et al. The impact of screening and genetic registration on mortality and colorectal cancer incidence in familial adenomatous polyposis. Gut 2010;59(10):1378–82.
53. Spigelman AD, Williams CB, Talbot IC, et al. Upper gastrointestinal cancer in patients with familial adenomatous polyposis. Lancet 1989;2(8666):783–5.
54. Sinha A, Tekkis PP, Gibbons DC, et al. Risk factors predicting desmoid occurrence in patients with familial adenomatous polyposis: a meta-analysis. Colorectal Dis 2010;13(11):1222–9.
55. Nieuwenhuis MH, Lefevre JH, Bülow S, et al. Family history, surgery, and APC mutation are risk factors for desmoid tumors in familial adenomatous polyposis: an international cohort study. Dis Colon Rectum 2011;54(10):1229–34.
56. Church J, Xhaja X, LaGuardia L, et al. Desmoids and genotype in familial adenomatous polyposis. Dis Colon Rectum 2015;58(4):444–8.
57. Groen EJ, Roos A, Muntinghe FL, et al. Extra-intestinal manifestations of familial adenomatous polyposis. Ann Surg Oncol 2008;15(9):2439–50.
58. Kubo K, Miyatani H, Takenoshita Y, et al. Widespread radiopacity of jaw bones in familial adenomatosis coli. J Craniomaxillofac Surg 1989;17(8):350–3.
59. Balaguer F, Leoz M, Carballal S, et al. The genetic basis of familial adenomatous polyposis and its implications for clinical practice and risk management. Appl Clin Genet 2015;8:95–107.
60. Caspari R, Friedl W, Mandl M, et al. Familial adenomatous polyposis: mutation at codon 1309 and early onset of colon cancer. Lancet 1994;343(8898):629–32.
61. Nieuwenhuis MH, Vasen HFA. Correlations between mutation site in APC and phenotype of familial adenomatous polyposis (FAP): a review of the literature. Crit Rev Oncol Hematol 2007;61(2):153–61.
62. Ripa R, Bisgaard ML, Bülow S, et al. De novo mutations in familial adenomatous polyposis (FAP). Eur J Hum Genet 2002;10(10):631–7.
63. Ho JW, Chu KM, Tse CW. Phenotype and management of patients with familial adenomatous polyposis in Hong Kong: perspective of the hereditary gastrointestinal cancer registry. Hong Kong Med J 2002;8(5):342–7.
64. Bjork J, Akerbrant H, Iselius L, et al. Epidemiology of familial adenomatous polyposis in Sweden: changes over time and differences in phenotype between males and females. Scand J Gastroenterol 1999;34(12):1230–5.
65. Aretz S, Uhlhaas S, Goergens H, et al. MUTYH-associated polyposis: 70 of 71 patients with biallelic mutations present with an attenuated or atypical phenotype. Int J Cancer 2006;119(4):807–14.
66. Bussey H. Familial polyposis coli: family studies, histopathology, differential diagnosis, and results of treatment. Baltimore (MD): Johns Hopkins University Press; 1975.
67. Vasen HFA, Moslein G, Alonso A, et al. Guidelines for the clinical management of familial adenomatous polyposis (FAP). Gut 2008;57(5):704–13.
68. Herendeen JM, Lindley C. Use of NSAIDs for the chemoprevention of colorectal cancer. Ann Pharmacother 2003;37(11):1664.
69. Giardiello FM, Hamilton SR, Krush AJ. Treatment of colonic and rectal adenomas with sulindac in familial adenomatous polyposis. N Engl J Med 1993;328(18):1313–6.
70. Steinbach G, Lynch PM, Phillips RK, et al. The effect of celecoxib, a cyclooxygenase-2 inhibitor, in familial adenomatous polyposis. N Engl J Med 2000;342(26):1946–52.
71. Nugent KP, Farmer KC, Spigelman AD, et al. Randomized controlled trial of the effect of sulindac on duodenal and rectal polyposis and cell proliferation in patients with familial adenomatous polyposis. Br J Surg 1993;80(12):1618–9.

72. O'Brien D. Polyps in the ileal pouch. Clin Colon Rectal Surg 2008;21(04):300–3.
73. Samadder NJ, Neklason DW, Boucher KM, et al. Effect of sulindac and erlotinib vs placebo on duodenal neoplasia in familial adenomatous polyposis. JAMA 2016;315(12):1266.
74. Campos FG. Surgical treatment of familial adenomatous polyposis: dilemmas and current recommendations. World J Gastroenterol 2014;20(44):16620.
75. Lovegrove RE, Constantinides VA, Heriot AG, et al. A comparison of hand-sewn versus stapled ileal pouch anal anastomosis (IPAA) following proctocolectomy. Ann Surg 2006;244(1):18–26.
76. Chambers WM, McC Mortensen NJ. Should ileal pouch-anal anastomosis include mucosectomy? Colorectal Dis 2007;9(5):384–92.
77. Fazio VW, Kiran RP, Remzi FH, et al. Ileal pouch anal anastomosis. Ann Surg 2013;257(4):679–85.
78. Aziz O, Athanasiou T, Fazio VW, et al. Meta-analysis of observational studies of ileorectalversus ileal pouch–anal anastomosis for familial adenomatous polyposis. Br J Surg 2006;93(4):407–17.
79. Soravia C, Klein L, Berk T, et al. Comparison of ileal pouch-anal anastomosis and ileorectal anastomosis in patients with familial adenomatous polyposis. Dis Colon Rectum 1999;42(8):1028–33 [discussion1033–4].
80. Olsen KO, Juul S, Bülow S, et al. Female fecundity before and after operation for familial adenomatous polyposis. Br J Surg 2003;90(2):227–31.
81. Burt R, Neklason DW. Genetic testing for inherited colon cancer. Gastroenterology 2005;128(6):1696–716.
82. Rodriguez-Moranta F, Rodriguez-Alonso L, Guardiola Capon J. Serrated polyposis syndrome. Cir Esp 2014;92(10):643–4.
83. Rosty C, Parry S, Young JP. Serrated polyposis: an enigmatic model of colorectal cancer predisposition. Patholog Res Int 2011;2011(4):1–13.
84. Snover DC, Ahnen DJ, Burt RW, et al. Serrated polyps of the colon and rectum and serrated ("hyperplastic") pol-yposis. In: Bosman ST, Carneiro F, Hruban RH, et al, editors. WHO Classification of tumours of the digestive system. Berlin: Springer-Verlag; 2010.
85. Langner C. Serrated and non-serrated precursor lesions of colorectal cancer. Dig Dis 2015;33(1):28–37.
86. Kanth P, Bronner MP, Boucher KM, et al. Gene signature in sessile serrated polyps identifies colon cancer subtype. Cancer Prev Res (Phila) 2016;9(6):456–65.
87. Anderson JC. Pathogenesis and management of serrated polyps: current status and future directions. Gut Liver 2014;8(6):582–9.
88. Rosty C, Walsh MD, Walters RJ, et al. Multiplicity and molecular heterogeneity of colorectal carcinomas in individuals with serrated polyposis. Am J Surg Pathol 2013;37(3):434–42.
89. Elorza G, Enríquez-Navascués JM, Bujanda L, et al. Phenotype characteristics of patients with colonic serrated polyposis syndrome: a study of 23 cases. Cir Esp 2014;92(10):659–64.
90. Gala MK, Mizukami Y, Le LP, et al. Germline mutations in oncogene-induced senescence pathways are associated with multiple sessile serrated adenomas. Gastroenterology 2014;146(2):520–9.
91. Hui VW, Steinhagen E, Levy RA, et al. Utilization of colonoscopy and pathology reports for identifying patients meeting the world health organization criteria for serrated polyposis syndrome. Dis Colon Rectum 2014;57(7):846–50.

92. Butterly L, Robinson CM, Anderson JC, et al. Serrated and adenomatous polyp detection increases with longer withdrawal time: results from the New Hampshire colonoscopy registry. Am J Gastroenterol 2014;109(3):417–26.
93. Pohl H, Srivastava A, Bensen SP, et al. Incomplete polyp resection during colonoscopy: results of the complete adenoma resection (CARE) study. Gastroenterology 2013;144(1):74–80.e1.
94. Hassan C, Repici A, Rex DK. Serrated polyposis syndrome: risk stratification or reduction? Gut 2016;65(7):1070–2.

Dysplasia and Cancer in Inflammatory Bowel Disease

 CrossMark

Lyen C. Huang, MD[a], Amit Merchea, MD[b],*

KEYWORDS

- Inflammatory bowel disease • Ulcerative colitis • Crohn disease • Dysplasia
- Colorectal cancer • Colitis • Colitis-associated cancer

KEY POINTS

- Improved medical management and endoscopic surveillance of inflammatory bowel disease have reduced the incidence of cancer and its associated mortality.
- Surveillance should begin 6 to 10 years after initial diagnosis. Most societies recommend high-definition colonoscopy with chromoendoscopy and targeted biopsies when available.
- High-grade dysplasia or cancer are indications for surgical resection. Exceptions can be considered for lesions contained in discrete adenomalike polyps that can be removed completely.
- The management of low-grade dysplasia is controversial and the choice between continued surveillance versus colectomy should be discussed with patients.
- Most patients requiring surgery should undergo total proctocolectomy with end ileostomy or reconstruction with or without ileal pouch anal anastomosis.

INTRODUCTION

Inflammatory bowel disease (IBD) is associated with an increased risk of developing dysplasia and cancer.[1-3] Dysplasia and colitis-associated cancer (CAC) develop via a different pathway than sporadic cancer and are secondary to longstanding inflammation; they are linked to the duration and extent of disease.[4] Despite improvements in medical management and endoscopic surveillance, the optimal strategies for surveillance and decision for colectomy remain under debate. Herein we review the current literature regarding the risk of dysplasia and cancer in IBD patients, the

No relevant disclosures.

[a] Division of Colon & Rectal Surgery, Mayo Clinic, Rochester, MN, USA; [b] Division of Colon & Rectal Surgery, Mayo Clinic, 4500 San Pablo Road, Jacksonville, FL 32224, USA
* Corresponding author.
E-mail address: Merchea.Amit@mayo.edu

pathogenesis of dysplasia and cancer, current surveillance guidelines, and best practices for managing these patients.

EPIDEMIOLOGY AND CANCER RISK

Cancer risk is increased in both ulcerative colitis (UC) and Crohn disease (CD) compared with the general population. A previously published population-based study over a 35-year period demonstrated an incidence of CAC to be 95 per 100,000.[5] It is, however, believed that this risk has decreased, particularly in UC. Whether this decrease has been due to improved surveillance techniques and technology or improved medical management of disease is unclear.[5,6]

It is generally believed that the risk of disease is related to the extent and duration of disease; however, reported data vary. Eaden and colleagues[7] performed a metaanalysis of 116 studies examining the risk of CRC in UC patients demonstrated the overall prevalence of CRC to be 3.7%. They reported cumulative incidence rate of 2% at 10 years, 8% at 20 years, and 18% at 30 years. In comparison, an analysis of a colonoscopic surveillance program in patients with UC found the cumulative incidence of CRC in UC to be 2.5% at 20 years, 7.6% at 30 years, and 10.8% at 40 years.[8] Similar findings have been noted in CD, with a reported incidence of 8% at 22 years, and a median duration of disease before a diagnosis of cancer (15 years for CD and 18 years for UC).[9,10]

A population-based study over a 60-year period from Olmsted County, Minnesota, demonstrated no significant increase of CAC in UC patients overall compared with the general population (standardized incidence ratio [SIR], 1.1; 95% confidence interval [CI], 0.4–2.4). However, there did seem to be a trend toward increased risk in those with extensive colitis. This study reported a cumulative incidence of CRC in UC patients of 0% at 5 years, 0.4% at 15 years, and 2% at 25 years after diagnosis of UC.[11] In those patients with CD, there also seemed to be a trend toward an increased incidence of CAC and there was a nearly 40-fold increase in risk of small bowel cancer (SIR, 40.6; 95% CI, 8.4–118). The cumulative risk of CRC in CD was reported as 0.3% at 5 years, 1.6% at 15 years, and 2.4% at 25 years after diagnosis.[11] The CESAME (Cancers Et Surrisque Associé aux Maladies Inflammatoires Intestinales En France) Study Group published an observational study of 19,486 patients with IBD and reported an SIR of 2.2 for all IBD patients. There was no increased risk in patients with limited disease (SIR, 1.1; 95% CI, 0.6–1.8). However, those with extensive colitis (>10 years and >50% of the colon involved) had a far greater risk of CAC (SIR, 7.0; 95% CI, 4.4–10.5).[12] Finally, a Manitoba Health study of 5529 patients observed over a 14-year period demonstrated an increased risk of colon cancer in UC (SIR, 2.8; 95% CI, 1.9–4.0) and CD (SIR, 2.6; 95% CI, 1.7–4.2). A nearly 2-fold increase in risk of rectal cancer was demonstrated only in the UC population and a 17-fold increase in risk of small bowel cancer was noted in the CD population.[13]

Other non–IBD-related risk factors for development of cancer exist, primarily a concomitant diagnosis of primary sclerosing cholangitis and a family history of CRC. Numerous studies have demonstrated an increased risk of CRC in patients with IBD and primary sclerosing cholangitis.[14] A metaanalysis found that the development of carcinoma or dysplasia in patients with UC and primary sclerosing cholangitis was increased (odds ratio [OR], 4.8; 95% CI, 3.6–6.4).[15] This risk has been reported to increase after liver transplantation.[16] Much like the general population, a family history of CRC imparts an increased risk of cancer in IBD. Askling and colleagues[17] reported that IBD patients with a positive family history of CRC had an increased relative risk compared with those with no family history of CRC (SIR, 31 [95% CI, 16–52] vs SIR,

14 [95% CI, 12–16]). This was also significantly greater if the patient was diagnosed before 50 years of age.

PATHOGENESIS

The pathogenesis of CAC seems to follow a different pathway from that of sporadic CRC. Colorectal dysplasia can be classified into 4 histologic criteria: negative for dysplasia, indefinite, low-grade dysplasia (LGD), or high-grade dysplasia (HGD).[18] In sporadic CRC, cancer typically develops within an adenoma and is believed to progress in an orderly fashion from LGD, to HGD, and finally to carcinoma. In contrast, the carcinogenic process in CAC seems to be driven by cellular damage from chronic inflammation and does not necessarily follow such an orderly fashion.[19] IBD patients may develop occult cancers in the absence of dysplasia,[20] or with only indefinite or LGD.[21,22]

Sporadic CRC commonly involves mutations the APC tumor suppressor gene or KRAS oncogene. IBD-related CRC have typically demonstrated early mutations in DCC, p53, IDH1, and MYC genes. Alterations in KRAS and APC seem to arise later if at all.[23,24] Whole-exome sequencing comparing sporadic and IBD-related CRC support these previous models, with sporadic tumors demonstrating altered WNT pathway genes (typically APC) and IBD-related tumors showing SOX9 inactivating mutations (which antagonize WNT/beta-catenin signaling).[23] In summary, the sequence from dysplasia to cancer in IBD patients is less predictable, and may occur at a rate faster than what is seen with the traditional adenoma to carcinoma sequence.

SCREENING AND SURVEILLANCE

Most current guidelines recommend starting surveillance colonoscopy 6 to 10 years after the diagnosis of IBD.[14] Recommended surveillance intervals vary by society, with some accounting for patient risk factors and others leaving it to clinician discretion (**Table 1**). The rate of missed malignancy in IBD patients is not insignificant and underscores the importance of an effective surveillance program, which depends on many factors: patient compliance, adequate bowel preparation, adequate mucosal sampling, and appropriate recognition of abnormal lesions. Wang and colleagues[25] reported a Surveillance, Epidemiology, and End Results database study on missed CRC with and without IBD and found that the rate of missed CRC was 5.8% for non-IBD patients compared with 15.1% for CD and 15.8% for UC ($P<.001$). Given these disparities and the relatively young age that CAC develops, continued efforts to improve surveillance techniques should be pursued.

The most common method of surveillance is traditional white-light endoscopy with random biopsies. General recommendations have been for biopsies in 4 quadrants every 10 cm with additional targeted biopsies of visible mucosal lesions. It has been reported previously that an estimated minimum of 33 biopsies from a single colonoscopy are needed to detect dysplasia with a greater than 90% probability.[26] As improvements in imaging technology have occurred and high-definition endoscopy has become more prevalent, it is believed that most dysplasia is, in fact, endoscopically visible and random biopsy may be low yield and less effective than a more targeted approach.[27,28] A recent retrospective review demonstrated that a median of 29 biopsies (range, 15–36) was obtained during surveillance colonoscopy in a population of UC patients and that only 0.2% of the specimens demonstrated dysplasia. This study also noted that UC-associated neoplasia was visible macroscopically in 94% of colonoscopies.[29] A recently published randomized trial compared the traditional strategy of random biopsies with targeted-only biopsies directly and found

Table 1
Comparison of IBD screening recommendations by society

Society, References	Timing and Indications of First Surveillance	Frequency of Surveillance	Surveillance Technique
American College of Gastroenterology[58,59]	8–10 y UC: Left-sided or extensive colitis; patients with proctitis or proctosigmoiditis alone are not at increased risk of cancer risk CD: Surveillance guidelines not yet determined	Every 1–2 y	Multiple biopsies at regular intervals Routine use of CE in low-risk patients awaits additional information regarding longer term follow-up Consider CE in "higher risk" patients (indefinite or known dysplasia not proceeding to colectomy) and to ensure adequacy of previous resection of polypoid or minimally raised lesions
American Gastroenterological Association[60]	8 y UC: All patients regardless of the extent of disease at initial diagnosis CD: Patients with disease affecting at least one-third of the colon	Extensive or left sided colitis: every 1–2 y After 2 negative examinations: consider every 1–3 y After 20 y of disease: consider every 1–2 y on an individualized based on risk factors PSC: every 1 y History of CRC in first-degree relatives; ongoing active endoscopic or histologic inflammation; anatomic abnormalities such as a foreshortened colon, stricture, or multiple inflammatory pseudopolyps: consider more frequent examinations	Multiple biopsies throughout the colon should be done at the first examination to assess the microscopic extent of inflammation Minimum of 33 biopsy specimens in patients with pancolitis CE with targeted biopsies is recommended if the endoscopist has sufficient experience
American Society of Colon and Rectal Surgeons[61]	8 y UC: All patients CD: No guidelines published	Patients with extensive colitis (disease proximal to the splenic flexure): every 1–2 y Patients with 2 successive negative colonoscopies: consider every 1–3 y PSC: annual	Minimum of 32 random biopsies (2 sets of 4-quadrant in each colonic segment) CE shows some promise but needs more research

American Society for Gastrointestinal Endoscopy[62]	8–10 y	Every 1–3 y	Colonoscopy with CE with resection or targeted biopsy of visible lesions is the preferred technique, consider 2 biopsies from each colonic segment for histologic staging
	UC: Patients with macroscopic or histologic evidence of inflammation within and proximal to the sigmoid colon	High risk (active inflammation, anatomic abnormality, stricture, multiple pseudopolyps), history of dysplasia, family history of CRC in first-degree relative, PSC): annual	Alternatively, random biopsies with targeted biopsies of suspicious lesions is reasonable
	CD: Patients with >1 segment and/or one-third of colonic involvement	Patients with ≥2 negative colonoscopies, the surveillance interval can be lengthened	Patients with pancolitis should have 4-quadrant biopsies every 10 cm, minimum 33 biopsies
			Patients without pancolitis should have 4 quadrant biopsies every 10 cm limited to greatest extent of involvement documented by any colonoscopy
European Cancer Organisation[63]	8 y	Low risk: schedule subsequent examination in 5 y	Colonoscopy with CE and targeted biopsies
	UC, CD: onset of colitic symptoms to all patients	Intermediate risk (extensive colitis with mild or moderate active inflammation; postinflammatory polyps or a family history of CRC in a first-degree relative at ≥50 y): schedule next examination in 2–3 y	If the appropriate expertise with CE is not available, random biopsies (4 every 10 cm) should be performed; however, this is inferior to CE in the detection rate of neoplastic lesions
		High risk (stricture or dysplasia detected within the past 5 y; PSC; extensive colitis with severe active inflammation; family history of CRC in a first degree relative <50 y): schedule next examination in 1 y	

(continued on next page)

Table 1
(continued)

Society, References	Timing and Indications of First Surveillance	Frequency of Surveillance	Surveillance Technique
NHS National Institute for Health and Clinical Excellence[64]	10 y UC: Patients with more involvement than proctitis CD: colitis involving >1 segment of colon	Low risk (extensive but quiescent UC; left-sided UC [but not proctitis alone] or Crohn's colitis of a similar extent): every 5 y Intermediate risk (extensive ulcerative or Crohn's colitis with mild active inflammation confirmed endoscopically or histologically; postinflammatory polyps; family history of CRC in a first-degree relative aged ≥50 y): every 3 y High risk (extensive ulcerative or Crohn's colitis with moderate or severe active inflammation confirmed endoscopically or histologically; PSC [before or after liver transplantation]; colonic stricture in the past 5 y; any grade of dysplasia in the past 5 y; family history of colorectal cancer in a first-degree relative <50 y): annual	Colonoscopy with CE

Abbreviations: CD, Crohn disease; CE, chromoendoscopy; CRC, colorectal cancer; IBD, inflammatory bowel disease; PSC, primary sclerosing cholangitis; UC, ulcerative colitis.
Data from Refs.[58–64]

that targeted biopsy was as effective as a random biopsy approach for detecting neoplasia. The proportion of dysplasia was found to be higher in the targeted biopsy arm, causing the authors to suggest that the increased time performing random biopsies may result in suspicious lesions being overlooked owing to bleeding or distraction of the endoscopist.[30]

Chromoendoscopy (CE) uses a dye, such as methylene blue or indigo carmine, to stain the mucosa. This enhances the visualization of the mucosal surface to better detect abnormal areas. A metaanalysis of 6 studies, included 1277 patients comparing white-light endoscopy with CE, found a 7% differential in favor of CE for dysplasia detection, a 44% increase in lesion detection by targeted biopsy, and a 27% increase in proportion of flat dysplastic lesions detected.[31] Given the improved detection rate noted with CE, most societies recommend its use combined with targeted biopsies whenever the technology and expertise are available.[14]

Narrow band imaging uses blue and green wavelength light to better delineate mucosal vasculature. It does not seem to impart any significant increase in neoplasia detection rates when compared with standard or high-definition white-light endoscopy.[32,33]

Another promising technology is confocal laser endomicroscopy (CLE), which uses fluorescent agents to allow in vivo histologic examination. The correlation of CLE with histopathology is very high ($\kappa = 0.91–0.94$)[34] and a randomized trial found CE and CLE detected nearly 5 times more dysplasia then conventional colonoscopy with random biopsies.[35] The main limitations of CLE are limited equipment availability and increased procedure times (approximately double that of conventional colonoscopy).[34]

MANAGEMENT OF DYSPLASIA AND CANCER

The management of dysplasia in the setting of IBD is largely predicated on the likelihood for an underlying malignancy and the risk of future progression to malignancy. When patients have biopsies showing HGD, their risk of harboring an invasive malignancy is high (>40% as reported by Bernstein and colleagues[21]), and there is little debate about the seriousness of this situation. However, in patients with LGD, the risk of HGD or cancer is more variable and ranges from 10% to 50%.[21,22,36–38] There is likely minimal difference in the predictive value of dysplasia in patients with CD compared with UC. The presence of synchronous dysplasia in CD patients with CRC is nearly ubiquitous.[39] However, in CD patients without CRC, only 2% of colectomy specimens demonstrated dysplasia.[40]

The optimal management of LGD continues to be debated. Reported rates of progression to HGD or CRC are variable, ranging from zero to greater than 50%.[37,38,41] A metaanalysis of endoscopic surveillance of LGD in a UC population reported a significant increase in the risk of developing CRC (OR, 9.0; 95% CI, 4.0–20.5) or a more advanced lesion, such as HGD or CRC (OR, 11.9; 95% CI, 5.2–27).[42] Befrits and colleagues[41] have reported a lesser risk of progression to more advanced disease. In their study of 60 patients, LGD was found at several endoscopic examinations in various segments of the colon in 73% of patients. However, only 2 patients (both of whom had a dysplasia-associated lesion or mass [DALMs]) progressed to more advanced lesions in 10 years of follow-up.

Although some controversy remains regarding the management of unifocal LGD, some risk factors may exist that predict which of these lesions will progress to a more advanced lesion. Choi and colleagues[43] reported that lesions that are nonpolypoid, endoscopically invisible, 1 cm or larger, or preceded by indefinite dysplasia are likely at increased risk for progression and should be considered for colectomy. These varied reports underscore the need to counsel patients regarding outcomes of continued surveillance versus surgery in the setting of LGD.[37]

The finding of HGD or CRC usually warrants surgical resection. Patients with UC should undergo total proctocolectomy with end ileostomy or ileal pouch anal anastomosis (IPAA). Approximately 12% to 55% of patients have been found to have an occult or synchronous cancer[21,43,44] and 48% have synchronous dysplasia.[44] Removal of the rectum is generally recommended because the rectum remains at risk, even if the dysplasia or cancer is located in the colon. However, it can be preserved in select patients with a plan for intensive surveillance. Approximately 2% of patients who have a retained rectal stump or who undergo ileorectal anastomoses develop cancer in their rectum.[45]

The type of lesion where the dysplasia is detected may also affect the risk of finding malignancy. Traditionally, lesions have been divided into endoscopically undetectable ("flat") and detectable ("elevated") lesions, with the latter also commonly referred to as DALMs.[2] DALMs are further classified into adenoma-like (polypoid) and nonadenoma-like (nonpolypoid). Adenoma-like DALMs, even those arising in areas of inflammation, behave like sporadic adenomas and can be safely treated with polypectomy and continued surveillance.[2] In contrast, nonadenoma-like DALMs can appear as velvety patches, plaques, irregular bumps and nodules, wartlike thickenings, stricturing lesions, or broad-based masses. Nonadenoma-like DALMs are generally not amenable to endoscopic removal techniques, and thus these patients should be referred for surgical resection.[2]

Patients found to have HGD arising in an adenoma-like DALM that is completely resected may be eligible for close follow-up with colonoscopy in 6 months in lieu of colectomy.[2] This is based on evidence showing that most dysplasia in IBD arises in detectable lesions amenable to endoscopic surveillance.[27] No head-to-head comparisons of polypectomy versus colectomy have been completed, but a small retrospective series found no progression to cancer after polypectomy for HGD with endoscopic follow-up after 6 years.[46] Additionally, a recently published metaanalysis of 10 studies including 376 patients examining endoscopic resection of adenoma-like DALMs found that progression to CRC was low (2.4% of patients after an average follow-up of 54 months). However, there was a 10-fold increased risk of developing dysplasia.[47] **Fig. 1** provides an algorithm for the management of dysplasia in the setting for IBD.[48]

In patients with UC, the presence of dysplasia or cancer is not a contraindication to reconstruction with IPAA. There is generally no impact to performance of restorative proctocolectomy in the setting of colon cancer. However, IPAA in the setting of locally advanced rectal cancer may lead to worse outcome, because preoperative pelvic radiation can impact pouch-related sepsis and long-term pouch function. Postoperative pelvic radiation after IPAA is an even more risky situation, and rarely allows for acceptable pouch function. Taylor and colleagues[49] reported on 17 patients who underwent IPAA in the setting of CRC. These patients had acceptable functional results; however, the use of adjuvant radiation did impact overall function. Another case series reported on 9 patients who underwent IPAA after pelvic radiation, 7 of which were due to rectal cancer,[50] and the pouch failure rate for this small group was 44%. Finally, Merchea and colleagues[51] published a series of UC patients with rectal cancer, including 11 patients undergoing IPAA. Two patients had a failed pouch, one of which was secondary to radiation enteritis. This paper concluded that patients with stage 1 rectal cancer not requiring neoadjuvant chemoradiotherapy can undergo restorative proctocolectomy with good functional results.

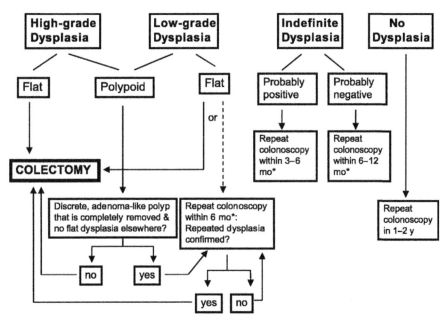

Fig. 1. Algorithm for the management of dysplasia in inflammatory bowel disease. *Duration of short-term surveillance has not been determined. (*From* Itzkowitz SH, Harpaz N. Diagnosis and management of dysplasia in patients with inflammatory bowel diseases. Gastroenterology 2004;126:1642; with permission.)

The most common method of creating IPAA is a double-stapled technique with a distal rectal anastomosis, preserving the anal transition zone. Compared with mucosectomy and a hand-sewn ileoanal anastomosis, a stapled IPAA leaves behind a small rim of at-risk mucosa. It is likely that a double-stapled technique has improved long-term functional outcomes compared with a hand-sewn technique; however, conflicting studies have been published.[52–54] Overall, metachronous cancers within the pouch or the anal transitional zone are rare, with one 2011 review demonstrating 43 known cases, including 30 patients with mucosectomy and 13 with a stapled anastomosis.[54]

Derikx and colleagues[45] reported the incidence of neoplasia after colectomy in IBD and found that, in the setting of IPAA, the prevalence of carcinoma in the pouch to be 0.5%. Limited evidence exists on the need for routine pouch surveillance. However, patients should be counseled to the potential risk of pouch carcinoma and occasional surveillance every few years, or when symptomatic, should be offered.[55]

Patients with CD and HGD, multifocal LGD, or invasive cancer should undergo total proctocolectomy. Approximately 40% of CD patients undergoing segmental resection or subtotal colectomy develop metachronous cancers, with 50% dying from the subsequent disease.[56] Furthermore, it has been reported that up to 44% of the patients with known malignancy will have multifocal disease in the final specimen and 40% may have evidence of dysplasia remote from the cancer site.[57] Because of the poor function associated with CD and IPAA, these patients typically require a permanent end ileostomy. In highly selected patients who are not willing have a permanent end ileostomy, and have "rectal sparing" with no active inflammation or dysplasia within the rectum, a total abdominal colectomy with ileorectal anastomosis can be considered as long as there is intense postoperative surveillance.

SUMMARY

Improvements in the medical management and endoscopic surveillance of IBD have reduced the incidence of cancer and its associated mortality. However, further research is needed to fully understand the molecular and genetic pathways unique to IBD-related dysplasia. Great debate still exists regarding the optimal strategy for determining which patients with early dysplasia can be managed endoscopically and which require radical surgery.

REFERENCES

1. Ekbom A, Helmick C, Zack M, et al. Ulcerative colitis and colorectal cancer. A population-based study. N Engl J Med 1990;323(18):1228–33.
2. Farraye FA, Odze RD, Eaden J, et al. AGA technical review on the diagnosis and management of colorectal neoplasia in inflammatory bowel disease. Gastroenterology 2010;138(2):746–74.
3. Weedon DD, Shorter RG, Ilstrup DM, et al. Crohn's disease and cancer. N Engl J Med 1973;289(21):1099–103.
4. Romano M, DE Francesco F, Zarantonello L, et al. From inflammation to cancer in inflammatory bowel disease: molecular perspectives. Anticancer Res 2016;36(4):1447–60.
5. Soderlund S, Brandt L, Lapidus A, et al. Decreasing time-trends of colorectal cancer in a large cohort of patients with inflammatory bowel disease. Gastroenterology 2009;136(5):1561–7.
6. Jess T, Simonsen J, Jorgensen KT, et al. Decreasing risk of colorectal cancer in patients with inflammatory bowel disease over 30 years. Gastroenterology 2012; 143(2):375–81.
7. Eaden JA, Abrams KR, Mayberry JF. The risk of colorectal cancer in ulcerative colitis: a meta-analysis. Gut 2001;48(4):526–35.
8. Rutter MD, Saunders BP, Wilkinson KH, et al. Thirty-year analysis of a colonoscopic surveillance program for neoplasia in ulcerative colitis. Gastroenterology 2006;130(4):1030–8.
9. Gillen CD, Walmsley RS, Prior P, et al. Ulcerative colitis and Crohn's disease: a comparison of the colorectal cancer risk in extensive colitis. Gut 1994;35(11):1590–2.
10. Choi PM, Zelig MP. Similarity of colorectal cancer in Crohn's disease and ulcerative colitis: implications for carcinogenesis and prevention. Gut 1994;35(7):950–4.
11. Jess T, Loftus EV Jr, Velayos FS, et al. Risk of intestinal cancer in inflammatory bowel disease: a population-based study from Olmsted County, Minnesota. Gastroenterology 2006;130(4):1039–46.
12. Beaugerie L, Svrcek M, Seksik P, et al. Risk of colorectal high-grade dysplasia and cancer in a prospective observational cohort of patients with inflammatory bowel disease. Gastroenterology 2013;145(1):166–75.
13. Bernstein CN, Blanchard JF, Kliewer E, et al. Cancer risk in patients with inflammatory bowel disease: a population-based study. Cancer 2001;91(4):854–62.
14. Gaidos JK, Bickston SJ. How to optimize colon cancer surveillance in inflammatory bowel disease patients. Inflamm Bowel Dis 2016;22(5):1219–30.
15. Soetikno RM, Lin OS, Heidenreich PA, et al. Increased risk of colorectal neoplasia in patients with primary sclerosing cholangitis and ulcerative colitis: a meta-analysis. Gastrointest Endosc 2002;56(1):48–54.

16. Bleday R, Lee E, Jessurun J, et al. Increased risk of early colorectal neoplasms after hepatic transplant in patients with inflammatory bowel disease. Dis Colon Rectum 1993;36(10):908–12.

17. Askling J, Dickman PW, Karlen P, et al. Family history as a risk factor for colorectal cancer in inflammatory bowel disease. Gastroenterology 2001;120(6):1356–62.

18. Riddell RH, Goldman H, Ransohoff DF, et al. Dysplasia in inflammatory bowel disease: standardized classification with provisional clinical applications. Hum Pathol 1983;14(11):931–68.

19. O'Connor PM, Lapointe TK, Beck PL, et al. Mechanisms by which inflammation may increase intestinal cancer risk in inflammatory bowel disease. Inflamm Bowel Dis 2010;16(8):1411–20.

20. Taylor BA, Pemberton JH, Carpenter HA, et al. Dysplasia in chronic ulcerative colitis: implications for colonoscopic surveillance. Dis Colon Rectum 1992;35(10): 950–6.

21. Bernstein CN, Shanahan F, Weinstein WM. Are we telling patients the truth about surveillance colonoscopy in ulcerative colitis? Lancet 1994;343(8889):71–4.

22. Ullman T, Croog V, Harpaz N, et al. Progression of flat low-grade dysplasia to advanced neoplasia in patients with ulcerative colitis. Gastroenterology 2003; 125(5):1311–9.

23. Robles AI, Traverso G, Zhang M, et al. Whole-exome sequencing analyses of inflammatory bowel disease-associated colorectal cancers. Gastroenterology 2016;150(4):931–43.

24. Yaeger R, Shah MA, Miller VA, et al. Genomic alterations observed in colitis-associated cancers are distinct from those found in sporadic colorectal cancers and vary by type of inflammatory bowel disease. Gastroenterology 2016;151(2): 278–87.

25. Wang YR, Cangemi JR, Loftus EV Jr, et al. Rate of early/missed colorectal cancers after colonoscopy in older patients with or without inflammatory bowel disease in the United States. Am J Gastroenterol 2013;108(3):444–9.

26. Rubin CE, Haggitt RC, Burmer GC, et al. DNA aneuploidy in colonic biopsies predicts future development of dysplasia in ulcerative colitis. Gastroenterology 1992; 103(5):1611–20.

27. Rutter MD, Saunders BP, Wilkinson KH, et al. Most dysplasia in ulcerative colitis is visible at colonoscopy. Gastrointest Endosc 2004;60(3):334–9.

28. Rubin DT, Rothe JA, Hetzel JT, et al. Are dysplasia and colorectal cancer endoscopically visible in patients with ulcerative colitis? Gastrointest Endosc 2007; 65(7):998–1004.

29. van den Broek FJ, Stokkers PC, Reitsma JB, et al. Random biopsies taken during colonoscopic surveillance of patients with longstanding ulcerative colitis: low yield and absence of clinical consequences. Am J Gastroenterol 2014;109(5): 715–22.

30. Watanabe T, Ajioka Y, Mitsuyama K, et al. Comparison of targeted vs random biopsies for surveillance of ulcerative colitis-associated colorectal cancer. Gastroenterology 2016;151(6):1122–30.

31. Subramanian V, Mannath J, Ragunath K, et al. Meta-analysis: the diagnostic yield of chromoendoscopy for detecting dysplasia in patients with colonic inflammatory bowel disease. Aliment Pharmacol Ther 2011;33(3):304–12.

32. van den Broek FJ, Fockens P, van Eeden S, et al. Narrow-band imaging versus high-definition endoscopy for the diagnosis of neoplasia in ulcerative colitis. Endoscopy 2011;43(2):108–15.

33. Ignjatovic A, East JE, Subramanian V, et al. Narrow band imaging for detection of dysplasia in colitis: a randomized controlled trial. Am J Gastroenterol 2012; 107(6):885–90.

34. Gunther U, Kusch D, Heller F, et al. Surveillance colonoscopy in patients with inflammatory bowel disease: comparison of random biopsy vs. targeted biopsy protocols. Int J Colorectal Dis 2011;26(5):667–72.

35. Kiesslich R, Goetz M, Lammersdorf K, et al. Chromoscopy-guided endomicroscopy increases the diagnostic yield of intraepithelial neoplasia in ulcerative colitis. Gastroenterology 2007;132(3):874–82.

36. Gorfine SR, Bauer JJ, Harris MT, et al. Dysplasia complicating chronic ulcerative colitis: is immediate colectomy warranted? Dis Colon Rectum 2000;43(11): 1575–81.

37. Ullman TA, Loftus EV Jr, Kakar S, et al. The fate of low grade dysplasia in ulcerative colitis. Am J Gastroenterol 2002;97(4):922–7.

38. Lim CH, Dixon MF, Vail A, et al. Ten year follow up of ulcerative colitis patients with and without low grade dysplasia. Gut 2003;52(8):1127–32.

39. Richards ME, Rickert RR, Nance FC. Crohn's disease-associated carcinoma. A poorly recognized complication of inflammatory bowel disease. Ann Surg 1989; 209(6):764–73.

40. Warren R, Barwick KW. Crohn's colitis with carcinoma and dysplasia. Report of a case and review of 100 small and large bowel resections for Crohn's disease to detect incidence of dysplasia. Am J Surg Pathol 1983;7(2):151–9.

41. Befrits R, Ljung T, Jaramillo E, et al. Low-grade dysplasia in extensive, longstanding inflammatory bowel disease: a follow-up study. Dis Colon Rectum 2002;45(5):615–20.

42. Thomas T, Abrams KA, Robinson RJ, et al. Meta-analysis: cancer risk of lowgrade dysplasia in chronic ulcerative colitis. Aliment Pharmacol Ther 2007; 25(6):657–68.

43. Choi CH, Ignjatovic-Wilson A, Askari A, et al. Low-grade dysplasia in ulcerative colitis: risk factors for developing high-grade dysplasia or colorectal cancer. Am J Gastroenterol 2015;110(10):1461–71.

44. Kiran RP, Khoury W, Church JM, et al. Colorectal cancer complicating inflammatory bowel disease: similarities and differences between Crohn's and ulcerative colitis based on three decades of experience. Ann Surg 2010;252(2):330–5.

45. Derikx LA, Nissen LH, Smits LJ, et al. Risk of neoplasia after colectomy in patients with inflammatory bowel disease: a systematic review and meta-analysis. Clin Gastroenterol Hepatol 2016;14(6):798–806.

46. Blonski W, Kundu R, Furth EF, et al. High-grade dysplastic adenoma-like mass lesions are not an indication for colectomy in patients with ulcerative colitis. Scand J Gastroenterol 2008;43(7):817–20.

47. Wanders LK, Dekker E, Pullens B, et al. Cancer risk after resection of polypoid dysplasia in patients with longstanding ulcerative colitis: a meta-analysis. Clin Gastroenterol Hepatol 2014;12(5):756–64.

48. Itzkowitz SH, Harpaz N. Diagnosis and management of dysplasia in patients with inflammatory bowel diseases. Gastroenterology 2004;126(6):1634–48.

49. Taylor BA, Wolff BG, Dozois RR, et al. Ileal pouch-anal anastomosis for chronic ulcerative colitis and familial polyposis coli complicated by adenocarcinoma. Dis Colon Rectum 1988;31(5):358–62.

50. Wu XR, Kiran RP, Remzi FH, et al. Preoperative pelvic radiation increases the risk for ileal pouch failure in patients with colitis-associated colorectal cancer. J Crohns Colitis 2013;7(10):e419–26.

51. Merchea A, Wolff BG, Dozois EJ, et al. Clinical features and oncologic outcomes in patients with rectal cancer and ulcerative colitis: a single-institution experience. Dis Colon Rectum 2012;55(8):881–5.
52. Reilly WT, Pemberton JH, Wolff BG, et al. Randomized prospective trial comparing ileal pouch-anal anastomosis performed by excising the anal mucosa to ileal pouch-anal anastomosis performed by preserving the anal mucosa. Ann Surg 1997;225(6):666–76.
53. Luukkonen P, Jarvinen H. Stapled vs hand-sutured ileoanal anastomosis in restorative proctocolectomy. A prospective, randomized study. Arch Surg 1993;128(4): 437–40.
54. Um JW, M'Koma AE. Pouch-related dysplasia and adenocarcinoma following restorative proctocolectomy for ulcerative colitis. Tech Coloproctol 2011;15:7–16.
55. Herline AJ, Meisinger LL, Rusin LC, et al. Is routine pouch surveillance for dysplasia indicated for ileoanal pouches? Dis Colon Rectum 2003;46(2):156–9.
56. Maser EA, Sachar DB, Kruse D, et al. High rates of metachronous colon cancer or dysplasia after segmental resection or subtotal colectomy in Crohn's colitis. Inflamm Bowel Dis 2013;19(9):1827–32.
57. Kiran RP, Nisar PJ, Goldblum JR, et al. Dysplasia associated with Crohn's colitis: segmental colectomy or more extended resection? Ann Surg 2012;256(2):221–6.
58. Lichtenstein GR, Hanauer SB, Sandborn WJ. Management of Crohn's disease in adults. Am J Gastroenterol 2009;104(2):465–83.
59. Kornbluth A, Sachar DB. Ulcerative colitis practice guidelines in adults: American College of Gastroenterology, Practice Parameters Committee. Am J Gastroenterol 2010;105(3):501–23.
60. Farraye FA, Odze RD, Eaden J, et al. AGA medical position statement on the diagnosis and management of colorectal neoplasia in inflammatory bowel disease. Gastroenterology 2010;138(2):738–45.
61. Ross H, Steele SR, Varma M, et al. Practice parameters for the surgical treatment of ulcerative colitis. Dis Colon Rectum 2014;57(1):5–22.
62. Shergill AK, Lightdale JR, Bruining DH, et al. The role of endoscopy in inflammatory bowel disease. Gastrointest Endosc 2015;81(5):1101–21.
63. Annese V, Daperno M, Rutter MD, et al. European evidence based consensus for endoscopy in inflammatory bowel disease. J Crohns Colitis 2013;7(12): 982–1018.
64. Colonoscopic surveillance for prevention of colorectal cancer in people with ulcerative colitis, Crohn's disease or adenomas. London: National Institute for Health and Clinical Excellence: Guidance; 2011. Available at: http://www.nice.org.uk/guidance/CG118.

Atypical Colorectal Neoplasms

Michael G. Porter, MD*, Scott M. Stoeger, MD, PhD

KEYWORDS

- Colorectal • Carcinoid • Lymphoma • Neuroendocrine • GIST

KEY POINTS

- Atypical colorectal tumors are rare tumors accounting for less than 10% of all colorectal tumors.
- Primary colorectal lymphomas are primarily of the B-cell lineage, most commonly arising from the right side of the colon, and despite multimodality therapy have a relatively poor prognosis.
- Carcinoids have been reclassified as neuroendocrine tumors (NETs). NETs of the colon and rectum rarely present with carcinoid syndrome and are commonly advanced at diagnosis.
- Appendiceal NETs, depending on size and location, may be treated with appendectomy alone. Larger appendiceal NETs or those with ominous characteristics require an oncologic operation.
- Gastrointestinal stromal tumors are the most common mesenchymal tumor of the gastrointestinal system, possessing gain-of-function mutations in c-Kit. Tyrosine kinase inhibitors have greatly improved their treatment.

INTRODUCTION

Colorectal cancer is the third most common cancer diagnosed in the United States, as well as the third leading cause of cancer related deaths in 2016.[1] Adenocarcinoma is the predominant malignancy found in the colon and rectum. Atypical colorectal neoplasms are rare, and their management is often different than the approach to adenocarcinoma. Although primary colorectal lymphoma (PCL), carcinoids (neuroendocrine tumors [NETs]), and gastrointestinal stromal tumors (GISTs) account for a small fraction of colorectal malignancies, the surgeon needs to be aware of the specific characteristics that dictate their diagnosis and management.

Disclosures: The authors have nothing to disclose.
Department of Surgery, University of Kansas School of Medicine – Wichita, 929 North St. Francis, Wichita, KS 67214, USA
* Corresponding author.
E-mail address: mporter@kumc.edu

Surg Clin N Am 97 (2017) 641–656
http://dx.doi.org/10.1016/j.suc.2017.01.011
0039-6109/17/© 2017 Elsevier Inc. All rights reserved.

LYMPHOMA
Introduction: Nature of the Problem

Primary lymphoma of the gastrointestinal system is rare, accounting for approximately 10% of patients with lymphoma.[2] The most common location is the stomach. PCL accounts for 10% to 20% of gastrointestinal lymphoma and comprises less than 1% of all colorectal malignancies.[3] The average age at presentation is approximately 55, with a 2:1 male to female ratio.[4]

Relevant Anatomy and Pathophysiology

PCL can be found throughout the colon and rectum. The right colon is involved most commonly. The cecum accounts for more than 50% and the ascending colon an additional 20% of all PCLs. It is hypothesized that the right colon predominance is due to the greater amount of lymphoid tissue present relative to the rest of the colon.[3]

A vast majority of PCLs are non-Hodgkin lymphomas of the B-cell lineage.[2] However, a study from China demonstrated a higher percentage of T-cell PCLs than those found in data from Western studies.[5] Of the B-cell lineage PCLs, diffuse large B-cell lymphoma is the most common, with follicular, mucosa-associated lymphoid tissue lymphoma, and mantle cell lymphoma, small lymphocytic also identified.[6,7]

Clinical Presentation and Examination

Patients with PCL present with expected signs and symptoms of colorectal malignancy. Abdominal pain is the most frequent complaint. In addition, patients may have weight loss, a palpable abdominal mass, and hematochezia. Perforation can occur as well, presenting as a surgical emergency.[6] Apart from weight loss, patients with PCL typically do not demonstrate the symptoms of night sweats and fevers commonly seen with lymphoma in other locations.[8] Because of the nonspecific nature of the symptoms, presentation is commonly late in the disease course. Immunosuppression, such as with human immunodeficiency virus infection, transplantation, or inflammatory bowel disease, has been linked to the development of colorectal lymphoma. However, a definitive connection has not been elucidated.[9]

Diagnostic Procedures

The diagnostic evaluation is similar for PCL as for other colonic tumors. Computed tomography (**Fig. 1**A) is the imaging method of choice. Findings are typically variable and may include a mass lesion or narrowing of the lumen.[10] Regional lymph nodes may be enlarged. Colonoscopy (see **Fig. 1**B) may show variable morphology as well, with ulceration, infiltration, and a mass lesion.[5] Colonoscopy also allows for obtaining of tissue for pathologic diagnosis.

Diagnosis

To diagnose PCL accurately, secondary colorectal involvement from another primary site must be excluded. To accomplish this, Dawson and colleagues[11] set forth a specific set of guidelines: (1) no peripheral lymphadenopathy, (2) absence of enlarged mediastinal lymph nodes, (3) white blood cell count and differential within normal limits, (4) primary involvement of the bowel with only proximal lymphadenopathy, and (5) lack of involvement of liver and spleen.

On biopsy, the tumor demonstrates findings indicative of non-Hodgkin's lymphoma, with large populations of lymphoid cells present (see **Fig. 1**C). Evaluation of CD20 typically ensures the diagnosis (see **Fig. 1**D). Further evaluation of other markers, such as Bcl-6, Bcl-2, MUM-1, and Ki67 can help to define prognosis.[12]

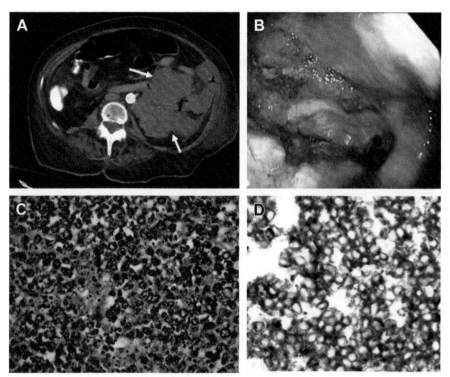

Fig. 1. (*A*) Computed tomography scan of a patient with a sigmoid primary colorectal lymphoma (PCL) with the mass in the left lower quadrant (*arrows*). (*B*) Colonoscopy demonstrating a primary colonic lymphoma. (*C*) Histologic finding of PCL on hematoxylin and eosin staining. (*D*) PCL stained for CD20.

The Ann Arbor staging system is used to describe the extent of the disease. Stage I is limited to 1 lymph node region. Stage II involves more than 1 lymph node region on the same side of the diaphragm, and stage III involved lymph node regions on both sides of the diaphragm. Stage IV demonstrates diffuse extralymphatic involvement. The designation "E" at any stage indicates extranodal involvement.[13]

Treatment

Owing to the rarity of PCL, to date, the only prospective controlled studies are for the medical treatment of PCL. There are no prospective, randomized controlled studies regarding surgery for PCL. Although chemotherapy and radiation remain the mainstay in the overall treatment regimen, surgery does provide an integral component to PCL treatment.

Surgery for PCL often is performed either in an emergent fashion for bowel perforation or as part of the therapeutic treatment for PCL. Although perforation is not common with PCL, it may occur either spontaneously or after chemotherapy.[4] Given the predominance of PCL in the right colon, a right hemicolectomy is often performed.[14] Surgery is combined commonly with adjuvant chemotherapy, although no specific guidelines have been defined. Reports show that survival is improved with the combined approach[15–18] compared with surgery or chemotherapy alone.

Chemotherapy for PCL is very similar to other primary non-Hodgkin's lymphomas, consisting of the CHOP (cyclophosphamide, hyroxydaunorubicin, vincristine (Oncovin), and prednisolone) regimen.[19] There are other combinations in use, but less frequently than CHOP. Recently, R-CHOP, with the addition to rituximab, an anti-CD20 monoclonal antibody, to the standard CHOP, has been evaluated. The addition of rituximab provided an additional survival benefit.[20,21]

Outcomes

The literature regarding PCL is limited primarily to retrospective reviews of patient populations. There is considerable variability in the data presented, such as the chemotherapy regimens used, complication rate, and, in particular, the type and stage of the PCLs examined. One of the more extensive studies, by Kim and colleagues,[22] examined 95 patients in Korea and included patients in all stages of disease. Sixty percent of patients underwent combined surgery and chemotherapy, 10% surgery alone, and the remaining 30% receiving chemotherapy and/or radiation. Survival at 1 and 5 years of 78% and 55%, respectively, was reported. The data were evaluated across all patients in the study and were not broken down by treatment regimen. In addition, they failed to comment on the chemotherapy regimens used or complications encountered. Similarly, Aviles and colleagues[23] evaluated 53 patients, all receiving surgery and chemotherapy, with a 10-year survival rate of 83%. All the patients in the study were stage 1E B cell lymphomas, limiting the data to those with early disease.

Survival for PCL is low, with reports indicating long-term survival rates of less than 60% demonstrated in multiple studies. The type/stage of the lymphomas was variable among the studies.[3,16,22,24] Drolet and colleagues[15] demonstrated survival for rectal lymphoma was even lower than colonic, with a median survival of 42 months versus 110 months. Among variables examined, only age greater than 60 years at time of diagnosis demonstrated a significant difference, with older age having far poorer outcomes. Another group demonstrated that the histologic grade was the only variable that affected outcome.[16]

CARCINOIDS (NEUROENDOCRINE TUMORS)
Introduction: Nature of the Problem

Carcinoids were originally described as benign because of their slow growth, but these tumors can behave aggressively. To reduce confusion, "carcinoid" is no longer used to describe these lesions, which are instead referred to as NETs.[25] Although these tumors are found most commonly in the bronchopulmonary system, around 25% occur in the gastrointestinal system. NETs account for less than 1% of colonic tumors; 20% of gastrointestinal NETs are found in the rectum, accounting for 1% of rectal tumors.[25,26] Colorectal NETs are more commonly found in African Americans and Asians than Caucasians.[27] Females are more commonly affected than males. Colon NETs primarily present around age 65, whereas rectal NETs are diagnosed 10 years earlier.[28]

Relevant Anatomy and Pathophysiology

NETs arise from the enterochromaffin cells or Kluchitschky cells within the crypts of Lieberkühn in the colon, whereas in the rectum, they arise from L cells.[29] These cells secrete a variety of bioactive molecules, including serotonin, kallikrein, bradykinin, histamine, and prostaglandins. Colonic NETs are primarily right-sided tumors[30]; in addition, they are the most common tumor of the appendix.[31] Appendiceal NETs are the most common epithelial tumor of the gastrointestinal system in children, with a majority found at the tip of the appendix.[32] Involvement of the base of the appendix, tumor size greater than 2 cm, and involvement of the mesoappendix or lymphovascular invasion are high-risk features that may require more extensive resection.[33]

Clinical Presentation and Examination

Like other colorectal tumors, NETs can present with nonspecific symptoms. These include obstruction, hematochezia, pain, weight loss, and changes in bowel habits.[34] Given that most colonic NETs are right sided, they may grow considerably before symptoms appear. Rectal NETs may produce bleeding, constipation, tenesmus, or pain.[35]

Carcinoid syndrome, characterized by flushing, diarrhea, pain, and cardiac symptoms, is uncommon. Fewer than 5% of patients with colorectal NETs develop this syndrome, usually in the presence of hepatic metastasis.[27,36,37]

Diagnostic Procedures

NETs are frequently found incidentally during routine endoscopy. Colonic NETs may appear as a discrete polyp (**Fig. 2**A), however, they can appear as large tumors during colonoscopy because they often present late. Rectal NETs may appear as focal thickening or as smooth, round submucosal nodules.[36] Higher grade tumors may demonstrate scarring, bleedings, or ulceration.[38] Endoscopic ultrasound examination can aid in assessing rectal tumors as well as assisting in evaluation of lymph node status.[39]

Several imaging modalities are useful in the evaluation of patients with NETs. Computed tomography scanning (see **Fig. 2**B) is used for staging, particularly for evaluation of metastatic spread.[40] MRI can aid in the determination of invasion of rectal NETs, helping to determine spread of disease.[41] Octreotide scan has been used for localization of NETs in other anatomic locations; however, its usefulness in colorectal NETs has not been determined.

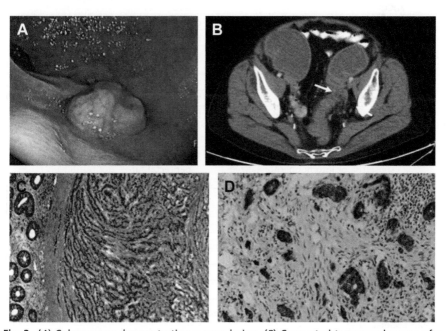

Fig. 2. (*A*) Colonoscopy demonstrating a mass lesion. (*B*) Computed tomography scan of a patient with a sigmoid stricture (*arrows*) resulting from a neuroendocrine tumor (NET). (*C*) Histologic finding of NET. (*D*) Appendiceal NET, stained with chromogranin A.

Diagnosis

Although the primary identification of NETs initially is through endoscopy and imaging, laboratory testing also aids in the diagnosis of NETs (see **Fig. 2**C). Urinary 5-hydroxyindolacetic acid (5-HIAA) is highly specific for NETs, although it lacks sensitivity. Chromogranin A (see **Fig. 2**D) is a much more sensitive marker than 5-HIAA; however, it lacks specificity.[42] Rectal NETs may also produce carcinoembryonic antigen and prostate specific antigen. Although these are much less useful in the diagnosis, they could play a role in surveillance after treatment.[43]

The grade of NETs is determined by microscopic examination of mitotic rate (mitoses per 10 high-power fields) and percentage of Ki67 staining. Grade 1 demonstrates a mitotic count of less than 2 and/or Ki67 of less than 2%. Grade 2 shows a mitotic count of 2 to 20 and/or Ki67 staining of 3% to 20%. Finally, grade 3 has a mitotic count of greater than 20 and/or Ki67 staining of greater than 20%.[44] If the mitotic count and Ki67 are not concordant for the same grade, the higher grade is assigned. Grades 1 and 2 describe well-differentiated tumors whereas grade 3 tumors are referred to as neuroendocrine carcinomas, which are typically poorly differentiated.[41]

There are several tumor, node(s), metastasis (TNM) staging systems for NETs, produced by the American Joint Cancer Committee and the European Neuroendocrine Tumour Society. **Table 1** summarizes the 2 TNM systems for colorectal NETs, and **Table 2** shows the staging systems. Although the 2 systems differ slightly, both systems have been shown to discriminate in terms of prognosis.[45,46]

Table 1 AJCC and ENETS TNM system		
	AJCC	**ENETS**
TX	Cannot be assessed	Cannot be assessed
T0	No evidence of tumor	No evidence of tumor
T1	Invasion of lamina propria or submucosa and size <2 cm	Invasion of lamina propria or submucosa
T1a	Tumor <1 cm	Tumor <1 cm
T1b	Tumor 1–2 cm	Tumor 1–2 cm
T2	Invasion of muscularis propria or size >2 cm with invasion of lamina propria or submucosa	Invasion of muscularis propria or size >2 cm
T3	Invasion through muscularis propria into subserosa or into nonperitonealized pericolic or perinectal tissue	Tumor invades subserosa, pericolic, or perirectal fat
T4	Tumor invades peritoneum or other organs	Tumor invades other organs and/or perforates visceral peritoneum
NX	Cannot be assessed	Cannot be assessed
N0	No region lymph nodes	No region lymph nodes
N1	Regional lymph node metastasis	Regional lymph node metastasis
M0	No distant metastasis	No distant metastasis
M1	Distant metastasis	Distant metastasis

Abbreviations: AJCC, American Joint Cancer Committee; ENETS, European Neuroendocrine Tumour Society.

From Anthony LB, Strosberg JR, Klimstra DS, et al. The NANETS consensus guidelines for the diagnosis and management of gastrointestinal neuroendocrine tumors (nets): well-differentiated nets of the distal colon and rectum. Pancreas 2010; 39(6):770; with permission.

Table 2				
AJCC and ENETS staging system				
	AJCC			ENETS
I	T1N0M0		IA	T1aN0M0
			IB	T1bN0M0
IIA	T2N0M0		IIA	T2N0M0
IIB	T3N0M0		IIB	T3N0M0
IIIA	T4N0M0		IIIA	T4N0M0
IIIB	T1-4N1M0		IIIB	T1-4N1M0
IV	T1-4N0-1M1		IV	T1-4N0-1M1

Abbreviations: AJCC, American Joint Cancer Committee; ENETS, European Neuroendocrine Tumour Society.

From Anthony LB, Strosberg JR, Klimstra DS, et al. The NANETS consensus guidelines for the diagnosis and management of gastrointestinal neuroendocrine tumors (nets): well-differentiated nets of the distal colon and rectum. Pancreas 2010; 39(6):770; with permission.

Treatment

Treatment for NETs depends on the location and size of the tumor. The treatment of appendiceal NETs is based on tumor size and characteristics. Appendectomy alone may be sufficient for treatment of small appendiceal NETs located at the tip of the appendix. However, tumors greater than 2 cm, or those involving the base of the appendix, mesoappendix, or with lymphovascular spread necessitate a right hemicolectomy and regional lymphadenectomy.[47] Positive margins after appendectomy also requires return to the operating room for a right hemicolectomy. Several studies have evaluated the surgical approach to appendiceal NETs. In the pediatric population, there is a growing consensus that a right hemicolectomy may be too aggressive an approach, despite the presence of the aforementioned ominous findings.[48,49]

Classically, the treatment for colonic NETs was similar to colonic adenocarcinoma, with segmental resection and lymphadenectomy.[50] Recent findings indicate that smaller tumors may be amenable to endoscopic mucosal resection.[51] The rate of metastasis for tumors less than 1 cm is less than 5%, indicating that limited resection is feasible.[52] Similarly, transanal endoscopic microsurgery can be used for rectal lesions, with success even after incomplete excision at the time of endoscopy.[53]

Chemotherapy and radiation play a minor role in the treatment of colorectal NETs, with the exception of poorly differentiated or metastatic tumors.[54] The evaluation of molecular targets is limited for NETs, although mammalian target of rapamycin has been studied in the RADIANT-2 and -3 trials (Everolimus Plus Octreotide Long-acting Repeatable for the Treatment of Advanced Neuroendocrine Tumours Associated with Carcinoid Syndrome).[55,56] No current recommendations for anti-mammalian target of rapamycin agents are available. Sunitinib, a nonspecific tyrosine kinase inhibitor, demonstrated improved progression-free survival in pancreatic NETs, but data for colorectal NETs are limited to a case report for its use in salvage therapy.[57]

Outcomes

The overall survival for NETs is quite variable. The best outcomes are found in pediatric appendiceal NETs, with a 5-year survival of 100% in multiple studies.[58–60] Historically, survival for nonappendiceal NETs in adults was less than 50%. More recent studies have shown improvement to around 60% for colonic NETs and up to 87% for tumors at the rectosigmoid junction.[27]

GASTROINTESTINAL STROMAL TUMORS OF THE COLON
Introduction: Nature of the Problem

GISTs, although the most common mesenchymal tumor, are exceedingly rare, with an annual incidence of 7 to 20 new cases per million persons.[61] These tumors originate in the interstitial cells of Cajal, which serve as pacemakers for smooth muscle contraction in the gastrointestinal system.[62] The average age at diagnosis is 60 years and men are affected more frequently than women.[63,64]

Relevant Anatomy and Pathophysiology

GISTs arise in the submucosal layer of the gastrointestinal system. The most common location for GISTs is the stomach.[65] Colorectal GISTs account for 5% to 10%, with colonic GISTs representing 1% of all GISTs.[61] The hallmark of the tumor is gain-of-function mutation in the tyrosine kinase gene c-KIT.[62,66] These tumors are found most commonly in the transverse and descending colon.[67] GISTs most commonly metastasize to the liver and peritoneum, with rare metastasis to the lung, bone, and lymph nodes.[68]

Clinical Presentation and Examination

As with other atypical colorectal tumors, the symptoms of GISTs are nonspecific. Most commonly, GISTs of the colon and rectum present with bleeding. Other symptoms include abdominal pain, obstruction, palpable mass, or perforation.[67,69]

Diagnostic Procedures

Colonoscopy may demonstrate an intraluminal or bulging mass (**Fig. 3**A). If the level of suspicion for GIST is high, biopsy is not necessary and reserved for large or potentially metastatic lesions.[70] There is concern for potential spillage of tumor during biopsy.

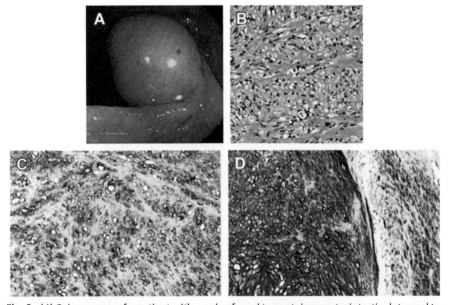

Fig. 3. (A) Colonoscopy of a patient with a polyp found to contain a gastrointestinal stromal tumor (GIST) in the proximal ascending colon. (B) Histologic finding of a patient with GIST. (C) Colonic GIST, with immunostaining for c-KIT. (D) Colonic GIST, with immunostaining for DOG1.

Computed tomography scanning commonly shows a large, exophytic tumor with inhomogenous enhancement.[71] Biopsy primarily is used to rule out other diagnoses of the tumor to plan neoadjuvant chemotherapy. Endoscopic ultrasound examination plays a limited role in the workup.

Diagnosis

GIST tumors demonstrate uniform spindle-shaped cells, small nuclei, and indistinct cytoplasm (see **Fig. 3**B). Although c-KIT positivity is a hallmark of GISTs (see **Fig. 3**C), it is not 100% specific. Other non-GIST tumors that may harbor c-KIT mutations include melanoma, primary clear cell tumor, sarcomas, and extramedullary myeloid tumor.[72–74] Similarly, there are tumors that morphologically can be classified as GISTs, but do not express c-KIT. These tumors can be confirmed by other markers, such as protein kinase C-theta or DOG-1 (see **Fig. 3**D).[75,76]

The prognosis for colorectal GISTs is based on tumor mitotic rates. Small tumors (<2 cm) with low mitotic rate (<5 per 50 high-power fields) demonstrate low clinical progression. However, mitotic rates of greater than 5 per 50 high-power fields are associated with a greater than 50% metastasis rate.[77] **Table 3** shows a breakdown of risk based on size and mitotic count.[78] The TNM classification was updated in 2010 and is summarized in **Table 4**.[79] In addition, the risk of progressive disease was formulated by analysis of more than 1800 GISTs, including rectal tumors by the Armed Forces Institute of Pathology (summarized in **Table 5**).[80]

Treatment

Treatment for colonic GISTs requires a multimodality approach, with surgery and chemotherapy with tyrosine kinase inhibitors as the mainstays of treatment. Progress has been made in improving the overall survival in patients with GISTs.

The goal of surgery for GIST is removal of the tumor with the pseudocapsule intact. Rupture of the pseudocapsule can lead to spillage of tumor and bleeding. Lymphadenectomy is not necessary because GISTs rarely spread to the lymphatics.[81] The abdominal contents should be evaluated, because GISTs do metastasize to the liver and peritoneum. Depending on the size of the tumor, segmental bowel resection may be adequate. Large tumors, especially those in the rectum may require more aggressive surgical resections, including abdominoperineal resection or possibly pelvic exenteration.[82] If more than 1 organ is involved, the resection is performed en bloc.

In a study from Memorial Sloan Kettering, colonic and rectal GIST patients, survival was predicated on tumor size, not microscopic margins. Invasion through the bowel

Table 3
GIST NIH risk assessment

Risk	Size (cm)	Mitotic Count per High-Powered Field
Very low	<2	<5/50
Low	2–5	<5/50
Intermediate	<5	6–10/50
	5–10	<5/50
High	>5	>5/50
	>10	Any
	Any	>10/50

Abbreviations: GIST, gastrointestinal stromal tumor; NIH, National Institutes of Health.
From Fletcher CD, Berman JJ, Corless C, et al. Diagnosis of gastrointestinal stromal tumors: a consensus approach. Hum Pathol 2002;33(5):459–65; with permission.

Table 4
GIST 2010 TNM classification

TNM Classification			Staging
T1	≤2 cm	I	T1-2N0M0, low mitotic rate
T2	2–5 cm	II	T3N0M0, low mitotic rate
T3	5–10 cm	IIIA	T1N0M0, high mitotic rate T4N0M0, low mitotic rate
T4	>10 cm	IIIB	T2-4N0M0, high mitotic rate
N0	No nodes	IV	T1-4N1-2M1
N1	Lymph node metastasis		
M0	No distant metastasis		
M1	Distant metastasis		

Abbreviation: GIST, gastrointestinal stromal tumor.
Data from Agaimy A. Gastrointestinal stromal tumors (GIST) from risk stratification systems to the new TNM proposal: more questions than answers? A review emphasizing the need for a standardized GIST reporting. Int J Clin Exp Pathol 2010;3(5):461–71 and Miettinen M, Lasota J. Gastrointestinal stromal tumors: pathology and prognosis at different sites. Semin Diagn Pathol 2006;23(2):70–83.

proper may be more significant than attaining an R0 resection, with complete microscopic removal of tumor.[83] Laparoscopic surgery can be used and is ideal for smaller tumors.[84] Again, careful handling of the tissue to prevent tumor rupture is critical.

Molecular target therapy has made considerable strides over the past decade. Specifically, in the treatment of GIST, the tyrosine kinase inhibitors imatinib mesylate and sunitinib malate have changed the course of chemotherapy for GIST. Previous chemotherapeutic options were poor, because GISTs had a very low response rate to traditional agents.[85] As mentioned, the vast majority of GISTs contain a mutation in c-KIT. Imatinib mesylate inhibits c-KIT signal transduction, as well as acting on structurally related tyrosine kinases, including PDGFRA and BCR-ABL. However, resistance can develop, and some mutations in c-KIT, especially on exon 9, are especially prone to resistance. Sunitinib malate acts on several tyrosine kinases, including several angiogenesis factors and has been shown to have an effect of some c-KIT mutations that confer resistance to imatinib.[86]

Recent studies have examined the neoadjuvant use of imatinib in phase II studies,[87,88] with additional studies also confirming tumor shrinkage.[89,90] By reducing

Table 5
GIST risk stratification

Mitotic Rate	Size (cm)	Risk for Progression (%)
<5/50	≤2	Low (0)
	2–5	Low (8.5)
	5–10	Insufficient data
	>10	High (57)
>5/50	≤2	High (54)
	2–5	High (52)
	5–10	Insufficient data
	>10	High (71)

Abbreviations: GIST, gastrointestinal stromal tumor.
Adapted from Miettinen M, Lasota J. Gastrointestinal stromal tumors: pathology and prognosis at different sites. Semin Diagn Pathol 2006;23(2):70–83; with permission.

tumor size, a less drastic resection can be undertaken, possibly preserving anal sphincter function in rectal tumors. The optimal dosing regimen has yet to be determined. Therefore, maximal response to treatment is determined by following serial computed tomographic imaging of the tumor.[91]

Imatinib was initially approved for treatment of GIST after resection. Two American College of Surgeons Oncology Group trials, Z9000 and Z9001, demonstrated improved recurrence-free survival in phase II and phase III trials, respectively.[92] Current recommendation is for a treatment course of 1 year after resection for intermediate- to high-risk patients.[93] However, the optimal duration of treatment is still under investigation.

Outcomes

Although treatment for GISTs has improved markedly, recurrence is still common and may occur a decade after the initial diagnosis and treatment. Metastases are most common to the liver and peritoneum for colonic tumors; rectal tumors also metastasize to the lung and bone.[77]

SUMMARY

Primary lymphomas, NETs, and GISTs are tumors found throughout the gastrointestinal system, but are quite uncommon in the colon and rectum. Although they may have a similar presentation in terms of symptoms, endoscopic findings, and imaging results to the more common adenocarcinoma, they are important to differentiate because their treatment and prognosis differ from the standard colorectal adenocarcinoma. For each of the atypical tumors reviewed, significant strides have been made in their treatment, with the potential of molecular target therapy, adding to the therapeutic armamentarium.

REFERENCES

1. American Cancer Society. Cancer facts & figures 2016. Atlanta (GA): American Cancer Society; 2016.
2. Koch P, del Valle F, Berdel WE, et al. Primary gastrointestinal non-Hodgkin's lymphoma: I. Anatomic and histologic distribution, clinical features, and survival data of 371 patients registered in the German Multicenter Study GIT NHL 01/92. J Clin Oncol 2001;19(18):3861–73.
3. Wong MT, Eu KW. Primary colorectal lymphomas. Colorectal Dis 2006;8(7): 586–91.
4. Zighelboim J, Larson MV. Primary colonic lymphoma. Clinical presentation, histopathologic features, and outcome with combination chemotherapy. J Clin Gastroenterol 1994;18(4):291–7.
5. Wang MH, Wong JM, Lien HC, et al. Colonoscopic manifestations of primary colorectal lymphoma. Endoscopy 2001;33(7):605–9.
6. Cai S, Cannizzo F Jr, Bullard Dunn KM, et al. The role of surgical intervention in non-Hodgkin's lymphoma of the colon and rectum. Am J Surg 2007;193(3): 409–12 [discussion: 412].
7. Tevlin R, Larkin JO, Hyland JM, et al. Primary colorectal lymphoma - a single centre experience. Surgeon 2015;13(3):151–5.
8. Zucca E, Roggero E, Bertoni F, et al. Primary extranodal non-Hodgkin's lymphomas. Part 1: gastrointestinal, cutaneous and genitourinary lymphomas. Ann Oncol 1997;8(8):727–37.

9. Jones JL, Loftus EV Jr. Lymphoma risk in inflammatory bowel disease: is it the disease or its treatment? Inflamm Bowel Dis 2007;13(10):1299–307.

10. Lee HJ, Han JK, Kim TK, et al. Primary colorectal lymphoma: spectrum of imaging findings with pathologic correlation. Eur Radiol 2002;12(9):2242–9.

11. Dawson IM, Cornes JS, Morson BC. Primary malignant lymphoid tumours of the intestinal tract. Report of 37 cases with a study of factors influencing prognosis. Br J Surg 1961;49:80–9.

12. Banks PM. Gastrointestinal lymphoproliferative disorders. Histopathology 2007; 50(1):42–54.

13. Carbone PP, Kaplan HS, Musshoff K, et al. Report of the committee on Hodgkin's disease staging classification. Cancer Res 1971;31(11):1860–1.

14. She WH, Day W, Lau PY, et al. Primary colorectal lymphoma: case series and literature review. Asian J Surg 2011;34(3):111–4.

15. Drolet S, Maclean AR, Stewart DA, et al. Primary colorectal lymphoma-clinical outcomes in a population-based series. J Gastrointest Surg 2011;15(10):1851–7.

16. Fan CW, Changchien CR, Wang JY, et al. Primary colorectal lymphoma. Dis Colon Rectum 2000;43(9):1277–82.

17. Kim SJ, Kang HJ, Kim JS, et al. Comparison of treatment strategies for patients with intestinal diffuse large B-cell lymphoma: surgical resection followed by chemotherapy versus chemotherapy alone. Blood 2011;117(6):1958–65.

18. Lee J, Kim WS, Kim K, et al. Prospective clinical study of surgical resection followed by CHOP in localized intestinal diffuse large B cell lymphoma. Leuk Res 2007;31(3):359–64.

19. Fisher RI, Gaynor ER, Dahlberg S, et al. Comparison of a standard regimen (CHOP) with three intensive chemotherapy regimens for advanced non-Hodgkin's lymphoma. N Engl J Med 1993;328(14):1002–6.

20. Morrison VA. Evolution of R-CHOP therapy for older patients with diffuse large B-cell lymphoma. Expert Rev Anticancer Ther 2008;8(10):1651–8.

21. Pettengell R, Linch D, Haemato-Oncology task force of the British Committee for Standards in Haematology. Position paper on the therapeutic use of rituximab in CD20-positive diffuse large B-cell non-Hodgkin's lymphoma. Br J Haematol 2003; 121(1):44–8.

22. Kim YH, Lee JH, Yang SK, et al. Primary colon lymphoma in Korea: a KASID (Korean Association for the Study of Intestinal Diseases) Study. Dig Dis Sci 2005;50(12):2243–7.

23. Aviles A, Neri N, Huerta-Guzman J. Large bowel lymphoma: an analysis of prognostic factors and therapy in 53 patients. J Surg Oncol 2002;80(2):111–5.

24. Gonzalez QH, Heslin MJ, Davila-Cervantes A, et al. Primary colonic lymphoma. Am Surg 2008;74(3):214–6.

25. Niederle MB, Hackl M, Kaserer K, et al. Gastroenteropancreatic neuroendocrine tumours: the current incidence and staging based on the WHO and European Neuroendocrine Tumour Society classification: an analysis based on prospectively collected parameters. Endocr Relat Cancer 2010;17(4):909–18.

26. Lawrence B, Gustafsson BI, Chan A, et al. The epidemiology of gastroenteropancreatic neuroendocrine tumors. Endocrinol Metab Clin North Am 2011; 40(1):1–18, vii.

27. Modlin IM, Lye KD, Kidd M. A 5-decade analysis of 13,715 carcinoid tumors. Cancer 2003;97(4):934–59.

28. Anthony LB, Strosberg JR, Klimstra DS, et al. The NANETS consensus guidelines for the diagnosis and management of gastrointestinal neuroendocrine tumors

(nets): well-differentiated nets of the distal colon and rectum. Pancreas 2010; 39(6):767–74.

29. Kloppel G, Perren A, Heitz PU. The gastroenteropancreatic neuroendocrine cell system and its tumors: the WHO classification. Ann N Y Acad Sci 2004;1014: 13–27.

30. Tsikitis VL, Wertheim BC, Guerrero MA. Trends of incidence and survival of gastrointestinal neuroendocrine tumors in the United States: a seer analysis. J Cancer 2012;3:292–302.

31. McCusker ME, Cote TR, Clegg LX, et al. Primary malignant neoplasms of the appendix: a population-based study from the surveillance, epidemiology and end-results program, 1973-1998. Cancer 2002;94(12):3307–12.

32. Mullen JT, Savarese DM. Carcinoid tumors of the appendix: a population-based study. J Surg Oncol 2011;104(1):41–4.

33. Volante M, Daniele L, Asioli S, et al. Tumor staging but not grading is associated with adverse clinical outcome in neuroendocrine tumors of the appendix: a retrospective clinical pathologic analysis of 138 cases. Am J Surg Pathol 2013;37(4): 606–12.

34. Murray SE, Lloyd RV, Sippel RS, et al. Clinicopathologic characteristics of colonic carcinoid tumors. J Surg Res 2013;184(1):183–8.

35. Yoon SN, Yu CS, Shin US, et al. Clinicopathological characteristics of rectal carcinoids. Int J Colorectal Dis 2010;25(9):1087–92.

36. Modlin IM, Kidd M, Latich I, et al. Current status of gastrointestinal carcinoids. Gastroenterology 2005;128(6):1717–51.

37. Thirlby RC, Kasper CS, Jones RC. Metastatic carcinoid tumor of the appendix. Report of a case and review of the literature. Dis Colon Rectum 1984;27(1):42–6.

38. Jetmore AB, Ray JE, Gathright JB Jr, et al. Rectal carcinoids: the most frequent carcinoid tumor. Dis Colon Rectum 1992;35(8):717–25.

39. Kobayashi K, Katsumata T, Yoshizawa S, et al. Indications of endoscopic polypectomy for rectal carcinoid tumors and clinical usefulness of endoscopic ultrasonography. Dis Colon Rectum 2005;48(2):285–91.

40. Sundin A, Vullierme MP, Kaltsas G, et al. ENETS consensus guidelines for the standards of care in neuroendocrine tumors: radiological examinations. Neuroendocrinology 2009;90(2):167–83.

41. Caplin M, Sundin A, Nillson O, et al. ENETS Consensus Guidelines for the management of patients with digestive neuroendocrine neoplasms: colorectal neuroendocrine neoplasms. Neuroendocrinology 2012;95(2):88–97.

42. Eriksson B, Oberg K, Stridsberg M. Tumor markers in neuroendocrine tumors. Digestion 2000;62(Suppl 1):33–8.

43. Federspiel BH, Burke AP, Sobin LH, et al. Rectal and colonic carcinoids. A clinicopathologic study of 84 cases. Cancer 1990;65(1):135–40.

44. Strosberg JR, Nasir A, Hodul P, et al. Biology and treatment of metastatic gastrointestinal neuroendocrine tumors. Gastrointest Cancer Res 2008;2(3):113–25.

45. Fahy BN, Tang LH, Klimstra D, et al. Carcinoid of the rectum risk stratification (CaRRs): a strategy for preoperative outcome assessment. Ann Surg Oncol 2007;14(5):1735–43.

46. Jann H, Roll S, Couvelard A, et al. Neuroendocrine tumors of midgut and hindgut origin: tumor-node-metastasis classification determines clinical outcome. Cancer 2011;117(15):3332–41.

47. Moertel CG, Weiland LH, Nagorney DM, et al. Carcinoid tumor of the appendix: treatment and prognosis. N Engl J Med 1987;317(27):1699–701.

48. Wu H, Chintagumpala M, Hicks J, et al. Neuroendocrine tumor of the appendix in children. J Pediatr Hematol Oncol 2016. [Epub ahead of print].

49. Henderson L, Fehily C, Folaranmi S, et al. Management and outcome of neuroendocrine tumours of the appendix-a two centre UK experience. J Pediatr Surg 2014;49(10):1513–7.

50. Plockinger U, Rindi G, Arnold R, et al. Guidelines for the diagnosis and treatment of neuroendocrine gastrointestinal tumours. A consensus statement on behalf of the European Neuroendocrine Tumour Society (ENETS). Neuroendocrinology 2004;80(6):394–424.

51. Zhou PH, Yao LQ, Qin XY, et al. Advantages of endoscopic submucosal dissection with needle-knife over endoscopic mucosal resection for small rectal carcinoid tumors: a retrospective study. Surg Endosc 2010;24(10):2607–12.

52. Al Natour RH, Saund MS, Sanchez VM, et al. Tumor size and depth predict rate of lymph node metastasis in colon carcinoids and can be used to select patients for endoscopic resection. J Gastrointest Surg 2012;16(3):595–602.

53. Kumar AS, Sidani SM, Kolli K, et al. Transanal endoscopic microsurgery for rectal carcinoids: the largest reported United States experience. Colorectal Dis 2012; 14(5):562–6.

54. Pavel M, Baudin E, Couvelard A, et al. ENETS Consensus Guidelines for the management of patients with liver and other distant metastases from neuroendocrine neoplasms of foregut, midgut, hindgut, and unknown primary. Neuroendocrinology 2012;95(2):157–76.

55. Pavel ME, Hainsworth JD, Baudin E, et al. Everolimus plus octreotide long-acting repeatable for the treatment of advanced neuroendocrine tumours associated with carcinoid syndrome (RADIANT-2): a randomised, placebo-controlled, phase 3 study. Lancet 2011;378(9808):2005–12.

56. Yao JC, Shah MH, Ito T, et al. Everolimus for advanced pancreatic neuroendocrine tumors. N Engl J Med 2011;364(6):514–23.

57. Blesa JM, Pulido EG. Colorectal cancer: response to sunitinib in a heavily pretreated colorectal cancer patient. Anticancer Drugs 2010;21(Suppl 1):S23–6.

58. Navalkele P, O'Dorisio MS, O'Dorisio TM, et al. Incidence, survival, and prevalence of neuroendocrine tumors versus neuroblastoma in children and young adults: nine standard SEER registries, 1975-2006. Pediatr Blood Cancer 2011; 56(1):50–7.

59. Boxberger N, Redlich A, Boger C, et al. Neuroendocrine tumors of the appendix in children and adolescents. Pediatr Blood Cancer 2013;60(1):65–70.

60. Virgone C, Cecchetto G, Alaggio R, et al. Appendiceal neuroendocrine tumours in childhood: Italian TREP project. J Pediatr Gastroenterol Nutr 2014;58(3):333–8.

61. Miettinen M, Lasota J. Gastrointestinal stromal tumors–definition, clinical, histological, immunohistochemical, and molecular genetic features and differential diagnosis. Virchows Arch 2001;438(1):1–12.

62. Hirota S, Isozaki K, Moriyama Y, et al. Gain-of-function mutations of c-kit in human gastrointestinal stromal tumors. Science 1998;279(5350):577–80.

63. Ueyama T, Guo KJ, Hashimoto H, et al. A clinicopathologic and immunohistochemical study of gastrointestinal stromal tumors. Cancer 1992;69(4):947–55.

64. Miettinen M, Sarlomo-Rikala M, Lasota J. Gastrointestinal stromal tumors: recent advances in understanding of their biology. Hum Pathol 1999;30(10):1213–20.

65. Edge SB, Compton CC. The American Joint Committee on Cancer: the 7th edition of the AJCC Cancer Staging Manual and the future of TNM. Ann Surg Oncol 2010;17(6):1471–4.

66. Heinrich MC, Rubin BP, Longley BJ, et al. Biology and genetic aspects of gastrointestinal stromal tumors: KIT activation and cytogenetic alterations. Hum Pathol 2002;33(5):484–95.

67. Caterino S, Lorenzon L, Petrucciani N, et al. Gastrointestinal stromal tumors: correlation between symptoms at presentation, tumor location and prognostic factors in 47 consecutive patients. World J Surg Oncol 2011;9:13.

68. Miettinen M, Lasota J. Gastrointestinal stromal tumors: review on morphology, molecular pathology, prognosis, and differential diagnosis. Arch Pathol Lab Med 2006;130(10):1466–78.

69. Stamatakos M, Douzinas E, Stefanaki C, et al. Gastrointestinal stromal tumor. World J Surg Oncol 2009;7:61.

70. Lamba G, Gupta R, Lee B, et al. Current management and prognostic features for gastrointestinal stromal tumor (GIST). Exp Hematol Oncol 2012;1(1):14.

71. Sandrasegaran K, Rajesh A, Rushing DA, et al. Gastrointestinal stromal tumors: CT and MRI findings. Eur Radiol 2005;15(7):1407–14.

72. Miettinen M, Sobin LH, Sarlomo-Rikala M. Immunohistochemical spectrum of GISTs at different sites and their differential diagnosis with a reference to CD117 (KIT). Mod Pathol 2000;13(10):1134–42.

73. Montone KT, van Belle P, Elenitsas R, et al. Proto-oncogene c-kit expression in malignant melanoma: protein loss with tumor progression. Mod Pathol 1997; 10(9):939–44.

74. Arber DA, Tamayo R, Weiss LM. Paraffin section detection of the c-kit gene product (CD117) in human tissues: value in the diagnosis of mast cell disorders. Hum Pathol 1998;29(5):498–504.

75. Motegi A, Sakurai S, Nakayama H, et al. PKC theta, a novel immunohistochemical marker for gastrointestinal stromal tumors (GIST), especially useful for identifying KIT-negative tumors. Pathol Int 2005;55(3):106–12.

76. West RB, Corless CL, Chen X, et al. The novel marker, DOG1, is expressed ubiquitously in gastrointestinal stromal tumors irrespective of KIT or PDGFRA mutation status. Am J Pathol 2004;165(1):107–13.

77. Miettinen M, Furlong M, Sarlomo-Rikala M, et al. Gastrointestinal stromal tumors, intramural leiomyomas, and leiomyosarcomas in the rectum and anus: a clinicopathologic, immunohistochemical, and molecular genetic study of 144 cases. Am J Surg Pathol 2001;25(9):1121–33.

78. Fletcher CD, Berman JJ, Corless C, et al. Diagnosis of gastrointestinal stromal tumors: a consensus approach. Hum Pathol 2002;33(5):459–65.

79. Agaimy A. Gastrointestinal stromal tumors (GIST) from risk stratification systems to the new TNM proposal: more questions than answers? A review emphasizing the need for a standardized GIST reporting. Int J Clin Exp Pathol 2010;3(5): 461–71.

80. Miettinen M, Lasota J. Gastrointestinal stromal tumors: pathology and prognosis at different sites. Semin Diagn Pathol 2006;23(2):70–83.

81. Hohenberger P, Ronellenfitsch U, Oladeji O, et al. Pattern of recurrence in patients with ruptured primary gastrointestinal stromal tumour. Br J Surg 2010; 97(12):1854–9.

82. Gervaz P, Huber O, Morel P. Surgical management of gastrointestinal stromal tumours. Br J Surg 2009;96(6):567–78.

83. DeMatteo RP, Lewis JJ, Leung D, et al. Two hundred gastrointestinal stromal tumors: recurrence patterns and prognostic factors for survival. Ann Surg 2000; 231(1):51–8.

84. Chang SC, Ke TW, Chiang HC, et al. Laparoscopic excision is an alternative method for rectal gastrointestinal stromal tumor. Surg Laparosc Endosc Percutan Tech 2010;20(4):284–7.

85. Edmonson JH, Marks RS, Buckner JC, et al. Contrast of response to dacarbazine, mitomycin, doxorubicin, and cisplatin (DMAP) plus GM-CSF between patients with advanced malignant gastrointestinal stromal tumors and patients with other advanced leiomyosarcomas. Cancer Invest 2002;20(5–6):605–12.

86. Demetri GD, van Oosterom AT, Garrett CR, et al. Efficacy and safety of sunitinib in patients with advanced gastrointestinal stromal tumour after failure of imatinib: a randomised controlled trial. Lancet 2006;368(9544):1329–38.

87. Eisenberg BL, Harris J, Blanke CD, et al. Phase II trial of neoadjuvant/adjuvant imatinib mesylate (IM) for advanced primary and metastatic/recurrent operable gastrointestinal stromal tumor (GIST): early results of RTOG 0132/ACRIN 6665. J Surg Oncol 2009;99(1):42–7.

88. McAuliffe JC, Hunt KK, Lazar AJ, et al. A randomized, phase II study of preoperative plus postoperative imatinib in GIST: evidence of rapid radiographic response and temporal induction of tumor cell apoptosis. Ann Surg Oncol 2009;16(4):910–9.

89. Machlenkin S, Pinsk I, Tulchinsky H, et al. The effect of neoadjuvant Imatinib therapy on outcome and survival after rectal gastrointestinal stromal tumour. Colorectal Dis 2011;13(10):1110–5.

90. Fiore M, Palassini E, Fumagalli E, et al. Preoperative imatinib mesylate for unresectable or locally advanced primary gastrointestinal stromal tumors (GIST). Eur J Surg Oncol 2009;35(7):739–45.

91. Bonvalot S, Eldweny H, Pechoux CL, et al. Impact of surgery on advanced gastrointestinal stromal tumors (GIST) in the imatinib era. Ann Surg Oncol 2006;13(12):1596–603.

92. DeMatteo RP. Nanoneoadjuvant therapy of gastrointestinal stromal tumor (GIST). Ann Surg Oncol 2009;16(4):799–800.

93. Demetri GD, von Mehren M, Antonescu CR, et al. NCCN Task Force report: update on the management of patients with gastrointestinal stromal tumors. J Natl Compr Canc Netw 2010;8(Suppl 2):S1–41 [quiz: S42–4].

Resection of the Primary Tumor in Stage IV Colorectal Cancer: When Is It Necessary?

CrossMark

Leandro Feo, MD[a], Michael Polcino, MD[b], Garrett M. Nash, MD, MPH[c],*

KEYWORDS

- Metastatic colorectal cancer • Primary tumor resection • Survival
- Palliative treatment

KEY POINTS

- The cornerstones in the management of metastatic colorectal cancer are accurate staging and multidisciplinary treatment planning.
- Treatment options are tailored to the patient's burden of disease, performance status, goals of care, and expected survival.
- Staged resection, with either colon or liver resection first, and synchronous resection are options for the management of resectable liver metastases.
- Unresectable metastases with an asymptomatic primary tumor should be initially managed with systemic chemotherapy, avoiding futile interventions.
- Additional therapies for local control at the primary tumor site include colonic stenting, fulguration, and laser therapy.

INTRODUCTION

Approximately 20% of patients with colorectal cancer present with metastatic disease, which can be challenging to manage.[1] Within this subpopulation, there are many different clinical scenarios, leading to a potentially complex decision-making process for selecting a treatment plan. Despite considerable advances in the treatment of metastatic colorectal cancer, in most cases the disease is not curable. Therefore, the treatment goal for most patients is to extend survival and improve the quality of life. Treatment options are tailored to the patient's performance status,

Disclosures: The authors have nothing to disclose.
[a] Colorectal Service, Department of Surgery, Catholic Medical Center, 100 McGregor Street, Suite 3100, Manchester, NH 03102, USA; [b] Division of Colorectal Surgery, St. Barnabas Hospital, 4422 Third Avenue, Bronx, NY 10457, USA; [c] Colorectal Service, Department of Surgery, Memorial Sloan Kettering Cancer Center, 1233 York Avenue, New York, NY 10065, USA
* Corresponding author.
E-mail address: nashg@mskcc.org

Surg Clin N Am 97 (2017) 657–669
http://dx.doi.org/10.1016/j.suc.2017.01.012
0039-6109/17/© 2017 Elsevier Inc. All rights reserved.
surgical.theclinics.com

comorbidities, disease burden, and the presence or absence of symptoms such as bowel obstruction.[2]

For patients with minimal primary tumor symptoms and acceptable performance status, the standard treatment according to the National Comprehensive Cancer Network guidelines is systemic chemotherapy, which has been shown to increase survival.[3,4] Over the last 10 years, the overall survival (OS) rate has improved from 9 to 24 months (and in some series up to 36 months), which is possibly the result of the addition of multiagent chemotherapy.[5,6] First-line chemotherapy with LV5FU2 plus oxaliplatin (FOLFOX) or folinic acid, fluorouracil, irinotecan (FOLFIRI) produces major responses in most previously untreated patients.[7] Systemic therapy alone rarely cures the disease; however, in patients with resectable disease, effective chemotherapy combined with complete resection of metastatic disease maximizes the possibility of a cure.

In this context, several important questions arise. Is the metastatic disease resectable? If so, should the resection be synchronous or staged and, if staged, in what order? If the metastatic disease is not resectable, is resection of the primary tumor indicated? These and related questions are matters of considerable debate, reflecting the complexity of the management of metastatic colorectal cancer. This article reviews the published literature with the goal of developing an evidence-based approach to managing various clinical scenarios associated with metastatic colorectal cancer.

EVALUATION

The evaluation of colorectal cancer is based on the principles of accurate staging and multidisciplinary treatment planning. After a thorough history is taken and a physical examination is performed, the disease is staged. Accurate staging includes tissue diagnosis; carcinoembryonic antigen measurement; and cross-sectional imaging of the chest, abdomen, and pelvis. In addition, rectal cancer requires rectal MRI and/or endorectal ultrasound for local staging. Several imaging modalities, including MRI, computed tomography (CT), and positron emission tomography (PET), are available to identify metastatic disease and facilitate differentiation from other conditions such as hemangiomas, focal nodular hyperplasia, or cysts in patients with liver metastases. Carcinoembryonic antigen levels greater than 20 ng/mL warrant a high degree of suspicion for systemic disease.[8]

SYMPTOMATIC PRIMARY TUMOR

One of the more disagreed on treatment decisions in metastatic colorectal cancer relates to the appropriate time and indication for resection of the primary tumor. Traditionally, symptomatic primary tumors warranted resection but, in reality, the degree of symptoms is variable, and tumors that are mildly symptomatic may become less troublesome after systemic therapy.

Without question, perforated primary tumors with associated peritonitis warrant exploration and resection when feasible. In cases of complete bowel obstruction, the need for urgent or emergency surgery is also straightforward. However, the incidence of this presentation is difficult to measure because cases of complete obstruction are commonly reported together with cases of partial obstruction. Patients with partial or complete bowel obstruction represent between 8% and 29% of all patients with colorectal cancer.[9] Patients with a complete obstruction typically have either stage III or stage IV disease.[10] Complete colonic obstruction requires urgent intervention by stenting, resection, or diversion to relieve this life-threatening condition, which can otherwise lead to perforation, peritonitis, or sepsis. Severe, massive bleeding from the tumor site, though less common, is another indication to pursue resection. Surgical intervention is performed using oncological principles as long as the preoperative circumstances allow it.[11] The risks and benefits of primary anastomosis must be discussed in detail so that the patient understands the risks of anastomotic leak, including death or possible delay in the initiation of chemotherapy.[12]

ASYMPTOMATIC PRIMARY TUMOR WITH RESECTABLE METASTATIC DISEASE

Excluding the scenarios previously described, the management of the primary tumor in patients with stage IV colorectal cancer depends on whether the metastatic disease is resectable. The most common site of colorectal cancer metastasis is the liver. Approximately 25% of patients with colorectal cancer present with liver metastasis at the time of diagnosis.[13] Among patients with stage IV colorectal cancer, those with liver metastasis have the greatest chance of complete resection and cure. In borderline resectable cases, induction chemotherapy may improve the likelihood of resection. The European Organisation for Research and Treatment of Cancer (EORTC) Chemotherapy + Local Ablation Versus Chemotherapy (CLOCC) trial[14,15] was the first prospective randomized trial to demonstrate a survival benefit from resection or ablation plus chemotherapy versus systemic treatment alone. The 8-year OS was 36% for the combination treatment and 9% for systemic therapy alone. Furthermore, progression-free survival was 16.8 and 9.9 months, respectively. For patients with apparently resectable disease, induction chemotherapy may be omitted (this decision-making process is outside the scope of this article).

Staged Resection

Historically, the preferred operative approach for stage IV colorectal cancer with liver metastasis began with resection of the primary tumor, followed by chemotherapy, and then liver resection 2 to 3 months later. The proponents of this strategy based their argument on the hypothesis that the primary tumor may seed metastatic disease in an ongoing manner. Furthermore, there was concern that the primary tumor would progress to complete colonic obstruction, perforation, or hemorrhage. Additionally, complications from colorectal resection, such as anastomotic leak, may be exacerbated by the perioperative effects of hepatic resection. It is believed that the low-flow state or temporary changes in portal blood circulation could affect oxygenation of the bowel anastomosis.[16]

On the other hand, there are arguments for not resecting the primary tumor first. One such argument is based on the fact that induction chemotherapy with fluorouracil-based regimens can produce a significant response in both the primary tumor and hepatic metastases. Another argument is that complications associated with resection at the primary site can delay further treatment and thereby promote metastasis progression. Given that the presence of systemic metastasis is among the main determinants of survival, many physicians prioritize the treatment of metastatic lesions.[17]

Simultaneous Resection

With the recent advances in liver resection techniques and the associated perioperative care, outcomes for patients who undergo simultaneous resection of the primary tumor and the metastasis have improved. Cumulative morbidity and mortality rates have been similar to or better than those for patients who have undergone staged procedures.[18,19]

Some investigators recommend that the simultaneous approach be used only when the liver resection is minor, because major liver resections are thought to be associated with relatively high morbidity.[20] However, recent data indicate that combining a major liver resection with resection of the primary colorectal tumor is safe, leading to more centers favoring the simultaneous approach.[21] Silberhumer and colleagues[22] reported that the 1-year and 5-year OS rates for simultaneous resection were similar to those for the staged approach (90.5% vs 92.6% at 1 year and 38.5% vs 38.9% at 5 years, respectively). The 5-year rates of disease-free survival were also similar (25.3% vs 24.3%, respectively). In a multicenter analysis, Mayo and colleagues[23] also found that the staged approach and the simultaneous approach produced similar oncological outcomes.

As shown in **Table 1**, many other studies found no significant differences between simultaneous resection and staged resection (regardless of whether the primary tumor or the metastasis was resected first). The choice of the approach should therefore be based on the expertise available at different institutions.

ASYMPTOMATIC PRIMARY TUMOR WITH UNRESECTABLE METASTATIC DISEASE

Traditionally, prophylactic resection of the primary tumor in asymptomatic patients with unresectable metastatic disease has been performed for many patients, with the goal of avoiding late complications such as obstruction, perforation, or hemorrhage. Most of the evidence supporting this strategy is from the era of fluoropyrimidine monotherapy, which was the standard of care during the 1990s. In those years, more than two-thirds of patients with synchronous colorectal cancer metastasis underwent upfront resection of the primary tumor, with the goal of preventing future hypothetical complications and eliminating chemoresistance thought to be associated with the primary tumor.[30,31] However, there was little evidence to support this approach because the few studies on outcomes in subjects with an intact primary tumor treated with fluoropyrimidine monotherapy showed that the risk of needing urgent palliative resection was 9% to 29% **(Table 2)**.

Ruo and colleagues[34] reported that of 103 subjects treated with fluorouracil monotherapy between 1996 and 1999, 30 required surgical palliative intervention, even though 23 subjects with rectal cancer received radiation therapy upfront (see **Table 2**). Another, prospective study showed a similar rate of palliative surgical intervention (25%) in 24 subjects treated with fluoropyrimidine monotherapy[33] (see **Table 2**). It can be concluded from these studies that approximately 4 in 5 patients with metastatic colorectal cancer treated upfront with single-agent chemotherapy will not experience complications associated with primary tumor requiring palliative surgical intervention.

Some recent findings support primary tumor resection in patients with unresectable colorectal cancer metastasis, including patients treated with FOLFOX or FOLFIRI in addition to biologic agents. In a Canadian study of subjects with stage IV colorectal cancer diagnosed from 2006 to 2010,[36] 199 subjects who received chemotherapy underwent upfront resection and 127 other subjects who also received chemotherapy did not undergo upfront resection. Ninety-one percent of subjects received FOLFIRI or FOLFOX, and 67% received a biologic agent. The median OS was 27 months in the resection group and 14 months in the nonresection group. These findings seem to suggest that primary tumor resection may improve outcomes. However, the longer OS could be a result of selection bias: 54% of the subjects in the nonresection group had stage IVb disease compared with 40% in the resection group, and performance status in the nonresection group was poorer (48%) than in the resection group (25%).

Table 1
Studies comparing simultaneous resection versus staged resection

Author, Year	N	Simultaneous n =	Staged n =	Rate of Simultaneous Resection (%)	Major Hepatectomy in Simultaneous vs Staged Resection (%)[a]	Morbidity Simultaneous/ Staged (%)	Mortality Simultaneous/ Staged (%)
Weber et al,[24] 2003	97	35	62	36	11 (31)	23/32	0/0
Martin et al,[18] 2003	240	134	106	56	34 (72)	49/67	2.2/2.8
Tanaka et al,[20] 2004	91	41	50[b]	47	6 (15)	28/16	0/0
Capussotti et al,[25] 2007	127	70	57	55	24 (34)	35.7/36.8	0/0
Turrini et al,[26] 2007	119	57	62	48	NA	21/31	3.5/5
Reddy et al,[27] 2007	610	135	475	28	36 (27)	36.3/38.6	1/0.5
Martin et al,[21] 2009	230	70	160	30	32 (33)	56/55	1.4/1.9
Luo et al,[19] 2010	405	129	276	31	44 (34)	47.3/54.3	1.5/2
Abbott et al,[28] 2012	144	60	84	42	20 (33)	38.3/40.5	3.3/1.2
Yoshioka et al,[29] 2014	150	127	23	85	18 (14)	61.4	0
Silberhumer et al,[22] 2016	429	320	109	74.6	58 (43)	NA	0

NA, not available.
[a] Major hepatectomy was defined as hepatic resection of 3 or more Couinaud segments.
[b] 13 subjects were excluded because they underwent 2-stage hepatectomy procedures.
Data from Yoshioka R, Hasegawa K, Mise Y, et al. Evaluation of the safety and efficacy of simultaneous resection of primary colorectal cancer and synchronous colorectal liver metastases. Surgery 2014;155:478–85.

Table 2
Published series of palliation of the primary tumor after upfront fluorouracil-based chemotherapy

Study	Study Period	N	Need for Palliative Surgery	Need for Radiation Therapy	Need for Colonic Stent
Scoggins et al,[32] 1999	1985–1997	23[a]	2 (9%)	—	—
Sarela et al,[33] 2001	1997–2000	24	6 (25%)	—	2 (8%)
Ruo et al,[34] 2003	1996–1999	103[b]	30 (29%)	—	—
Tebbutt et al,[35] 2003	1990–2000	82	8 (10%)	11 (13%)	—
Total	—	232	46 (20%)	—	—

[a] 10 of 23 patients received upfront radiation therapy to the primary tumor.
[b] 23 of 103 patients received upfront radiation therapy to the primary tumor.
Data from Poultsides GA, Paty PB. Reassessing the need for primary tumor surgery in unresectable metastatic colorectal cancer: overview and perspective. Ther Adv Med Oncol 2011;3:35–42.

A meta-analysis of 21 studies including 44,226 subjects[37] found that subjects with metastasis who underwent resection of the primary tumor had a lower risk of death than subjects who received chemotherapy alone, with a difference in mean OS of 6.4 months (95% CI 5.0–7.9; $P<.001$). However, selection bias may have played a significant role in these findings as well. Subjects who underwent resection were more likely to have colon rather than rectal cancer and most of the resection subjects had a single metastasis confined to the liver.

A pooled post hoc analysis of 4 randomized trials including 816 subjects[38–42] **(Table 3)** found that primary tumor resection was independently associated with longer OS (median, 19.2 vs 13.3 months) in multivariate analysis (Kaplan-Meier curve). The association of OS with resection of the primary tumor did not differ significantly between the trials or between the types of chemotherapy received. Selection bias seems to be the most common limitation across the 4 studies. For example, in 1 of the trials[38] the decision to resect the primary tumor was made before randomization. Also, no tumor-specific mutation markers (eg, RAS or BRAF) were available when these studies were conducted, which, in addition to other unmeasured factors, may explain the lower survival in the nonresection group. Finally, despite the adjustments for known potential confounders, it remains likely that resections were more likely to be performed in patients with better prognoses, leading to longer OS.

A retrospective analysis of 2 randomized trials conducted by the Dutch Colorectal Cancer Group (CAIRO [Sequential versus combination chemotherapy with capecitabine, irinotecan, and oxaliplatin in advanced colorectal cancer (CAIRO): a phase III randomised controlled trial] and CAIRO-2) compared 547 subjects who underwent a primary tumor resection and 310 subjects who received upfront chemotherapy.[43–45] As a prognostic factor, primary tumor resection was associated with a significantly longer median OS (CAIRO, 16.7 vs 11.4 months; CAIRO-2, 20.7 vs 13.4 months). A similar association was found for progression-free survival. The subjects in the 2 trials received capecitabine, oxaliplatin, and irinotecan regimens as well as biologic therapy. Selection bias also seems to have affected the results of these studies because the subjects who underwent resection had, on average, better performance status and lower disease burden than nonresection subjects, and the proportion of subjects with colon, rather than rectal, cancer was higher in the resection group. In contrast, Poultsides and colleagues[46] reported a median OS of 18 months among 233 subjects who did not undergo initial resection of the primary tumor, which is comparable to the median OS for resection subjects in the meta-analysis.

Table 3
Characteristics of the 4 randomized trials

	FFCD-9601	FFCD-2000-05	ML-16987	ACCORD-13
Accrual period	1997–2001	2002–2006	2003–2004	2006–2008
Line	First-line	First-line	First-line	First-line
Phase	III	III	III	II
Number of patients	294	410	306	145
Primary endpoint	Progression-free survival	Progression-free survival after second-line	Overall response rate	6 mo progression-free survival
Treatment allocated by randomization (number of patients on this arm)	LV5FU2 (N = 74) LV5FU2 with low dose LV (N = 75) Bolus 5FU (N = 73) Raltitrexed (N = 72)	LV5FU2 followed by FOLFOX at progression then third-line FOLFIRI (N = 205) FOLFIRI followed by FOLFIRI at progression (N = 205)	FOLFOX (N = 150) XELOX (N = 156)	Bevacizumab + FOLFIRI (N = 73) Bevacizumab + XELIRI (N = 72)
More than 1 metastatic site	39%	57%	52%	51%
At least 1 unresectable site[a]	35%	41%	42%	28%
Subsequent Surgery	4% had surgery	3% curative intent resection	No data available	14% curative intent resection

Abbreviations: ACCORD, Actions Concertees dan les cancers ColoRectaux et Digestifs; FFCD, Federation Francophone de Cancerologie Digestive; FOLFIRI, irinotecan plus bolus and infusional FU and LV; FOLFOX, oxaliplatin plus bolus and infusional FU and LV; FU, fluorouracil; LV, leucovorin; LV5FU2, bolus and infusional FU and LV; XELIRI, capecitabine and irinotecan; XELOX, capecitabine and oxaliplatin.

[a] Defined by the presence of metastasis in 1 of the following sites: bone, retroperitoneal nodes, supraclavicular nodes, brain, pleura, peritoneum.

Data from Faron M, Pignon JP, Malka D, et al. Is primary tumor resection associated with survival improvement in patients with colorectal cancer and unresectable synchronous metastases? A pooled analysis of individual data from four randomized trials. Eur J Cancer 2015;51:166–76.

In summary, retrospective studies that argue for resection of an asymptomatic primary tumor in subjects with metastatic colon cancer must be interpreted with caution because they are compromised by selection bias and, therefore, cannot be used to conclude that upfront resection is beneficial. Prospective randomized clinical trials such as CAIRO 4, CAIRO 5, and the French Research Group of Rectal Cancer Surgery (GRECCAR) 8 trial are currently being conducted in Europe to explicitly address this question.

CHEMOTHERAPY AS INITIAL TREATMENT

With the advent of fluorouracil-based combination regimens, survival and the quality of life have improved in patients with metastatic colorectal cancer. In the United States, Asia, and Europe, many centers are avoiding futile interventions by resecting only symptomatic primary tumors.[47] Matsumoto and colleagues[48] reported that approximately 75% of patients with metastatic colorectal cancer can be spared surgery for an asymptomatic primary tumor. Another study suggested that in 68% to 91% of the patients, resection of the primary tumor is not required.[49]

Poultsides and colleagues[46] also addressed this issue when they reported the frequency of interventions necessary to palliate the primary tumor among 233 subjects receiving upfront combination chemotherapy without prophylactic surgery. Ninety-three percent of the subjects did not experience complications associated with primary tumor requiring surgery. In the remaining 7%, surgery was performed at a median of 7 months (range, 1–27 months) after initiation of chemotherapy. In addition, 4% of the 233 subjects required nonoperative intervention (stenting or radiotherapy) at a median of 12 months (range, 1–36 months) after initiation of chemotherapy. Given the wide range of time points, no specific trend in the timing of primary tumor complications can be discerned. Nevertheless, the overall need for intervention was very low. Seo and colleagues[50] reported a similar, 5% rate of emergency surgical interventions in 83 subjects treated with first-line chemotherapy between 2001 and 2008. Four percent of the subjects in that study needed colonic stenting to manage symptoms related to primary tumor.

Some investigators have argued for upfront resection of the primary tumor based on bevacizumab-associated bowel perforation. Bevacizumab, an antiangiogenic agent, has been found in prospective clinical trials to be associated with a 1% to 2% incidence of gastrointestinal perforation.[5,51–53] The multicenter Bevacizumab Regimens' Investigation of Treatment Effects (BRiTE) registry study found that in subjects with an intact primary tumor, the risk of perforation was higher than in subjects in whom the primary tumor had been resected (3 vs 1.7%).[51] These findings indicate that resection of the primary tumor does not eliminate the risk of perforation. Interestingly, perforations were seen not just at the primary tumor site but throughout the entire gastrointestinal tract. In another study, half of the subjects received bevacizumab (n = 112); of the 5 subjects with perforations at the primary tumor site, only 2 received bevacizumab at the time of the perforation.[46]

A phase II, prospective, single-arm study of primary systemic chemotherapy with mFOLFOX-6 and bevacizumab in subjects with unresectable stage IV colorectal cancer also found that an asymptomatic primary tumor may not need to be resected.[54] Eighty-six subjects from 29 institutions were evaluated. With a median follow-up of 20.7 months, most subjects were managed successfully without the need to resect the primary tumor. The median OS was 19.9 months, and the primary-tumor-associated morbidity rate was 16.3% at 24 months. The investigators concluded that this is an acceptable complication rate and that prophylactic resection is therefore unnecessary. Because the risk of perforation associated with bevacizumab is to some extent counterbalanced by the risk of anastomotic leak after resection, the risk of bevacizumab-associated perforation should not be used as the sole justification for upfront resection.

NONSURGICAL APPROACHES

Emergency operations for colorectal cancer are associated with high complication rates and often result in irreversible stomas, which have significant quality-of-life implications. One study found that surgery was associated with a complication rate of 30% and a hospital mortality rate of 8.5%.[55] When faced with a symptomatic, obstructing tumor in the setting of unresectable metastatic disease, clinicians must consider whether the morbidity of surgery can be avoided with less invasive techniques. Endoluminal therapy has the advantage of shorter hospital stay and less morbidity than resection or diversion.

Both laser therapy and fulguration have been used to palliate primary tumors. Laser therapy has been shown to be appropriate for rectosigmoid cancers. One study had an 85% success rate and a 2% complication rate in a series of 272 subjects.[56] In that series, subjects had functional improvement for an average of 10.1 months. One of the major disadvantages of laser therapy is that it is time-intensive and requires multiple treatments. Fulguration, another endoluminal technique, can also reduce the size of a distal tumor that is not amenable to resection and provide symptomatic relief.

Over the past 20 years, due to mixed results obtained with laser therapy and fulguration, colonic stents have become the preferred endoluminal therapy for obstructing or near-obstructing tumors. Colonic stents were first introduced in 1991 and have proven to be useful in patients who have unresectable metastatic disease or who need decompression of obstructed bowel as a bridge to resection.[57] Some investigators argue that stenting should not be performed for palliative decompression in patients receiving or expected to receive antiangiogenic therapy (eg, bevacizumab)[58] but this argument remains speculative.

One of the advantages of colonic stenting is that the procedure can be done under sedation. In addition to their effectiveness for rectosigmoid tumors, colonic stents have been shown to be effective for tumors in the ascending and transverse portions of the colon.[59] However, because colonic stenting requires special expertise, which is not universally available, resection remains an appropriate treatment of tumors obstructing the right colon.

Stenting is often not feasible for tumors obstructing the rectum because it may result in pain, tenesmus, and incontinence. Furthermore, due to the anatomy of the rectum, possible distal stent migration can result in significant symptoms and this risk usually precludes rectal stenting. Some initial studies on colonic stenting reported high rates of stent-associated perforation, and an earlier randomized controlled study was closed early due to a high perforation rate.[60] However, a more recent study reported a relatively low perforation rate of 5.2%.[61] This low rate may be due to better patient selection, improved technique, and/or the knowledge gained from early missteps.

In sum, endoluminal therapy, particularly colonic stenting, is an important alternative for treatment of obstructing or near-obstructing colorectal tumors when surgery is not desirable. Nevertheless, surgery remains the first-line treatment if an obstruction causes systemic toxicity with suspicion for peritonitis, bowel ischemia, or high-grade bowel obstruction with massive colonic distention.

SUMMARY

The decision of whether to resect the primary tumor in patients with stage IV colorectal cancer is multifactorial and includes the presence of symptoms and the resectability of metastatic disease. With the advent of modern therapeutic regimens, resection of the primary tumor does not seem to provide a survival benefit if the patient is asymptomatic. For symptomatic primary tumors, options include resection, diversion, and endoluminal therapy.

REFERENCES

1. Jemal A, Murray T, Ward E, et al. Cancer statistics, 2005. CA Cancer J Clin 2005; 55(1):10–30.
2. Ault GT, Cologne KG. Colorectal cancer: management of stage IV disease. In: Steele SR, Hull TL, Read ThE, et al, editors. The ASCRS textbook of colon and rectal surgery, vol. 1, 3rd edition. New York: Springer; 2016. p. 589–616.
3. Nordic Gastrointestinal Tumor Adjuvant Therapy Group. Expectancy or primary chemotherapy in patients with adjuvant asymptomatic colorectal cancer: a randomized trial. J Clin Oncol 1992;10:904–11.
4. Scheithauer W, Rosen H, Kornek GV, et al. Randomized comparison of combination chemotherapy plus supportive care alone in patients with metastatic colorectal cancer. Br Med J 1993;306:752–5.
5. Hurwitz H, Fehrenbacher L, Novotny W, et al. Bevacizumab plus irinotecan, fluorouracil, and leucovorin for metastatic colorectal cancer. N Engl J Med 2004;350: 2335–42.
6. Bokemeyer C, Bondarenko I, Makhson A, et al. Fluorouracil, leucovorin, and oxaliplatin with and without cetuximab in the first line treatment of metastatic colorectal cancer. J Clin Oncol 2009;27:663–71.
7. Tournigand C, André T, Achille E, et al. FOLFIRI followed by FOLFOX6 or the reverse sequence in advanced colorectal cancer: a randomized GERCOR study. J Clin Oncol 2004;22:229–37.
8. Chen CC, Yang SH, Lin JK, et al. Is it reasonable to add preoperative serum level of CEA and CA19-9 to staging for colorectal cancer? J Surg Res 2005;124: 169–74.
9. Deans GT, Krukowski ZH, Irwin ST. Malignant obstruction of the left colon. Br J Surg 1994;81:1270–6.
10. Van Hooft JE, Bemelman WA, Fockens P. A study of the value of colonic stenting as a bridge to elective surgery for the management of acute left-sided malignant colonic obstruction: the STENT-IN 2 study. Ned Tijdschr Geneeskd 2007;151: 1249–51 [in Dutch].
11. Chang GJ, Kaiser AM, Mills S, et al, Standards Practice Task Force of The American Society of Colon and Rectal Surgeons. Practice parameters for the management of colon cancer. Dis Colon Rectum 2012;55:831–43.
12. Smithers BM, Theile DE, Cohen JR, et al. Emergency right colectomy in colon carcinoma: a prospective study. Aust N Z J Surg 1986;56:749–52.
13. Leporrier J, Maurel J, Chiche L, et al. A population-based study of the incidence, management and prognosis of hepatic metastases from colorectal cancer. Br J Surg 2006;93:465–74.
14. Ruers T, Punt C, Van Coevorden F, et al. Radiofrequency ablation combined with systemic treatment versus systemic treatment alone in patients with nonresectable colorectal liver metastases: a randomized EORTC Intergroup phase II study (EORTC 40004). Ann Oncol 2012;23:2619–26.

15. Ruers T, Punt C, van Coevorden F, et al. Radiofrequency ablation (RFA) combined with chemotherapy for unresectable colorectal liver metastases (CRC LM): long-term survival results of a randomized phase II study of the EORTC-NCRI CCSG-ALM Intergroup 40004 (CLOCC). J Clin Oncol 2015;33;(suppl; abstr 3501).

16. Kimura F, Miyazaki M, Suwa T, et al. Reduced hepatic acute-phase response after simultaneous resection for gastrointestinal cancer with synchronous liver metastases. Br J Surg 1996;83:1002–6.

17. Lam VW, Laurence JM, Pang T, et al. A systematic review of a liver-first approach in patients with colorectal cancer and synchronous colorectal liver metastases. HPB (Oxford) 2014;16:101–8.

18. Martin R, Paty P, Fong Y, et al. Simultaneous liver and colorectal resections are safe for synchronous colorectal liver metastasis. J Am Coll Surg 2003;197:233–41.

19. Luo Y, Wang L, Chen C, et al. Simultaneous liver and colorectal resections are safe for synchronous colorectal liver metastases. J Gastrointest Surg 2010;14:1974–80.

20. Tanaka K, Shimada H, Matsuo K, et al. Outcome after simultaneous colorectal and hepatic resection for colorectal cancer with synchronous metastases. Surgery 2004;136:650–9.

21. Martin RCG 2nd, Augenstein V, Reuter NP, et al. Simultaneous versus staged resection for synchronous colorectal cancer liver metastases. J Am Coll Surg 2009;208:842–50.

22. Silberhumer GR, Paty PB, Denton B, et al. Long-term oncologic outcomes for simultaneous resection of synchronous metastatic liver and primary colorectal cancer. Surgery 2016;160:67–73.

23. Mayo SC, Pulitano C, Marques H, et al. Surgical management of patients with synchronous colorectal liver metastasis: a multicenter international analysis. J Am Coll Surg 2013;216:707–18.

24. Weber JC, Bachellier P, Oussoultzoglou E, et al. Simultaneous resection of colorectal primary tumour and synchronous liver metastases. Br J Surg 2003;90:956–62.

25. Capussotti L, Vigano L, Ferrero A, et al. Timing of resection of liver metastases synchronous to colorectal tumor: proposal of prognosis-based decisional model. Ann Surg Oncol 2007;14:1143–50.

26. Turrini O, Viret F, Guiramand J, et al. Strategies for the treatment of synchronous liver metastases. Eur J Surg Oncol 2007;33:735–40.

27. Reddy SK, Pawlik TM, Zorzi D, et al. Simultaneous resections of colorectal cancer and synchronous liver metastases: a multi-institutional analysis. Ann Surg Oncol 2007;14:3481–91.

28. Abbott DE, Cantor SB, Hu CY, et al. Optimizing clinical and economic outcomes of surgical therapy for patients with colorectal cancer and synchronous liver metastases. J Am Coll Surg 2012;215:262–70.

29. Yoshioka R, Hasegawa K, Mise Y, et al. Evaluation of the safety and efficacy of simultaneous resection of primary colorectal cancer and synchronous colorectal liver metastases. Surgery 2014;155:478–85.

30. Temple LK, Hsieh L, Wong WD, et al. Use of surgery among elderly patients with stage IV colorectal cancer. J Clin Oncol 2004;22:3475–84.

31. Cook AD, Single R, McCahill LE. Surgical resection of primary tumors in patients who present with stage IV colorectal cancer: an analysis of surveillance, epidemiology, and end results data, 1988 to 2000. Ann Surg Oncol 2005;12:637–45.

32. Scoggins CR, Meszoely IM, Blanke CD, et al. Nonoperative management of primary colorectal cancer in patients with stage IV disease. Ann Surg Oncol 1999;6: 651–7.

33. Sarela AI, Guthrie JA, Seymour MT, et al. Non-operative management of the primary tumor in patients with incurable stage IV colorectal cancer. Br J Surg 2001; 88:1352–6.

34. Ruo L, Gougoutas C, Paty PB, et al. Elective bowel resection for incurable stage IV colorectal cancer: prognostic variables for asymptomatic patients. J Am Coll Surg 2003;196:722–8.

35. Tebbutt NC, Norman AR, Cunningham D, et al. Intestinal complications after chemotherapy for patients with unresected primary colorectal cancer and synchronous metastases. Gut 2003;52:568–73.

36. Ahmed S, Leis A, Chandra-Kanthan S, et al. Surgical management of the primary tumor in stage IV colorectal cancer: a confirmatory retrospective cohort study. J Cancer 2016;7:837–45.

37. Clancy C, Burke JP, Barry M, et al. A meta-analysis to determine the effect of primary tumor resection for stage IV colorectal cancer with unresectable metastases on patient survival. Ann Surg Oncol 2014;21:3900–8.

38. Ducreux M, Bouche O, Pignon JP, et al. Randomized trial comparing three different schedules of infusional 5FU and raltitrexed alone as first-line therapy in metastatic colorectal cancer. Final results of the Federation Francophone de Cancerologie Digestive (FFCD) 9601 trial. Oncology 2006;70:222–30.

39. Ducreux M, Malka D, Mendiboure J, et al. Sequential versus combination chemotherapy for the treatment of advanced colorectal cancer (FFCD 2000-05): an open-label, randomized, phase 3 trial. Lancet Oncol 2011;12:1032–44.

40. Ducreux M, Adenis A, Mendiboure J, et al. Efficacy and safety of bevacizumab (BEV)-based combination regimens in patients with metastatic colorectal cancer (mCRC): randomized phase II study of BEV+FOLFIRI versus BEV+XELIRI (FNCLCC ACCORD-13/0503). Abstr Annu Meet Am Soc Clin Oncol 2009;27: 4086.

41. Ducreux M, Bennouna J, Hebbar M, et al. Capecitabine plus oxaliplatin (XELOX) versus 5-fluorouracil/leucovorin plus oxaliplatin (FOLFOX-6) as first-line treatment for metastatic colorectal cancer. Int J Cancer 2011;128:682–90.

42. Faron M, Pignon JP, Malka D, et al. Is primary tumor resection associated with survival improvement in patients with colorectal cancer and unresectable synchronous metastases? A pooled analysis of individual data from four randomized trials. Eur J Cancer 2015;51:166–76.

43. Koopman M, Antonini NF, Douma J, et al. Sequential versus combination therapy with capecitabine, irinotecan, and oxaliplatin in advanced colorectal cancer (CAIRO): a phase III randomized controlled trial. Lancet 2007;370:135–42.

44. Tol J, Koopman M, Rodenburg CJ, et al. A randomized phase III study on capecitabine, oxaliplatin and bevacizumab with or without cetuximab in first-line advanced colorectal cancer: the CAIRO2 study of the Dutch Colorectal Cancer Group (DCCG). An interim analysis of toxicity. Ann Oncol 2008;19:734–8.

45. Venderbosch S, de Wilt JH, Teerenstra S, et al. Prognostic value of resection of primary tumor in patients with stage IV colorectal cancer: retrospective analysis of two randomized studies and a review of literature. Ann Surg Oncol 2011;18: 3252–60.

46. Poultsides GA, Servais EL, Saltz LB, et al. Outcome of primary tumor in patients with synchronous stage IV colorectal cancer receiving combination chemotherapy without surgery as initial treatment. J Clin Oncol 2009;27:3379–84.

47. Van Steenbergen LN, Elferink MA, Krijnen P, et al. Improved survival of colon cancer due to improved treatment and detection: a nationwide population-base study in the Netherlands, 1989-2006. Ann Oncol 2010;21:2206–12.

48. Matsumoto T, Hasegawa S, Matsumoto S, et al. Overcoming the challenges of primary tumor management in patients with metastatic colorectal cancer unresectable for cure and an asymptomatic primary tumor. Dis Colon Rectum 2014; 57:679–86.

49. Liu SK, Church JM, Lavery IC, et al. Operation in patients with incurable colon cancer—is it worthwhile? Dis Colon Rectum 1997;40:11–4.

50. Seo GJ, Park JW, Yoo SB, et al. Intestinal complications after palliative treatment for asymptomatic patients with unresectable stage IV colorectal cancer. J Surg Oncol 2010;102:94–9.

51. Kozloff M, Yood MU, Berlin J, et al. Clinical outcomes associated with bevacizumab-containing treatment of metastatic colorectal cancer: the BRiTE observational cohort study. Oncologist 2009;14:862–70.

52. Saltz LB, Clarke S, Diaz-Rubio E, et al. Bevacizumab in combination with oxaliplatin-based chemotherapy as first-line therapy in metastatic colorectal cancer: a randomized phase III study. J Clin Oncol 2008;26:2013–9.

53. Giantonio BJ, Catalano PJ, Meropol NJ, et al. Bevacizumab in combination with oxaliplatin, fluorouracil, and leucovorin (FOLFOX 4) for previously treated metastatic colorectal cancer: results from the Eastern Cooperative Oncology Group Study E3200. J Clin Oncol 2007;25:1539–44.

54. McCahill LE, Yothers G, Sharif S, et al. Primary mFOLFOX6 plus bevacizumab without resection of the primary tumor for patients presenting with surgically unresectable metastatic colon cancer and an intact asymptomatic colon cancer: definitive analysis of NSABP trial C-10. J Clin Oncol 2012;30:3223–8.

55. Vemulapalli R, Lara LF, Sreenarasimhaiah J, et al. A comparison of palliative stenting or emergent surgery for obstructing incurable colon cancer. Dig Dis Sci 2010;55:1732–7.

56. Brunetaud JM, Maunoury V, Cochelard D. Lasers in rectosigmoid tumors. Semin Surg Oncol 1995;11:319–27.

57. Salvati EP, Rubin RJ, Eisenstat TE, et al. Electrocoagulation of selected carcinoma of the rectum. Surg Gynecol Obstet 1988;166:393–6.

58. Van Hooft JE, Van Halsema EE, Vanbiervliet G, et al. Self-expandable metal stents for obstructing colonic and extracolonic cancer: European Society of Gastrointestinal Endoscopy (ESGE) Clinical Guideline. Gastrointest Endosc 2014;80: 747–61.e1-75.

59. Dronamraju SS, Ramamurthy S, Kelly SB, et al. Role of self-expanding metallic stents in the management of malignant obstruction of the proximal colon. Dis Colon Rectum 2009;52:1657–61.

60. Van Hooft JE, Fockens P, Marinelli AW, et al. Early closure of a multicenter randomized clinical trial of endoscopic stenting versus surgery for stage IV left-sided colorectal cancer. Endoscopy 2008;40:184–91.

61. Choi JH, Lee YJ, Kim ES, et al. Covered self-expandable metal stents are more associated with complications in the management of malignant colorectal obstruction. Surg Endosc 2013;27:3220–7.

Cytoreduction and Hyperthermic Intraperitoneal Chemotherapy in the Management of Colorectal Peritoneal Metastasis

Bradley Hall, MD[a], James Padussis, MD[b], Jason M. Foster, MD[b],*

KEYWORDS

- Peritoneal metastasis (PM) • Cytoreductive surgery (CRS)
- Hyperthermic intraperitoneal chemotherapy (HIPEC)
- Intraperitoneal chemotherapy (IP) • Peritoneal carcinoma index (PCI)
- CC score • R score

KEY POINTS

- Patients with peritoneal metastasis have poor prognosis and symptoms due to untreated peritoneal disease are common.
- Outcomes compared with patients with hematogenous metastasis receiving the same systemic chemotherapy continue to demonstrate a worse prognosis.
- Published data in patients treated with CRS + HIPEC reveal a survival benefit similar that observed in the surgical management of hepatic metastasis.
- Clinical trials will continue help optimize the management of patients with peritoneal metastasis.

INTRODUCTION

Since the 1990s, increasing evidence supporting the surgical management of peritoneal metastasis (PM) with cytoreductive surgery (CRS) and hyperthermic intraperitoneal chemotherapy (HIPEC) has emerged, demonstrating improved survival and outcomes in highly-selected patients with several tumor histologies. The benefits of

Disclosures: The authors have nothing to disclose.
[a] Division of General Surgery, University of Nebraska Medical Center, 984030 Nebraska Medical Center, Omaha, NE 68198-4030, USA; [b] Division of Surgical Oncology, University of Nebraska Medical Center, 984030 Nebraska Medical Center, Omaha, NE 68198-4030, USA
* Corresponding author.
E-mail address: jfosterm@unmc.edu

Surg Clin N Am 97 (2017) 671–682
http://dx.doi.org/10.1016/j.suc.2017.01.013
0039-6109/17/© 2017 Elsevier Inc. All rights reserved.

CRS and HIPEC (CRS + HIPEC) for colorectal cancer (CRC) have recently become a central focus in the literature. This article provides an overview of the mechanism of PM, the utility of CRS + HIPEC in, and outcomes of patients with CRC with using chemotherapy therapy alone compared with CRS + HIPEC in conjunction with chemotherapy.

BACKGROUND

Distant CRC metastasis develops from either hematogenous dissemination or direct seeding of the peritoneal space. Metastasis is a complex process that involves cellular proliferation, immune system evasion, epithelial-mesenchymal transition and invasion, endothelial adhesion at metastatic sites, endothelial translocation, and growth at metastatic sites.[1] Although the liver is the most common site of metastasis, 15% to 25% of patients with stage IV CRC present with isolated PM (CRC-PM).[2] Although the cellular and biological events necessary to establish PM are similar to hematogenous metastasis, PM occurs after serosal disruption or perforation of the primary tumor (T4) or capsular disruption of nodal disease. This results in microscopic tumor shedding that disperses throughout the abdominal cavity. The capacity for tumors to grow on the surface of different abdominal organs is linked to specific biological changes of the tumor and the extent of disease can range from adjacent disease near the T4 site to extensive dissemination to all peritoneal surfaces.

The management of PM with CRS was initially established for appendiceal malignancies, peritoneal mesotheliomas, and ovarian cancers. High peritoneal recurrence rates in these patient populations fostered an interest in the development of intraperitoneal (IP) therapies, including HIPEC. In all of these tumors, data have demonstrated that CRS + HIPEC can decrease peritoneal recurrence and prolong overall survival (OS).

Hyperthermia alone is cytotoxic to cancer cells and its effect is potentiated when combined with chemotherapy.[3] Administering chemotherapy into the peritoneal cavity permits higher concentrations of the drug to be delivered directly to tumor cells with less systemic toxicity due to the peritoneal-plasma partition. This same partition may also be a factor in the reduced systemic chemotherapy (SC) response observed in patients with PM.[4] Overall, HIPEC permits administration of concentrated doses of chemotherapy 20 to 50 times more concentrated than serum levels seen with SC.[5] Heat also decreases interstitial pressure, allowing for optimal diffusion of chemotherapy and increases cytotoxicity, preferentially killing susceptible tumor cells. Penetration depths of 2 mm are common but 5 mm is possible with therapies such as oxaliplatin.

It has also been identified that some characteristics of tumor cells, such as mucin production, may be a factor in the chemotherapy refractory nature of PM relative to hematogenous metastasis. Mucins are glycoproteins that may support tumor cells survival in the peritoneal cavity with minimal vascular support and is a common feature in patients with PM. Animal models have been a major tool in studying the efficacy and mechanism of IP and HIPEC therapy.[6–9]

VALUE OF HYPERTHERMIC INTRAPERITONEAL CHEMOTHERAPY IN OTHER CANCERS

HIPEC has been used extensively in the management of appendiceal cancer with PM with a relatively large body of published data. Unfortunately, the low incidence of appendiceal tumors has been a barrier to conducting clinical trials. Evidence supporting the benefit of HIPEC in patients with low-grade pseudomyxoma peritonei was reported by Smeenk and colleagues.[10] The investigators reviewed the literature and compared the outcomes of patients treated with CRS alone versus CRS + HIPEC. The 10-year survival for CRS alone was 21% to 32% with 3% to 12% of patients free of disease, whereas in the CRS + HIPEC group 10-year survival was 60% to 80%, with 55% to 74% of patients free of disease.

HIPEC has been used in patients with advanced or recurrent ovarian cancer for many years, and randomized clinical trials (RCTs) have demonstrated both a progression free survival (PFS) and OS benefit compared with subjects who received intravenous chemotherapy only following optimal cytoreduction.[11–17] One of these RCTs, published in 2001, showed that IP chemotherapy prolonged PFS from 22.2 to 27.9 months and OS increased from 52.2 to 63.2 months compared with intravenous chemotherapy alone. Regardless of intervention, most patients with ovarian cancer present with advanced disease and 5-year OS is less than 50%.[14] **Table 1** summarizes relevant studies on CRS + HIPEC for patients with advanced ovarian cancer.

PATIENTS WITH COLORECTAL CANCER WITH PERITONEAL METASTASIS TREATED WITH CHEMOTHERAPY ALONE
Natural History

The EVOCAPE-1 study explored and reported the outcomes of subjects with peritoneal disease from gastrointestinal primary tumors. In subjects with CRC-PM who received no treatment, the median and mean survival was less than 6 months.[18] The cause of death in these subjects was due to bowel obstruction, fistula, or malnutrition; indirect consequences of PM and not directly due to overwhelming cancer burden. Thus an opportunity to extend survival in CRC-PM starts by controlling the peritoneal disease burden and reducing or delaying these events.

Table 1
Benefits of cytoreductive surgery and heated intraperitoneal chemotherapy in patients with advanced ovarian cancer

Authors	Number of Subjects	Treatment or Group	Median OS (mo)	Median PFS (mo)
Markman et al,[12] 2001	227	IV Paclitaxel, then IV cisplatin	52.2	22.2
	235	IV paclitaxel, then IV carboplatin and IV paclitaxel and IP cisplatin	63.2	27.9
Armstrong et al,[13] 2006	210	Paclitaxel IV followed IV cisplatin	49.7	18.3
	205	Paclitaxel IV followed IP cisplatin	65.5	23.8
Deraco et al,[15] 2011	26	CRS + HIPEC w/cisplatin and doxorubicin then IV carboplatin and paclitaxel	NA 60.7% (5-y survival)	30 (15.2% 5-y survival)
Bakrin et al,[16] 2013	474	Recurrent OEC CRS + HIPEC	45.7	NR
Spiliotis et al,[17] 2015	60	CRS + HIPEC + SC	26.7	NR
	60	CRS + SC	13.4	NR

Abbreviations: IV, intravenous; NA, not applicable; NR, not reported; OEC, ovarian epithelial cancer.
Data from Refs.[12,13,15–17]

Outcomes with Chemotherapy

Outcomes for CRC-PM subjects treated with SC are summarized in **Table 2**. Chemotherapy based on 5- fluorouracil (FU) alone or in combination with other agents has been the primary treatment option for patients with CRC-PM.[19] Current regimens include 5-FU and leucovorin combined with either oxaliplatin (FOLFOX) or irinotecan (FOLFIRI), as well as the possible addition of a biological agent such as bevacizumab or cetuximab. Clinical trials that established the benefit of these combinations have included both subjects with solid-organ metastases and with peritoneal disease. In general, survival has been shown to be worse for subjects with PM when compared with subjects who have solid-organ metastases and immeasurable peritoneal disease.[20–23] Both of these groups had improved survival when biological therapy was added.

CYTOREDUCTIVE SURGERY AND HYPERTHERMIC INTRAPERITONEAL CHEMOTHERAPY FOR COLORECTAL CANCER
Basic Principles

Patient selection for CRS + HIPEC is driven by the same principles in patient selection for the resection of metastatic disease to the liver. The 2 major factors include patient fitness for surgery and the ability to achieve a complete resection. To assess the overall burden of disease, scoring systems have been developed to help both select patients and help predict the relative benefit of CRS + HIPEC. The peritoneal carcinomatosis index (PCI) is a tool that measures disease burden. It can be determined radiographically before surgery with either computed tomography or MRI but is most accurately reported intraoperatively. The PCI divides the abdomen and pelvis into 13 domains, 4 of which are reserved for the small bowel. Disease severity in each domain is scored from 0 to 3, for a maximum score of 39, with higher scores associated with a worse prognosis. The PCI is predictive of long-term operative outcomes, and is used to select appropriate surgical candidates and evaluate response to chemotherapy.[24,25]

Once PCI is known, the next question is whether the tumor burden can be adequately cytoreduced. Two scoring systems commonly used are the completeness of cytoreduction score (CCS) and R score. The CCS was developed by Sugarbaker[25] as a scoring system for patients with PM. Scored CC-0 to 3, the CC score estimates the amount of residual disease at the completion of surgery. CC-0 denotes no visible residual disease, CC-1 if less than 2.5 mm in size, CC-2 for residual disease 2.5 mm to 2.5 cm in size, and CC-3 for anything larger than 2.5 cm.[25] R scoring is more widespread, with R0 indicating complete cytoreduction with negative margins, R1 indicating microscopically positive margins but no visible residual disease, and R2 indicating gross disease left behind. In the setting of residual disease, this is divided into R2a if less 5 mm, R2b if greater than 5 mm or less than 2 cm, and R2c if greater than 2 cm. Similar to the PCI, the CCS and R scores have been shown to be predictive of outcomes.[26]

Technical Details

CRS + HIPEC is typically performed for a highly selected group of patients. These patients typically have documented CRC and peritoneal carcinomatosis in the absence of solid-organ metastases. When these patients are identified, they will start with neoadjuvant SC, after which they are restaged to confirm there has not been any progression of disease. This prevents unnecessary operations for patients whose aggressive tumor biology negates the benefits of surgery.

Table 2
Outcomes with chemotherapy

Authors, Year	Subjects	Group	Treatment Regimen	PM (mo) Median OS	No PM (mo) Median OS
Klaver et al,[22] 2012 (CAIRO-1)	401	Sequential treatment	1st line: capecitabine 2nd line: irinotecan 3rd line: capecitabine + oxaliplatin	10.4	16.8
	402	Combination treatment	1st line: capecitabine + irinotecan 2nd line: capecitabine + oxaliplatin	7.8	17.9
Klaver et al,[22] 2012 (CAIRO-2)	192	Without cetuximab	Capecitabine + oxaliplatin + bevacizumab	15.2	21.4
	197	With cetuximab	Capecitabine + oxaliplatin + bevacizumab + cetuximab	13.9	20.4
Franko et al,[20] 2012 (N9741 and N9841)	2095	FU IFL or IRI IROX FOLFOX	Fluorouracil Irinotecan leucovorin, and fluorouracil or irinotecan Irinotecan and oxaliplatin IV 5-FU, leucovorin, and oxaliplatin	12.7	17.6

Data from Klaver YLB, Simkens LHJ, Lemmens VEPP, et al. Outcomes of colorectal cancer patients with peritoneal carcinomatosis treated with chemotherapy with and without targeted therapy. Eur J Surg Oncol 2012;38(7):617–23; and Franko J, Shi Q, Goldman, CD, et al. Treatment of colorectal peritoneal carcinomatosis with systemic chemotherapy: a pooled analysis of north central cancer treatment group phase III trials N9741 and N9841. J Clin Oncol 2012;30(3):263–7.

HIPEC can be administered through either an open or a closed approach. Both techniques involve placement of inflow and outflow catheters connected to a perfusion device. The perfusion device heats the solution and circulates the solution through the inflow tubes with passive outflow drainage. Typically, a volume of 3 to 5 L is used and the level of hyperthermia achieved in the solution is typically 39.5° to 42.5°C. Perfusion is typically performed for 60 to 120 minutes.

The open approach, although less common, allows the surgeon to manipulate internal organs to disperse chemotherapy throughout the peritoneal cavity and perform concomitant debulking. Although the open technique is safe, most institutions perform HIPEC with the closed technique. One concern many HIPEC providers have to consider when establishing the procedure at a new facility is the perceived potential for chemotherapy exposure. Stuart and colleagues[27] demonstrated that there is no significant risk of exposure with the open technique. The closed method does circumvent the theoretic exposure risk and it involves temporarily closing the skin before HIPEC administration with gentle external agitation of the abdomen to distribute the chemotherapy.

Agents Used

In the United States, mitomycin C (MMC) is the most common drug used during HIPEC. It can be administered in 2 ways. The first is a standard 30 mg dose for the first 60 minutes with an additional 10 mg given for the next 30 to 60 minutes. The second is based on body surface area and is commonly dosed at 15 mg/m^2. Oxaliplatin has recently become more prominent as monotherapy. It is typically dosed around 460 mg/m^2.[28]

OUTCOMES OF CYTOREDUCTIVE SURGERY AND HYPERTHERMIC INTRAPERITONEAL CHEMOTHERAPY IN COLORECTAL CANCER

Reports demonstrating the value of CRS + HIPEC in CRC-PM began to emerge in the 1990s. Most of the literature has emerged from a small group of highly specialized CRS + HIPEC enthusiasts. Results from the first RCT were published in 2003,[19] comparing CRS + HIPEC to SC alone (5-FU monotherapy). Palliative surgery for subjects in the SC-only arm was performed if needed, including bowel resection or stoma creation. HIPEC was performed in an open fashion over 90 minutes, with perfusate heated to 41° to 42°C, consisting of 17.5 mg/m^2 of MMC followed by 8.8 mg/m^2 every 30 minutes up to 70 mg. A minimum of 3L of perfusate was used with flow rates varying from 1 to 2 L/min. In this study of 105 subjects, SC median OS was 12.6 months and CRS + HIPEC improved the median OS to 22.4 months ($P = .032$). Completeness of cytoreduction and extent of disease were predictive of outcomes after CRS + HIPEC. Specifically, subjects in whom an R0/R1 resection was achieved had a 3-year survival of 95%.

In 2008, the investigators published 6-year follow-up data from the original study to report the long-term outcomes of CRS + HIPEC. The initial survival advantage was maintained with a 12.6 month median OS in the SC-only group and 22.2 months in the HIPEC group, identical to the previous results. In addition, the 5-year survival was 45% for an R0/R1 resection, demonstrating that the long-term survival benefits of CRS + HIPEC are similar to the outcomes reported in hepatic resection for CRC liver metastasis (LM).[29]

A 2009 retrospective case-control study focused on 48 CRS + HIPEC in CRC-PM subjects treated with contemporary chemotherapy regimens, including FOLFOX or FOLFIRI, and compared the outcomes to 48 historical controls with SC only. Optimal debulking was achieved in all 48 subjects. Although there were no significant differences in the chemotherapy regimens received, the CRS + HIPEC with SC group had a significantly longer survival with median OS of 62.7 months versus 23.9 months in subjects who received SC alone. Five-year survival rates were significantly higher in the CRS + HIPEC with SC group at 51% compared with 13% in the control arm (P<.05). No statistically significant differences in baseline subject characteristics were noted between the 2 arms other than there being older subjects in the control arm (51 years vs 46 years, P = .01). Tumors in the operative group were more frequently well-differentiated (P = .02).[28]

A 2010 multicenter French study analyzed 523 subjects who underwent CRS + HIPEC for CRC-PM, excluding appendiceal malignancies. For subjects undergoing CRS + HIPEC, median OS was 30.1 months with 5-year survival of 27%, comparable with previous studies. In this study, complete cytoreduction was obtained in 84% of subjects and predictors of a prolonged survival included complete cytoreduction, limited disease, no nodal involvement, and adjuvant SC.[30,31]

Outcomes for CRC-PM treated with CRS + HIPEC are outlined in **Table 3**. CRS + HIPEC has been shown to improve median OS by 12 to 40 months and it is associated with a 5-year OS of 27% to 45%, similar to survival rates reported for surgical resection of LM.[19,29,32–40]

The Role of Cytoreductive Surgery and Hyperthermic Intraperitoneal Chemotherapy in Patients with Both Peritoneal and Liver Metastasis

The liver is the most frequent site of metastasis in patients with CRC and patients with PM do present with synchronous LM. Few studies have investigated the utility of simultaneous resection of both LM and PM, and they have included a very small number of subjects because traditionally patients with solid-organ metastasis have been excluded from case series.

A 2013 systematic review demonstrated that survival for subjects treated with simultaneous resection for LM and PM (median OS 6–36 months) was shorter than subjects undergoing surgery for isolated PM (median OS 19–62.7 months). However,

Table 3
Outcomes for colorectal cancer present with isolated peritoneal metastasis treated with cytoreductive surgery and heated intraperitoneal chemotherapy

Author, Year	Number	Median OS (mo)	5-y Survival (%)
Verwaal et al,[19] 2003; Verwaal et al,[29] 2008	105	22	45
Glehen et al,[32] 2004	377	32	40
da Silva,[33] 2006	70	33	32
Shen et al,[34] 2008	121	34	26
Chua et al,[35] 2009	60	33	NA
Franko et al,[36] 2010	67	34	26
Elias et al,[30] 2010	523	30	27
Elias et al,[37] 2011	146	41	42
Ung et al,[38] 2013	211	47	42
Chua et al,[39] 2013	663	33	43
Esquivel et al,[40] 2014	705	41	58

Abbreviation: NA, not applicable.
Data from Refs.[19,29,30,32–40]

OS was superior to subjects who received SC only (median OS 5.2–23.9 months), demonstrating that simultaneous resection of LM and PM may be of benefit[41] for a highly selected group. Factors worthy of future investigation include the size, number, and location of lesions.[42]

Morbidity of Cytoreductive Surgery and Hyperthermic Intraperitoneal Chemotherapy

In general, CRS + HIPEC is a very complex procedure with high rates of associated complications, including major morbidity rates as high as 62% and mortality rates up to 10%.[43] This has limited the enthusiasm for CRS + HIPEC among some members of multidisciplinary cancer teams because the rewards from the procedure must obviously outweigh the risks. One of the oncologist's biggest fears is that patients who experience complications will require a significant break from SC, allowing for significant disease progression.

An up-to-date, single-center study from Roswell Park demonstrated that CRS + HIPEC can be safe overall when performed by experienced surgeons.[44] These investigators reported a 60-day mortality rate of 2.7% (3 out of 112 subjects). Although they did not report an overall morbidity rate, surgical site infection was encountered in 26% of subjects, with 5.3% having cardiopulmonary complications, and a 6.3% rate of unplanned return to the operating room. For subjects with CRC-PM, the investigators reported a 5-year OS of 38%.

A 2013 retrospective, single-center study from Wake Forest reported an overall morbidity of 62% with a mortality rate of 7.7%.[45] This group found that functional status, including Eastern Cooperative Oncology Group (ECOG) scores and health-related quality-of-life scores, was predictive of outcome. The same group looked at quality of life after CRS + HIPEC, demonstrating that emotional wellbeing is improved after surgery, despite high rates of morbidity, and that subjects return to their baseline level of function after 3 to 6 months.[46]

CONTROVERSIES AND ONGOING STUDIES

CRS + HIPEC is slowly gaining momentum as a viable treatment option for select patients with CRC-PM. However, there is still a great deal of variation in the components of HIPEC, including the chosen chemotherapeutic agents, dosage, the temperature of the circuit, and the duration of perfusion. Although most US centers use mitomycin as first-line therapy, oxaliplatin is still used in many European centers in conjunction with systemic administration of 5-FU.

To try and answer the question of which chemotherapy agent is more effective, the American Society of Peritoneal Surface Malignancies conducted a retrospective review of 15 international databases comparing the OS in patients who underwent CRS + HIPEC with oxaliplatin versus MMC. Although the median OS of the 539 subjects with complete cytoreduction was not significantly different between the oxaliplatin cohort versus the MMC cohort, subjects with low PCI scores had significantly longer survival in the MMC cohort (54.3 months vs 28.3 months, $P = .012$).[47] Given the retrospective nature of this study, further prospective studies comparing chemotherapy agents and duration of therapy are warranted.

Another area of debate is the value of HIPEC following optimal CRS, and whether every patient requires HIPEC. Recently, a French multicenter randomized controlled trial, Prodige 7, was designed to evaluate this question, randomizing subjects with complete cytoreduction to CRS alone versus CRS + HIPEC with oxaliplatin. This trial has recently met accrual and the outcomes are pending.

Another area of interest is defining the role of adjuvant CRS + HIPEC in patients with colon cancer at high risk of PM. One theory is by exploring high-risk patients with second-look surgery, occult disease may be identified and early CRS + HIPEC can be performed based on the detection of disease. Elias and colleagues[37] conducted an interesting prospective trial that conducted systematic second-look surgeries plus HIPEC in 41 asymptomatic subjects previously treated for their primary colorectal tumors who were deemed to be high risk for development of carcinomatosis. Subjects were considered high-risk if they met 1 of the following criteria found at the index operation: (1) macroscopically visible and completely resected carcinomatosis, (2) ovarian metastasis, or (3) perforated tumor. After surgical resection of the primary tumor, these subjects received adjuvant FOLFOX or FOLFIRI chemotherapy regimens for 6 months. After systemic therapy was complete, if there were no symptoms, nor radiologic evidence of recurrence, nor tumor marker elevation, subjects were taken for a second-look laparotomy. Remarkably, macroscopic peritoneal carcinomatosis (median PCI 7.8) was discovered in 56% of the cohort and an R0 resection with HIPEC was performed in all subjects. Long-term results have not yet been published but at a median follow-up of 30 months, 5-year OS was 90% and 5-year disease-free survival was 44%.[37]

A second theory is to treat all high-risk patients early, with no disease burden in high-risk patients, in an effort to prevent the establishment of bulky peritoneal disease. The ProphyloCHIP randomized controlled trial is currently being undertaken in France to evaluate whether systematic second-look surgery plus HIPEC improves disease-free survival and OS in high-risk patients. A similar trial, COLOPEC is a randomized trial currently being conducted at 9 Dutch HIPEC centers to investigate the effectiveness of adjuvant HIPEC in preventing the development of peritoneal carcinomatosis in patients who underwent curative resection for T4 or intra-abdominally perforated colon cancers. Subjects will be randomized to adjuvant HIPEC followed by routine SC in the experimental group versus routine SC in the control group. Primary endpoint is disease-free survival and diagnostic laparoscopy will be performed in all subjects at 18 months if no evidence of disease recurrence on clinical or radiographic examination.

SUMMARY

Similar to the management of hepatic metastasis, a subset of patients with PM can achieve long-term survival when complete resection of all visible disease is possible. CRS + HIPEC can be performed safely and the number of centers offering CRS + HIPEC is increasing worldwide. With increased adoption of CRS + HIPEC, multi-institutional research efforts to improve patient selection and optimize timing of intervention will improve outcomes for patients with CRC-PM.

REFERENCES

1. Jin K, Gao W, Lu Y, et al. Mechanisms regulating colorectal cancer cell metastasis into liver (Review). Oncol Lett 2012;3(1):11–5.
2. Siegel R, Naishadham D, Jemal A. Cancer statistics, 2012. CA Cancer J Clin 2012;62(1):10–29.
3. Pelz JO, Doerfer J, Hohenberger W, et al. A new survival model for hyperthermic intraperitoneal chemotherapy (HIPEC) in tumor-bearing rats in the treatment of peritoneal carcinomatosis. BMC cancer 2005;5(1):1.
4. Jacquet P, Sugarbaker PH. Clinical research methodologies in diagnosis and staging of patients with peritoneal carcinomatosis. In peritoneal carcinomatosis: principles of management. Springer US; Cancer Treat Res 1996;82:359–74.

5. Witkamp AJ, van Coevorden F, Kaag MM, et al. Dose finding study of hyperthermic intraperitoneal chemotherapy with mitomycin C in patients with carcinosis of colorectal origin. Eur J Surg Oncol 1998;24(214):18.

6. Ferron G, Gesson-Paute A, Classe JM, et al. Feasibility of laparoscopic peritonectomy followed by intra-peritoneal chemohyperthermia: an experimental study. Gynecol Oncol 2005;99(2):358–61.

7. Zeamari S, Floot B, Van der Vange N, et al. Pharmacokinetics and pharmacodynamics of cisplatin after intraoperative hyperthermic intraperitoneal chemoperfusion (HIPEC). Anticancer Res 2002;23(2B):1643–8.

8. Esquis P, Consolo D, Magnin G, et al. High intra-abdominal pressure enhances the penetration and antitumor effect of intraperitoneal cisplatin on experimental peritoneal carcinomatosis. Ann Surg 2006;244(1):106–12.

9. Facy O, Al Samman S, Magnin G, et al. High pressure enhances the effect of hyperthermia in intraperitoneal chemotherapy with oxaliplatin: an experimental study. Ann Surg 2012;256(6):1084–8.

10. Smeenk RM, Verwaal VJ, Antonini N, et al. Survival analysis of pseudomyxoma peritonei patients treated by cytoreductive surgery and hyperthermic intraperitoneal chemotherapy. Ann Surg 2007;245(1):104–9.

11. Alberts DS, Liu PY, Hannigan EV, et al. Intraperitoneal cisplatin plus intravenous cyclophosphamide versus intravenous cisplatin plus intravenous cyclophosphamide for stage III ovarian cancer. N Engl J Med 1996;335(26):1950–5.

12. Markman M, Bundy BN, Alberts DS, et al. Phase III trial of standard-dose intravenous cisplatin plus paclitaxel versus moderately high-dose carboplatin followed by intravenous paclitaxel and intraperitoneal cisplatin in small-volume stage III ovarian carcinoma: an intergroup study of the Gynecologic Oncology Group, Southwestern Oncology Group, and Eastern Cooperative Oncology Group. J Clin Oncol 2001;19(4):1001–7.

13. Armstrong DK, Bundy B, Wenzel L, et al. Intraperitoneal cisplatin and paclitaxel in ovarian cancer. N Engl J Med 2006;354(1):34–43.

14. Coleman RL, Monk BJ, Sood AK, et al. Latest research and treatment of advanced-stage epithelial ovarian cancer. Nat Rev Clin Oncol 2013;10(4): 211–24.

15. Deraco M, Kusamura S, Virzì S, et al. Cytoreductive surgery and hyperthermic intraperitoneal chemotherapy as upfront therapy for advanced epithelial ovarian cancer: multi-institutional phase-II trial. Gynecol Oncol 2011;122(2):215–20.

16. Bakrin N, Bereder JM, Decullier E, et al. Peritoneal carcinomatosis treated with cytoreductive surgery and Hyperthermic Intraperitoneal Chemotherapy (HIPEC) for advanced ovarian carcinoma: a French multicentre retrospective cohort study of 566 patients. Eur J Surg Oncol 2013;39(12):1435–43.

17. Spiliotis J, Halkia E, Lianos E, et al. Cytoreductive surgery and HIPEC in recurrent epithelial ovarian cancer: a prospective randomized phase III study. Ann Surg Oncol 2015;22(5):1570–5.

18. Sadeghi B, Arvieux C, Glehen O, et al. Peritoneal carcinomatosis from non-gynecologic malignancies. Cancer 2000;88(2):358–63.

19. Verwaal VJ, van Ruth S, de Bree E, et al. Randomized trial of cytoreduction and hyperthermic intraperitoneal chemotherapy versus systemic chemotherapy and palliative surgery in patients with peritoneal carcinomatosis of colorectal cancer. J Clin Oncol 2003;21(20):3737–43.

20. Franko J, Shi Q, Goldman CD, et al. Treatment of colorectal peritoneal carcinomatosis with systemic chemotherapy: a pooled analysis of north central cancer treatment group phase III trials N9741 and N9841. J Clin Oncol 2012;30(3):263–7.

21. Koopman M, Antonini NF, Douma J, et al. Sequential versus combination chemotherapy with capecitabine, irinotecan, and oxaliplatin in advanced colorectal cancer (CAIRO): a phase III randomised controlled trial. Lancet 2007;370(9582): 135–42.

22. Klaver YLB, Simkens LHJ, Lemmens VEPP, et al. Outcomes of colorectal cancer patients with peritoneal carcinomatosis treated with chemotherapy with and without targeted therapy. Eur J Surg Oncol 2012;38(7):617–23.

23. Tol J, Koopman M, Rodenburg CJ, et al. A randomised phase III study on capecitabine, oxaliplatin and bevacizumab with or without cetuximab in first-line advanced colorectal cancer, the CAIRO2 study of the Dutch Colorectal Cancer Group (DCCG). An interim analysis of toxicity. Ann Oncol 2008;2008(19):734–8.

24. Sugarbaker PH. Successful management of microscopic residual disease in large bowel cancer. Cancer Chemother Pharmacol 1999;43(1):S15–25.

25. Portilla AG, Sugarbaker PH, Chang D. Second-look surgery after cytoreduction and intraperitoneal chemotherapy for peritoneal carcinomatosis from colorectal cancer: analysis of prognostic features. World J Surg 1999;23(1):23–9.

26. Sugarbaker PH, Chang D. Results of treatment of 385 patients with peritoneal surface spread of appendiceal malignancy. Ann Surg Oncol 1999;6(8):727–31.

27. Stuart OA, Stephens AD, Welch L, et al. Safety monitoring of the coliseum technique for heated intraoperative intraperitoneal chemotherapy with mitomycin C. Ann Surg Oncol 2002;9(2):186–91.

28. Elias D, Lefevre JH, Chevalier J, et al. Complete cytoreductive surgery plus intraperitoneal chemohyperthermia with oxaliplatin for peritoneal carcinomatosis of colorectal origin. J Clin Oncol 2009;27(5):681–5.

29. Verwaal VJ, Bruin S, Boot H, et al. 8-year follow-up of randomized trial: cytoreduction and hyperthermic intraperitoneal chemotherapy versus systemic chemotherapy in patients with peritoneal carcinomatosis of colorectal cancer. Ann Surg Oncol 2008;15(9):2426–32.

30. Elias D, Gilly F, Boutitie F, et al. Peritoneal colorectal carcinomatosis treated with surgery and perioperative intraperitoneal chemotherapy: retrospective analysis of 523 patients from a multicentric French study. J Clin Oncol 2010;28(1):63–8.

31. Esquivel J. Cytoreductive surgery and hyperthermic intraperitoneal chemotherapy for colorectal cancer: survival outcomes and patient selection. J Gastrointest Oncol 2016;7(1):72–8.

32. Glehen O, Kwiatkowski F, Sugarbaker PH, et al. Cytoreductive surgery combined with perioperative intraperitoneal chemotherapy for the management of peritoneal carcinomatosis from colorectal cancer: a multi-institutional study. J Clin Oncol 2004;22(16):3284–92.

33. da Silva RG, Sugarbaker PH. Analysis of prognostic factors in seventy patients having a complete cytoreduction plus perioperative intraperitoneal chemotherapy for carcinomatosis from colorectal cancer. J Am Coll Surg 2006;203(6): 878–86.

34. Shen P, Thai K, Stewart JH, et al. Peritoneal surface disease from colorectal cancer: comparison with the hepatic metastases surgical paradigm in optimally resected patients. Ann Surg Oncol 2008;15(12):3422–32.

35. Chua TC, Yan TD, Ng KM, et al. Significance of lymph node metastasis in patients with colorectal cancer peritoneal carcinomatosis. World J Surg 2009;33(7): 1488–94.

36. Franko J, Ibrahim Z, Gusani NJ, et al. Cytoreductive surgery and hyperthermic intraperitoneal chemoperfusion versus systemic chemotherapy alone for colorectal peritoneal carcinomatosis. Cancer 2010;116(16):3756–62.

37. Elias D, Honore C, Dumont F, et al. Results of systematic second-look surgery plus HIPEC in asymptomatic patients presenting a high risk of developing colorectal peritoneal carcinomatosis. Ann Surg 2011;254(2):289–93.

38. Ung L, Chua TC, Morris DL. Peritoneal metastases of lower gastrointestinal tract origin: a comparative study of patient outcomes following cytoreduction and intraperitoneal chemotherapy. J Cancer Res Clin Oncol 2013;139(11):1899–908.

39. Chua TC, Esquivel J, Pelz JO, et al. Summary of current therapeutic options for peritoneal metastases from colorectal cancer. J Surg Oncol 2013;107(6):566–73.

40. Esquivel J, Lowy AM, Markman M, et al. The American Society of Peritoneal Surface Malignancies (ASPSM) multiinstitution evaluation of the Peritoneal Surface Disease Severity Score (PSDSS) in 1,013 patients with colorectal cancer with peritoneal carcinomatosis. Ann Surg Oncol 2014;21(13):4195–201.

41. De Cuba EMV, Kwakman R, Knol DL, et al. Cytoreductive surgery and HIPEC for peritoneal metastases combined with curative treatment of colorectal liver metastases: systematic review of all literature and meta-analysis of observational studies. Cancer Treat Rev 2013;39(4):321–7.

42. Delhorme JB, Dupont-Kazma L, Addeo P, et al. Peritoneal carcinomatosis with synchronous liver metastases from colorectal cancer: Who will benefit from complete cytoreductive surgery? Int J Surg 2016;25:98–105.

43. Halkia E, Kopanakis N, Nikolaou G, et al. Cytoreductive surgery and HIPEC for peritoneal carcinomatosis. A review on morbidity and mortality. J BUON 2015; 20(Suppl 1):S80–7.

44. Haslinger M, Francescutti V, Attwood K, et al. A contemporary analysis of morbidity and outcomes in cytoreduction/hyperthermic intraperitoneal chemoperfusion. Cancer Med 2013;2(3):334–42.

45. Ihemelandu CU, McQuellon R, Shen P, et al. Predicting postoperative morbidity following cytoreductive surgery with hyperthermic intraperitoneal chemotherapy (CS+HIPEC) with preoperative FACT-C (Functional Assessment of Cancer Therapy) and patient-rated performance status. Ann Surg Oncol 2013;20:3519–26.

46. Hill AR, McQuellon RP, Russell GB, et al. Survival and quality of lie following cytoreductive surgery plus hypothermic intraperitoneal chemotherapy for peritoneal carcinomatosis of colonic origin. Ann Surg Oncol 2011;18:3673–9.

47. Prada-Villaverde A, Esquivel J, Lowy AM, et al. The American Society of Peritoneal Surface Malignancies evaluation of HIPEC with Mitomycin C versus Oxaliplatin in 539 patients with colon cancer undergoing a complete cytoreductive surgery. J Surg Oncol 2014;110(7):779–85.

Molecular Markers for Colorectal Cancer

Moriah Wright, MD[a], Jenifer S. Beaty, MD[b,c], Charles A. Ternent, MD[b,c],*

KEYWORDS

- Colorectal neoplasm • Drug therapy • Antineoplastic combined chemotherapy
- Biomarkers • Tumor/genetics • Antibodies • Monoclonal/therapeutic use

KEY POINTS

- Colorectal carcinoma develops through 3 main pathways, including chromosomal instability, mismatch repair, and methylator phenotype.
- Microsatellite instability (MSI) is a marker of mismatch repair, which occurs from MLH1 gene mutation as in Lynch syndrome or from sporadic silencing of a normal MLH1 gene via promoter hypermethylation.
- Anti–vascular endothelial growth factor therapy is preferred over anti–epidermal growth factor receptor therapy for metastatic colorectal cancers with KRAS gene mutation.
- High MSI colorectal cancer with BRAF gene mutation is most likely associated with sporadic nature rather than with Lynch syndrome.
- Programmed cell death protein 1 receptors in T cells are used by colorectal cancer cells to downregulate the antitumor effects of the immune system.

INTRODUCTION

Colorectal cancer (CRC) is the third most common cancer in the world. There has been abundant research on its pathophysiology and treatment. CRC has variable genetic signatures, which can be as unique as the individual host. CRC develops through at least 3 major pathways, which include chromosomal instability, mismatch repair, and methylator phenotype. These pathways can coexist in a single CRC and result in neoplasms with distinct genotype and phenotype. These major pathways of tumorigenesis can be present in both sporadic and inherited CRC. In spite of the unique molecular and genetic signatures of individual CRCs, nonspecific chemotherapy based on the antineoplastic effects of 5-fluorouracil (5-FU) is the cornerstone of therapy for stage III and some stage II disease. More recently, 5-FU-leucovorin-oxaliplatin

Disclosures: The authors have nothing to disclose.
[a] Colon and Rectal Surgery, Inc, 9850 Nicholas Street, Suite 100, Omaha, NE 68114, USA;
[b] Department of Surgery, CHI Creighton University Medical Center Bergan Mercy, 7500 Mercy Road, Omaha, NE 68124, USA; [c] Department of Surgery, University of Nebraska Medical Center, S 42nd Street and Emile Street, Omaha, NE 68198, USA
* Corresponding author. 9850 Nicholas Street, Suite 100, Omaha, NE 68114.
E-mail address: Cat@colonrectalsurgeons.com

(FOLFOX) has become the standard of care for CRC adjuvant therapy. Additional therapies have emerged to treat CRC based on the specific molecular markers present. Techniques to recognize CRC at the molecular and genetic levels have facilitated the development of new signature drugs designed to inhibit the unique pathways of CRC growth and immunity. This article focuses on the new developments in molecular markers associated with CRC with emphasis on the clinical implications and relevance for the practicing physician.

DEVELOPMENT OF CARCINOMA PATHWAYS
Chromosomal Instability

Fearon and Vogelstein[1] first described the well-known adenoma-to-carcinoma sequence for CRC in 1990. This pathway details the multiple mutations required to progress from normal colonic mucosa to carcinoma. At the time of original introduction of the adenoma-to-carcinoma sequence, it was understood that the accumulation of genetic mutations is what actually leads to carcinogenesis, rather than the specific order of mutations. Therefore, this pathway for colorectal neoplasia was coined the chromosomal instability (CIN) pathway.[2] The adenoma-to-carcinoma sequence is generally described as a stepwise process starting with mutation of the adenomatous polyposis coli (APC) gene, a tumor suppressor gene, which regulates neoplasia prevention in its wild state. APC mutations are also the most common mutation in this CIN pathway, affecting up to 85% of patients with sporadic CRC.[3] APC mutations are generally followed by mutations in KRAS, deleted in CRC, and p53 genes on the path to carcinoma.[1] The accumulation of genetic mutations by the natural tendency of chromosomal instability, with loss of complementary chromosomal pairs known as loss of heterozygosity, leads to inherent risk of neoplasia. These deleterious genetic mutations can interfere with downstream cellular function pathways such as those associated with programmed cell death (apoptosis). Interference with apoptosis can result in immortal cells and neoplasms.

Adenomatous polyposis coli

APC gene mutations are present in most CRCs, giving rise to the APC gene tumor suppressor role as a gatekeeper mutation in CRC.[3] APC is part of the Wnt signaling pathway that regulates cytoplasmic levels of B-catenin, which is involved in cytoskeletal integrity.[3] The Wnt pathway is important in organ development, cellular proliferation, morphology, motility, and fate of embryonic stem cells.[4] Increased levels of B-catenin that result from APC mutation or enhanced expression can lead to increased levels of c-myc, a known factor in cell proliferation.[4] The relationship between APC, B-catenin, c-myc, and cytoskeleton integrity results in APC becoming part of the cell-cell adhesion complex. Therefore, mutations in APC may result in poor cell-cell adhesion and cell migration.[4]

When functioning appropriately, the APC gene is responsible for maintaining the normal direction of upward movement of specialized colonic epithelial cells toward the gut lumen.[4] Cells with mutations in APC tend to migrate aberrantly or less efficiently toward the crypt base where they accumulate and form neoplastic polyps.[4] APC gene mutations are, therefore, associated with the tendency to form adenomatous polyps in the gastrointestinal (GI) tract, which carry a risk of carcinoma.

KRAS

The next most common mutation in the traditional CIN pathway to neoplasia is KRAS, which is part of a mitogen-activated protein kinase (MAPK) pathway. Alterations in this pathway are generally found in both the tumor and its metastases, indicating that these mutations occur early in carcinogenesis.[5] MAPK forms major cell-proliferation signaling pathways from the cell surface to the nucleus which are basic to regulation of cell function.[6] There are 3 main MAPK pathways: extracellular-signal-related kinases (ERK MAPK, Ras/Raf1/Mek/Erk); c-Jun N-terminal (JNK) or stress-activated protein kinases; and MAPK14 (**Fig. 1**). It is well documented that these signaling cascades lead to altered gene expression.[7] The pathway most connected with the pathogenesis, progression, and oncogenic behavior of CRC is the ERK MAPK pathway.[6] This pathway is one of the most important for cell proliferation and is frequently stimulated by binding of the growth factors to receptors in the cell membrane.[6] One such receptor is epidermal growth factor receptor (EGFR).

The ERK pathway includes several proto-oncogenes and is deregulated in about 30% of CRC.[6] This cascade is involved in the control of growth signals and cell survival.[8] Ras is mutated in 36% of CRCs.[9] Oncogenic activation of KRAS mutations seems to consistently follow APC inactivation during tumor progression.[3] Mutation in KRAS confers elevated Ras activity that is accompanied by increased ERK activity uncoupled from EGFR stimulation.[6]

In cases of KRAS-mutated metastatic colorectal neoplasia, an anti-vascular endothelial growth factor (VEGF) agent used along with metastatic chemotherapy, such as

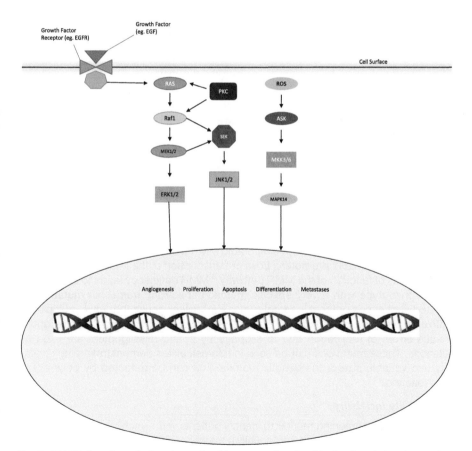

Fig. 1. MAPK signaling. Serine-threonine kinases are involved in 3 related signal transduction cascades activated by stimuli, such as growth factors, stress, and inflammation.

FOLFOX, provides added survival advantage. In wild-type KRAS gene status, adding an anti-EGFR therapy to the standard FOLFOX regimen provides targeted treatment. The anti-EGFR agent binds to EGFR preventing downstream activation of the ERK MAPK pathway, resulting in improved survival when combined with FOLFOX.

BRAF

BRAF, a serine-threonine kinase of the Raf family, is another member of the ERK MAPK pathway. Mutations in BRAF are present in 5% to 15% of CRCs[5] and are associated with increased kinase activity.[6] Mutations in BRAF have a less clear effect on responsiveness to anti-EGFR chemotherapy.[2] BRAF is, however, important in determining prognosis because mutations of this gene are associated with worsened survival and are a negative prognostic indicator.

P53

The final step in the adenoma-to-carcinoma sequence is mutation in p53. This protein preserves the cell cycle and genomic stability. P53 is a tumor suppressor gene that stops the cell cycle in the G1/S phase to allow repair of mutations or replications. If these errors cannot be repaired, then wild-type p53 will induce apoptosis. Therefore, p53 mutations will inhibit apoptosis. Mutations in p53 are rarely found in adenomas (5%) but are increasingly common in malignant polyps (50%) and invasive CRCs (75%).[10] P53 mutation is a key event in the pathogenesis of CRC, which results in tumor genomic chaos and conversion from benign to malignant cells.[3]

Mismatch Repair

Another well-known carcinogenesis pathway is the DNA mismatch repair (MMR) pathway. MMR genes code for proteins that band together to repair occurring DNA mutations. Genetic and epigenetic inactivation of MMR genes leads to multiple mutations and cancer development.[11] This pathway is associated with Lynch syndrome and microsatellite instability (MSI). Microsatellites are noncoding segments of DNA that contain repetitive sequences of 1 to 4 nucleotides. Microsatellites occur throughout the genome. About 15% of CRCs arise from this MMR pathway: 12% are sporadic from somatic mutations or epigenetic mechanisms and the remaining 3% are from germline mutations associated with Lynch syndrome.[2] There are 4 genes that are most associated with MMR: MLH1, MSH2, MSH6, and PMS2.[2]

Mismatch Repair Protein Deficiency

MLH1 is the most common source of sporadic MMR deficiency and is primarily due to methylation of the MLH1 promoter.[2] Loss of transcription of the MLH1 gene results in complete loss of function of the MMR pathway.[3] MMR deficiency leads to an elevated mutator phenotype with a very specific mutation spectrum: frameshift mutations in repeated sequences present in target tumor suppressor genes that have multiple repetitive sequences prone to DNA mismatch.[11] When the MMR mechanism fails, spontaneous errors of replication due to slippage by strand misalignment are fixed as mutations. These mutations can be seen in microsatellites demonstrating high instability and variable size of the genetic material that can be detected by polymerase chain reaction.[11]

Microsatellite Instability

MSI is useful as a screening marker to identify patients with Lynch syndrome. It is also a marker of better prognosis and potentially a marker of chemotherapy efficacy in sporadic and inherited CRC.[11] The standard MSI testing recommended by the National Cancer Institute is analysis of both the tumor and normal, noncancerous tissues by using 5 microsatellite markers, including 2 mononucleotide repeats (BAT26 and BAT25) and 3 dinucleotide repeats (D2S123, D5S346, and D17S250).[11] Tumors then fall into 3 groups: greater than 30% to 40% of markers showing instability (MSI-high [MSI-H]), less than 30% to 40% of the markers showing instability, and no instability (microsatellite stable [MSS]).[11]

Approximately 70% of MSI-H CRCs are proximal to the splenic flexure. MSI-H CRCs are more likely to contain mucin, be poorly differentiated, and possess subepithelial lymphoid aggregates and intraepithelial lymphocytes.[3,11] This immune response seems to be favorable for prognosis.[3,11] Sporadic CRC with MSI-H and Lynch syndrome-associated CRCs have similar morphologic features; however, mucin secretion, poor differentiation, tumor heterogeneity, and glandular serration with coexisting serrated polyps are more evident in sporadic CRC.[11]

An important factor when treating MSI-H tumors is whether or not a BRAF mutation is present; MMR proficient tumors that have a BRAF mutation have a substantially worse prognosis than BRAF wild-type tumors. The same applies to metastatic MMR-deficient tumors.[2] BRAF mutation is associated with high-risk characteristics: lymph node metastasis, high-grade T4 tumors, mucinous histology, MSI, and right-side location.[12,13]

CpG Island Methylator Phenotype

The final major pathway to carcinoma is the CpG Island Methylator Phenotype (CIMP) pathway. CpG islands are CG-rich stretches of DNA that occur in half of all gene promoters.[2] These islands are usually unmethylated in non-neoplastic cells; methylation silences the activity of these genes.[2] In mammals, methylation is essential for normal development; it is thought to have evolved to silence repetitive elements.[14] This pathologic methylation triggers the binding of methylated DNA-specific binding proteins to these CpG sites, which attracts histone-modifying enzymes that focally establish a silenced chromatin state.[14] CIMP is known to be present in multiple types of cancer; these cancer cells often have a loss of global methylation and a gain of methylation at the promoters of selected CpG islands.[14] This state results in the silencing of hundreds of nonmutated genes per cancer cell, some of which are tumor-suppressor genes.[14]

There is considerable overlap between CIMP and MSI-H pathways; CIMP has been proposed to explain the silencing of the MLH1 gene in sporadic cancers with MSI-H.[11] This proposal is supported by the observation that inhibition of methylation reversed the MMR defect in a colon cancer cell line.[14] CIMP CRCs are often defined by the presence of this excessive methylation; however, there are no universally accepted criteria to define a tumor as CIMP-high.

Investigators studying this pathway have used the presence of 3 or more from a selected panel of 5 genes (RUNX3, SOCS1, NEUROG1, CACNA1G, IGF2) to define the CIMP-high methylator phenotype.[3] CIMP-high CRC tends to occur in older patients, women, and in the proximal colon.[14] CIMP-high occurs in about 20% of sporadic CRCs, and these tumors demonstrate BRAF mutation and hypermethylation of MLH1 primarily.[3] CIMP-high in turn constitutes most MSI-H cancers. CIMP-H tumors have a paucity of p53 mutations and a high rate of KRAS or BRAF mutations.[14] This pattern is observed in the pathogenesis of sessile serrated adenomas.[3] However, CIMP status has not yet proved to be a useful clinical tool or biomarker.[3] Nevertheless, BRAF mutation can be used as a surrogate for CIMP-high.[11]

There is a strong correlation between CIMP and V600E mutation in BRAF.[2] This correlation can serve as a surrogate marker for MLH1 promoter methylation testing. Sixty percent of MSI-H with a V600E BRAF mutation is associated with sporadic CRC. Because of the ease of testing and the expression pattern, BRAF V600E testing may prove to be useful in the screening of Lynch syndrome families.[11] MSI-H CRC with a V600E BRAF mutation is considered more likely to be sporadic versus Lynch syndrome.

Serrated adenomas

The recognition of MSI-H CRC as a pathologically distinct pathway led investigators to reevaluate hyperplastic polyps and serrated adenomas.[14] Histologic similarities between these lesions, as well as co-occurrence of unusual tumors and compelling molecular data, have led to the identification of some hyperplastic polyps as precursors to serrated adenomas.[14] The evidence for hyperplastic polyps being precursors for CRC is derived from studies that show some of these lesions are associated with KRAS mutations.[15–17] When hyperplastic polyps contain focal areas of dysplasia they become serrated adenomas.[17] It has been shown that serrated adenomas and hyperplastic polyps are more likely to occur in patients with MSI-H tumors.[18] Hyperplastic polyps in patients with MSI-H are more likely to have loss of MLH1 protein expression, suggesting they may be important precursor lesions.[14,18] Remarkable similarities exist between proximal hyperplastic polyps, serrated adenomas, and CIMP-high CRC; these include high degree of methylation of multiple genes, frequent mutations in BRAF, and shared histologic features like serration.[14] Serrated adenomas are considered a higher-risk colorectal polyp, and closer surveillance is usually recommended.

SPREAD OF DISEASE AND CHEMOPREVENTION
Metalloproteinases and Metastasis

Matrix metalloproteinases (MMPs) are proteolytic enzymes; most are activated by serine proteases or by other activated MMPs.[19] They are essential in the interplay between tumor and stromal cells.[19] High levels of expression of multiple MMPs are reportedly correlated with advanced tumor stage, invasion, metastasis, and decreased survival in many tumors.[19] MMP-9 is produced by many tumor cells, including CRC, and is involved in tumor invasion and metastasis.[20] MMP-9 is capable of degrading the basement membrane and type IV collagen in the extracellular matrix, resulting in both tumor invasion and ability to metastasize.[20]

Tissue inhibitor of metalloproteases 1 (TIMP-1) is a glycoprotein found in the extracellular compartment that works as an endogenous inhibitor of MMPs.[21] This protein can have tumor-promoting effects, including the stimulation of cell proliferation, prevention of apoptosis, and support of angiogenesis.[21] TIMP-1 is known to bind MMP-9 in a 1:1 proportion, and increased expression correlates with overexpression of MMP-9.[20] High baseline plasma TIMP-1 levels have consistently been associated with poor prognosis in patients with primary or advanced CRC; any subsequent increase also has a poor prognosis. Tarpgaard and colleagues[21] tested interactions between plasma TIMP-1 levels and EGFR targeted treatment using data from the NORDIC VII study. They found no difference in baseline levels between those who benefitted from cetuximab treatment and those who did not. They did find an association between high plasma TIMP-1 levels and benefit from adding cetuximab to FOLFOX in patients with KRAS-mutated tumors. They also noted a strong prognostic effect of plasma TIMP-1 levels, irrespective of treatment.

Both MMP and TIMP have been proposed to play a role not only in colorectal tumor invasion and the initiation of metastasis but also in colorectal carcinogenesis.[20] The expression on MMP-9 is much higher in CRC than in adenomas or normal colonic tissue.[20]

Cyclooxygenase inhibitors

Cancer chemoprevention or cancer chemo-protection is defined as the inhibition, retardation, or reversal of carcinogenesis by chemical or pharmaceutical means.[22]

For many years, observational studies consistently reported a 40% to 50% lower CRC risk in people who regularly take aspirin or other nonsteroidal antiinflammatory medications (NSAIDs).[23–25] NSAIDs produce their analgesic, antipyretic, and antiinflammatory effects by inhibiting the enzyme cyclooxygenase (COX).[22] COX converts arachidonic acid found in the cell membrane to prostacyclin, thromboxanes, and various prostaglandins. Each of these compounds has its own effect on cell function and physiology. There are 2 isoforms of COX: COX-1 is expressed constitutively in most tissues and performs housekeeping and mediates physiologic functions; COX-2 is only expressed in certain tissues, such as the kidney, brain, and pancreatic islet cells. COX-2 can be induced in response to cytokines and growth factors in inflammatory conditions. Immunohistochemical studies have demonstrated that, apart from areas of inflammation, COX-2 is upregulated and overexpressed in 40% of colorectal adenomas and in 85% of CRCs.[26–28] Increased COX-2 expression and increased levels of prostaglandins, particularly prostaglandin E2, have been shown to stimulate cellular proliferation and angiogenesis.[29,30] These cells are also noted to be more attached to the extracellular matrix and, therefore, more resistant to apoptosis.[30] By inhibiting these mechanisms, COX-2 inhibitors are thought to exert a negative influence on carcinogenesis.

There is also evidence that COX inhibitors can inhibit tumorigenesis via antiproliferative and proapoptotic effects on cancer cells devoid of the COX-2 enzyme.[31] Based on this evidence, several clinical trials were performed using sulindac, a nonselective NSAID. These studies were conducted in patients with FAP, using change in degree of polyposis as a surrogate marker for COX-2 inhibition effects.[32–35] Giardiello and colleagues[34] were able to demonstrate regression of adenomatous polyps maximally after 6 months of treatment. There has also been a prospective randomized, double-blinded, placebo-controlled trial using the COX-2 inhibitor celecoxib. The purpose of this study was to determine the effect of celecoxib on the size and number of polyps in patients with FAP.[36] The study demonstrated a 28% reduction in mean polyp number and a 30% reduction in polyp burden in patients receiving 400 mg twice daily of celecoxib for 6 months.

Multiple pathways have been implicated in the protective effect of COX inhibitors. Sulindac sulfone induces apoptosis and demonstrates cancer chemopreventive activity; however, this is through activation of PKG, which then activates the Raf/SEK/JNK cascade and does not inhibit COX 1 or 2.[37] In addition, MAPK pathways are also involved in the expression of COX2, which is associated with a poor prognosis in CRC. MAPK pathways are also involved in the anticancer effects of COX inhibitors on CRC.[6] For example, salicylates promote apoptosis via a MAPK14-dependent mechanism.[38]

CHEMOTHERAPY AND CHEMORADIOTHERAPY
Predictors of Response

MSI-H, although generally thought to be a good prognostic indicator, actually predicts response to traditional chemotherapy regimens as well. Multiple studies support the notion of stage-adjusted prognosis being better for patients with MSI-H than for patients with MSS CRC; however, the difference is larger for patients with stage II disease than for patients with stage III disease.[39] Sargent and colleagues[40] advocate that patients with stage II MSI-H might be spared adjuvant treatment because of a lack of survival benefit.

KRAS mutation not only has prognostic effects but can also help determine which chemotherapy agents will provide benefit. Multiple phase II and III trials have demonstrated patients with a KRAS mutation usually do not benefit from anti-EGFR monoclonal antibody treatment.[41–43] However, the same clinical benefit is seen in both wild-type and mutated KRAS when treated with antibodies against VEGF.[43]

Neoadjuvant chemoradiotherapy (NACRT) for the treatment of locally advanced rectal cancer has become the standard of care. It is known to decrease local recurrence, and the overall prognosis is closely associated with degree of response.[44] Multiple studies have attempted to identify markers of response to NACRT, but no common markers seem to exist between studies.[44–46] One of the limitations when trying to validate these studies is the heterogeneity of treatment algorithms and patient populations.

Traditional Agent Therapies

5-FU has played an important role in the treatment of colorectal and other cancers since 1957.[47] Response rates to 5-FU are only 10% to 20% as a single agent, but responses increase up to 30% with the addition of leucovorin. Combining these two with oxaliplatin or irinotecan increases response rates even further, up to 60% in the postoperative adjuvant setting.[48–52] 5-FU inhibits thymidylate synthase, resulting in depletion of decreased DNA synthesis and increased DNA repair.[53–60]

Leucovorin, also known as folinic acid, is combined with 5-FU to potentiate its effects, allowing 5-FU to stay in the cells longer.[61,62] In a large meta-analysis, 5-FU and leucovorin (FOLFIRI) were found to have a much higher objective response (23%) versus 5-FU alone (11%).[63]

Oxaliplatin is the newest platinum derivative in standard chemotherapy for CRC.[64] In plasma, it rapidly undergoes nonenzymatic transformation in reactive compounds because of displacement of its oxalate group,[64] exerting its cytotoxic effect through DNA damage causing apoptosis.[64] Oxaliplatin exhibits synergism with other cytotoxic drugs, but the underlying mechanisms of action for these effects are not well understood.[65,66] Observation suggests that oxaliplatin can slow the catabolism of 5-FU.[66] Most cancers will eventually develop resistance to oxaliplatin. This resistance can be due to a variety of mechanisms, but one of the most important seems to be related to DNA repair: MMR or nucleotide excision repair.[67] The high activity of FOLFOX in 5-FU-refractory CRC has been confirmed,[68] which improves overall survival in patients with stage III CRC over 5-FU alone.[69]

Irinotecan is a topoisomerase inhibitor that inhibits DNA replication and transcription. Most cells have no way to detoxify the active metabolites of irinotecan, which contributes to its high cytotoxicity.[70] Irinotecan has been shown to increase survival in patients with stage IV colorectal cancer, often in combination with FOLFIRI.[71,72]

Current therapies targeting molecular markers of colorectal cancer

Bevacizumab is a recombinant monoclonal antibody approved for use as part of combination therapy with fluorouracil-based agents for metastatic CRC.[73] It targets VEGF and binds and inactivates all forms to inhibit angiogenesis and tumor growth and proliferation.[73] It neutralizes the ability of VEGF to bind to its receptor and activate the MAPK pathway. In practice, bevacizumab is added to infusion regimens of either FOLFOX or FOLFIRI.[73] Such regimens show improved overall survival (20.3 months vs 10.6 months) in the first- and second-line treatment of metastatic CRC.[74] Adverse events include thrombocytopenia, deep vein thrombosis, GI hemorrhage, hypertension, epistaxis, and proteinuria.[73]

Cetuximab is a monoclonal antibody against EGFR.[75] It stops the binding and activation of the downstream signaling pathways and prevents cell proliferation, invasion, metastasis, and neovascularization.[76] Panitumumab is another monoclonal antibody against EGFR, but it is entirely human, whereas cetuximab is chimeric.[76] Mutation in KRAS causes persistent activation of the ERK MAPK pathway, which does not respond to signaling from growth factor receptors.[76,77] Thus, EGFR inhibitors are only used in KRAS wild-type patients. The most common side effects are skin rash, hypomagnesemia, hypokalemia, and infusion reaction.[76]

IMMUNOTHERAPY
Immunity Checkpoints: Cytotoxic T-Lymphocyte-Associated Antigen 4 and Programmed Cell Death Protein 1

There is increasing evidence to suggest the immune system plays a role in regulating the development of CRC. Immune surveillance is defined as the capacity of the immune system to promote an effective response against tumor cell–specific neoantigens not expressed by normal cells before the clinical expression of cancer.[78] Tumor-associated antigens (TAAs) are molecules that are expressed by tumor cells and allow immune system recognition.[78] One such antigen in CRC is CEA, which is normally expressed in fetal tissue and is overexpressed in many CRCs.[78] CEA has been shown to have immunosuppressive effects in that T cells sensitized to the TAA are unable to initiate a cytotoxic response.[78,79]

Although immune checkpoints are a vital component of maintenance of self-tolerance, they also protect tissues from damage when the immune system is fighting a pathogen.[80] Tumor cells can dysregulate immune checkpoint proteins as an immune resistance mechanism.[80]

Most efforts to therapeutically manipulate antitumor immunity have been focused on T cells because of their capacity for selective recognition of peptides, their capacity to directly recognize and kill antigen-expressing cells, and their ability to orchestrate diverse immune responses.[80] Therefore, agonists of costimulatory receptors or antagonists of inhibitory signals, both resulting in amplification of the immune response, are the primary agents under investigation for this targeted therapy.[80]

The two immune checkpoints that have been studied the most are cytotoxic T-lymphocyte-associated antigen 4 (CTLA4) and programmed cell death protein 1 (PD-1).[81] CTLA4 is expressed on T cells exclusively; it regulates the amplitude of early stages of T-cell activation.[80] The primary function of CTLA4 is to counteract the activity of T-cell costimulatory receptor CD28.[82] It has been proposed that expression of CTLA4 on the cell surface dampens the activation of T cells by outcompeting CD28 in binding CD80 and CD86, in addition to delivering signals to inhibit the T cell.[83–87] CTLA4 blockade produces a broad enhancement of immune responses dependent on T helper cells.[80] The central role of CTLA4, keeping T-cell activation in check, is demonstrated by the lethal systemic immune hyperactivation phenotype of CTLA4-knockout mice.[88,89]

PD-1 is a cell surface receptor that limits the activity of T cells in the periphery at the time of an inflammatory response to infection to limit autoimmunity (**Fig. 2**).[90–96] PD-1 is a more broadly expressed cell surface antigen than CTLA4; it is induced on other activated non–T-lymphocyte subsets, such as B cells and natural killer cells, which limits their lytic activity.[97,98] Chronic antigen exposure, such as in chronic viral infection or cancer, can cause high levels of persistent PD-1 expression; this can induce a state of anergy among antigen-specific T cells. This state seems to be partially reversible by PD-1 blockade.[99] PD-1 is expressed on a large proportion of tumor-infiltrating lymphocytes from many different tumor types.[100,101] In an adaptive response, tumors express high levels of PD-1 ligands in an attempt to repress the cytotoxic T-cell response that the neoantigens ordinarily incite.[2] The primary ligand expressed on solid

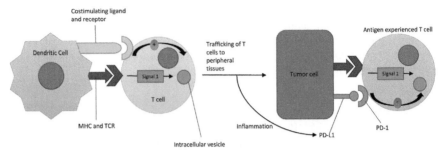

Fig. 2. The major role of the programmed death 1 protein (PD-1) is to regulate inflammatory responses in tissues by effector T cells recognizing antigen in peripheral tissues. Activated T cells will upregulate PD-1 and express it in tissues. Inflammatory signals in tissues
induce the expression of PD-1 ligands, such as PD-L1, which downregulate the activity of
T cells and limit collateral damage. MHC, major histocompatibility complex; TCR, T-cell receptor. (*Data from* Pardoll DM. The blockade of immune checkpoints in cancer immunotherapy. Nat Rev Cancer 2012;12(4):252–64.)

tumors is PD-L1.[80] Antitumor T-cell–mediated responses are inhibited by forced
expression of PD-L1 on mouse tumor cells.[102–104] These findings provide the basis
for PD-1 pathway blockade to enhance antitumor functions in the tumor microenviron-
ment. Expression patterns of PD-1 ligands may be crucial for determining the suit-
ability of therapeutic blockade of this pathway.[80]

Microsatellite instability

MSI has also been linked to immunogenic TAAs, and this has been observed in both
Lynch syndrome and sporadic tumors. The frameshift mutations seen in MSI create
novel proteins that are potentially immunogenic.[78] One of the purported reasons
behind the improvement in survival for MSI-H tumors and patients with Lynch syndrome is an increase in immune response to novel proteins. MSI-H is associated
with high levels of tumor-associated inflammation, which may be due to high levels
of non-self neoantigens.[2] High levels of PD-1–positive tumor-infiltrating lymphocytes
and high levels of PD-L1 are significantly more frequent in MSI-H CRC.[81]

Current Therapies Related to Programmed Cell Death Protein 1 and Cytotoxic
T-Lymphocyte-Associated Antigen 4

Pembrolizumab is a PD-1 inhibitor that manipulates the PD-1 pathway.[2] Pembrolizumab demonstrated a dramatic response in MMR-deficient tumors and no response in
MMR-proficient tumors in a small study on 32 patients.[2] In contrast to most currently
approved antibodies, these medications do not target tumor cells but rather lymphocyte receptors or their ligands to enhance endogenous antitumor activity.[80] There
have been few clinical trials evaluating objective response in the setting of metastatic
CRC. In a phase II trial, pembrolizumab was found to have a 40% objective response
rate in MSI-H metastatic CRC and 78% had no progression of disease at 12 weeks.
The MSS group had 0% objective response with 11% progression-free survival.[105]
Further studies are underway.

Ipilimumab and tremelimumab are fully human antibodies that target CTLA4. The Food
and Drug Administration has approved ipilimumab for the treatment of melanoma.[78] It is
thought to function by permitting the development of immune response to tumor self-
antigens presented by antigen-presenting cells.[78] Both antibodies produce about a
10% objective clinical response in patients with melanoma. Immune-related toxicities

were present in 25% to 30% of patients, and colitis was a particularly common event.[106–108] A phase II trial for tremelimumab was performed as a single-agent study in patients with metastatic CRC who had failed conventional treatment. This study was not able to demonstrate clinically meaningful activity in this patient population; however, there was one patient who showed a partial response.[109]

Vaccines
Development of vaccines represents 85% of current nonantibody clinical trials focusing on CRC. Whole tumor cell vaccines are different from those addressing a single peptide. These vaccines require a sample of tumor tissue that is lysed or irradiated, mixed with an immune adjuvant, and is reinjected into patients.[78] Previous clinical trials on whole tumor cell vaccines have demonstrated limited efficacy.[110,111] A peptide vaccine is based on the identification of a specific epitope that can induce a TAA-specific antitumor immune response.[78] These vaccines are also administered with adjuvants to help induce an immune response. These vaccines tend to induce a more specific antitumor response and are more economical.[78] TAAs that have been targeted in CRC include CEA and EGFR.[112–114] Peptide vaccines targeting these TAAs have been shown to induce an antigen-specific immune response, which was correlated with cytotoxic activity in CRC cell lines. This area is an active area of research with current phase I and II trials.

MARKERS OF COLORECTAL CANCER RECURRENCE RISK
Tumor Genotype

The premise of these studies is the behavior of a given tumor should be predictable based on its genetic fingerprint. The Oncotype DX test for colon cancer evaluates

Table 1
Molecular markers in colorectal cancer

Marker	Location	Clinical Relevance
KRAS	Cell cytoplasm	• MAPK pathway • Mutation is a poor prognostic indicator. • Mutation indicates it is unlikely to respond to cetuximab (Erbitux).
BRAF	Cell cytoplasm	• MAPK pathway • Mutation is a poor prognostic indicator. • V600E mutation is seen in sporadic MSI-H tumors. • It is associated with CIMP.
MLH1	Cell nucleus	• MMR pathway • Methylation by CIMP will silence gene. • Absence of expression will cause MSI-H.
TIMP-1	Extracellular fluid	• It is a metalloproteinase inhibitor. • It stimulates cell proliferation. • It may enhance metastatic capabilities.
PD-1	T-cell membrane	• Receptor • Binding by PD-L1 reduces T-cell cytotoxicity. • Tumor-infiltrating lymphocytes tend to express higher levels.
CEA	Extracellular fluid	• Tumor marker • It is normally expressed in the fetus but in low levels in normal adults. • Attempts at developing a vaccine have had limited success.

Table 2
Chemotherapeutic agents in colorectal cancer

Medication	Class	Mechanism of Action
5-FU	Cytotoxic chemotherapy	Inhibitor of thymidylate synthase, affecting DNA and RNA synthesis
Leucovorin	Cytotoxic chemotherapy	Potentiates the effect of 5-FU
Oxaliplatin	Platinum-based chemotherapy	Creates DNA lesions Inhibits catabolism of 5-FU
Irinotecan	Topoisomerase inhibitor	Inhibits DNA replication and transcription
Bevacizumab (Avastin)	Monoclonal antibody	Binds VEGF Prevents activation of MAPK pathway
Cetuximab (Erbitux)	Monoclonal antibody	Binds EGFR Prevents activation of MAPK pathway Cannot be used with KRAS mutation
Pembrolizumab	Monoclonal antibody	Binds PD-1 on the T cell Deactivates PD-1 Works well in MSI-H tumors
Ipilimumab	Monoclonal antibody	Binds CTLA4 Approved for use in melanoma Under study for CRC Improves T-cell response to tumor antigens

stage II and IIIA/B cancers to help guide further treatment based on the likelihood of recurrence and metastatic spread. Patients with stage II colon cancer stand to benefit the most from such prognostic information. Oncotype DX is a 12-gene assay evaluating 5 reference genes and 7 recurrence genes. The 7 recurrence genes are MKI67, MYC, MYBL2, FAP, BGN, INHBA, and GADD45B.[115] Oncotype DX has been shown to provide information about recurrence risk above and beyond clinical and pathologic markers, such as node positivity or lymphovascular invasion.[116] However, the recurrence score is not associated with responsiveness to chemotherapy agents, such as FOLFOX. Therefore, questions remain with regard to the prognostic implications based on tumor genotype.[116]

SUMMARY

Three main pathways exist that lead to neoplasia. These pathways can coexist and be part of sporadic and inherited neoplastic conditions. Each of these pathways, including CIN, MMR, and CIMP, have specific phenotypes and are associated with specific and recognizable molecular and genetic signatures. Molecular markers (**Table 1**) and affected genes in CRC can be identified and used to treat specific targets with pharmacologic agents (**Table 2**). Multiple ongoing areas of research into these specific therapies for CRC at the molecular level will likely continue to yield further novel therapies with the advantage of narrow targets and maximal antitumor effect while minimizing morbidity.

REFERENCES

1. Fearon ER, Vogelstein B. A genetic model for colorectal tumorigenesis. Cell 1990;61(5):759–67.

2. Nowak JA, Hornick JL. Molecular evaluation of colorectal adenocarcinoma: current practice and emerging concepts. Surg Pathol Clin 2016;9(3):427–39.

3. Carethers JM, Jung BH. Genetics and genetic biomarkers in sporadic colorectal cancer. Gastroenterology 2015;149(5):1177–90.e3.

4. Narayan S, Roy D. Role of APC and DNA mismatch repair genes in the development of colorectal cancers. Mol Cancer 2003;2:41.

5. Grellety T, Gros A, Pedeutour F, et al. Challenging a dogma: co-mutations exist in MAPK pathway genes in colorectal cancer. Virchows Arch 2016;469(4):459–64.

6. Fang JY, Richardson BC. The MAPK signalling pathways and colorectal cancer. Lancet Oncol 2005;6(5):322–7.

7. Hommes DW, Peppelenbosch MP, van Deventer SJ. Mitogen activated protein (MAP) kinase signal transduction pathways and novel anti-inflammatory targets. Gut 2003;52(1):144–51.

8. Watanabe M, Ishiwata T, Nishigai K, et al. Overexpression of keratinocyte growth factor in cancer cells and enterochromaffin cells in human colorectal cancer. Pathol Int 2000;50(5):363–72.

9. Andreyev HJ, Norman AR, Cunningham D, et al. Kirsten ras mutations in patients with colorectal cancer: the multicenter "RASCAL" study. J Natl Cancer Inst 1998;90(9):675–84.

10. Bahnassy AA, Zekri AR, Salem SE, et al. Differential expression of p53 family proteins in colorectal adenomas and carcinomas: prognostic and predictive values. Histol Histopathol 2014;29(2):207–16.

11. Imai K, Yamamoto H. Carcinogenesis and microsatellite instability: the interrelationship between genetics and epigenetics. Carcinogenesis 2008;29(4):673–80.

12. Ogino S, Liao X, Imamura Y, et al. Predictive and prognostic analysis of PIK3CA mutation in stage III colon cancer intergroup trial. J Natl Cancer Inst 2013;105(23):1789–98.

13. Andre T, de Gramont A, Vernerey D, et al. Adjuvant fluorouracil, leucovorin, and oxaliplatin in stage II to III colon cancer: updated 10-year survival and outcomes according to BRAF mutation and mismatch repair status of the MOSAIC Study. J Clin Oncol 2015;33(35):4176–87.

14. Issa JP. CpG island methylator phenotype in cancer. Nat Rev Cancer 2004;4(12):988–93.

15. Konishi M, Kikuchi-Yanoshita R, Tanaka K, et al. Molecular nature of colon tumors in hereditary nonpolyposis colon cancer, familial polyposis, and sporadic colon cancer. Gastroenterology 1996;111(2):307–17.

16. Otori K, Oda Y, Sugiyama K, et al. High frequency of K-ras mutations in human colorectal hyperplastic polyps. Gut 1997;40(5):660–3.

17. Longacre TA, Fenoglio-Preiser CM. Mixed hyperplastic adenomatous polyps/serrated adenomas. A distinct form of colorectal neoplasia. Am J Surg Pathol 1990;14(6):524–37.

18. Hawkins NJ, Ward RL. Sporadic colorectal cancers with microsatellite instability and their possible origin in hyperplastic polyps and serrated adenomas. J Natl Cancer Inst 2001;93(17):1307–13.

19. Buergy D, Fuchs T, Kambakamba P, et al. Prognostic impact of extracellular matrix metalloprotease inducer: immunohistochemical analyses of colorectal tumors and immunocytochemical screening of disseminated tumor cells in bone marrow from patients with gastrointestinal cancer. Cancer 2009;115(20):4667–78.

20. Mroczko B, Groblewska M, Okulczyk B, et al. The diagnostic value of matrix metalloproteinase 9 (MMP-9) and tissue inhibitor of matrix metalloproteinases 1 (TIMP-1) determination in the sera of colorectal adenoma and cancer patients. Int J Colorectal Dis 2010;25(10):1177–84.

21. Tarpgaard LS, Orum-Madsen MS, Christensen IJ, et al. TIMP-1 is under regulation of the EGF signaling axis and promotes an aggressive phenotype in KRAS-mutated colorectal cancer cells: a potential novel approach to the treatment of metastatic colorectal cancer. Oncotarget 2016;7(37):59441–57.

22. Tsu JHL, Ho JWC. COX-2 inhibitors and colorectal cancer chemoprevention. Ann Coll Surg 2002;6:31–5. H.K.

23. Thun MJ, Namboodiri MM, Heath CW Jr. Aspirin use and reduced risk of fatal colon cancer. N Engl J Med 1991;325(23):1593–6.

24. Giovannucci E, Egan KM, Hunter DJ, et al. Aspirin and the risk of colorectal cancer in women. N Engl J Med 1995;333(10):609–14.

25. Marnett LJ. Aspirin and related nonsteroidal anti-inflammatory drugs as chemopreventive agents against colon cancer. Prev Med 1995;24(2):103–6.

26. Sano H, Kawahito Y, Wilder RL, et al. Expression of cyclooxygenase-1 and -2 in human colorectal cancer. Cancer Res 1995;55(17):3785–9.

27. Eberhart CE, Coffey RJ, Radhika A, et al. Up-regulation of cyclooxygenase 2 gene expression in human colorectal adenomas and adenocarcinomas. Gastroenterology 1994;107(4):1183–8.

28. Kargman SL, O'Neill GP, Vickers PJ, et al. Expression of prostaglandin G/H synthase-1 and -2 protein in human colon cancer. Cancer Res 1995;55(12):2556–9.

29. Qiao L, Kozoni V, Tsioulias GJ, et al. Selected eicosanoids increase the proliferation rate of human colon carcinoma cell lines and mouse colonocytes in vivo. Biochim Biophys Acta 1995;1258(2):215–23.

30. Tsujii M, DuBois RN. Alterations in cellular adhesion and apoptosis in epithelial cells overexpressing prostaglandin endoperoxide synthase 2. Cell. 1995;83(3):493–501.

31. Williams CS, Tsujii M, Reese J, et al. Host cyclooxygenase-2 modulates carcinoma growth. J Clin Invest 2000;105(11):1589–94.

32. Waddell WR, Ganser GF, Cerise EJ, et al. Sulindac for polyposis of the colon. Am J Surg 1989;157(1):175–9.

33. Labayle D, Fischer D, Vielh P, et al. Sulindac causes regression of rectal polyps in familial adenomatous polyposis. Gastroenterology 1991;101(3):635–9.

34. Giardiello FM, Hamilton SR, Krush AJ, et al. Treatment of colonic and rectal adenomas with sulindac in familial adenomatous polyposis. N Engl J Med 1993;328(18):1313–6.

35. Nugent KP, Farmer KC, Spigelman AD, et al. Randomized controlled trial of the effect of sulindac on duodenal and rectal polyposis and cell proliferation in patients with familial adenomatous polyposis. Br J Surg 1993;80(12):1618–9.

36. Steinbach G, Lynch PM, Phillips RK, et al. The effect of celecoxib, a cyclooxygenase-2 inhibitor, in familial adenomatous polyposis. N Engl J Med 2000;342(26):1946–52.

37. Soh JW, Mao Y, Kim MG, et al. Cyclic GMP mediates apoptosis induced by sulindac derivatives via activation of c-Jun NH2-terminal kinase 1. Clin Cancer Res 2000;6(10):4136–41.

38. Schwenger P, Alpert D, Skolnik EY, et al. Cell-type-specific activation of c-Jun N-terminal kinase by salicylates. J Cell Physiol 1999;179(1):109–14.

39. Klingbiel D, Saridaki Z, Roth AD, et al. Prognosis of stage II and III colon cancer treated with adjuvant 5-fluorouracil or FOLFIRI in relation to microsatellite status: results of the PETACC-3 trial. Ann Oncol 2015;26(1):126–32.

40. Sargent DJ, Marsoni S, Monges G, et al. Defective mismatch repair as a predictive marker for lack of efficacy of fluorouracil-based adjuvant therapy in colon cancer. J Clin Oncol 2010;28(20):3219–26.

41. Amado RG, Wolf M, Peeters M, et al. Wild-type KRAS is required for panitumumab efficacy in patients with metastatic colorectal cancer. J Clin Oncol 2008; 26(10):1626–34.

42. Bokemeyer C, Bondarenko I, Makhson A, et al. Fluorouracil, leucovorin, and oxaliplatin with and without cetuximab in the first-line treatment of metastatic colorectal cancer. J Clin Oncol 2009;27(5):663–71.

43. Hurwitz HI, Yi J, Ince W, et al. The clinical benefit of bevacizumab in metastatic colorectal cancer is independent of K-ras mutation status: analysis of a phase III study of bevacizumab with chemotherapy in previously untreated metastatic colorectal cancer. Oncologist 2009;14(1):22–8.

44. Kalady MF. Lessons learned from the quest for gene signatures that predict treatment response in rectal cancer. Dis Colon Rectum 2016;59(9):898–900.

45. Perez RO, Habr-Gama A, Sao Juliao GP, et al. Should we give up the search for a clinically useful gene signature for the prediction of response of rectal cancer to neoadjuvant chemoradiation? Dis Colon Rectum 2016;59(9):895–7.

46. Lopes-Ramos C, Koyama FC, Habr-Gama A, et al. Comprehensive evaluation of the effectiveness of gene expression signatures to predict complete response to neoadjuvant chemoradiotherapy and guide surgical intervention in rectal cancer. Cancer Genet 2015;208(6):319–26.

47. Peters GJ, Kohna CH. Fluoropyrimidines as antifolate drugs. In: Jackman JL, editor. Antifolate drugs in cancer therapy. New York: Humana Press; 1999. p. 101–45.

48. Comella P, Casaretti R, De Vita F, et al. Concurrent irinotecan and 5-fluorouracil plus levo-folinic acid given every other week in the first-line management of advanced colorectal carcinoma: a phase I study of the Southern Italy Cooperative Oncology Group. Ann Oncol 1999;10(8):915–21.

49. Andre T, Louvet C, Maindrault-Goebel F, et al. CPT-11 (irinotecan) addition to bimonthly, high-dose leucovorin and bolus and continuous-infusion 5-fluorouracil (FOLFIRI) for pretreated metastatic colorectal cancer. GERCOR. Eur J Cancer 1999;35(9):1343–7.

50. Douillard JY, Cunningham D, Roth AD, et al. Irinotecan combined with fluorouracil compared with fluorouracil alone as first-line treatment for metastatic colorectal cancer: a multicentre randomised trial. Lancet 2000;355(9209):1041–7.

51. Giacchetti S, Perpoint B, Zidani R, et al. Phase III multicenter randomized trial of oxaliplatin added to chronomodulated fluorouracil-leucovorin as first-line treatment of metastatic colorectal cancer. J Clin Oncol 2000;18(1):136–47.

52. de Gramont A, Figer A, Seymour M, et al. Leucovorin and fluorouracil with or without oxaliplatin as first-line treatment in advanced colorectal cancer. J Clin Oncol 2000;18(16):2938–47.

53. Leichman CG, Lenz HJ, Leichman L, et al. Quantitation of intratumoral thymidylate synthase expression predicts for disseminated colorectal cancer response and resistance to protracted-infusion fluorouracil and weekly leucovorin. J Clin Oncol 1997;15(10):3223–9.

54. Salonga D, Danenberg KD, Johnson M, et al. Colorectal tumors responding to 5-fluorouracil have low gene expression levels of dihydropyrimidine

dehydrogenase, thymidylate synthase, and thymidine phosphorylase. Clin Cancer Res 2000;6(4):1322–7.

55. Davies MM, Johnston PG, Kaur S, et al. Colorectal liver metastasis thymidylate synthase staining correlates with response to hepatic arterial floxuridine. Clin Cancer Res 1999;5(2):325–8.

56. Lenz HJ, Leichman CG, Danenberg KD, et al. Thymidylate synthase mRNA level in adenocarcinoma of the stomach: a predictor for primary tumor response and overall survival. J Clin Oncol 1996;14(1):176–82.

57. Peters GJ, van der Wilt CL, van Groeningen CJ, et al. Thymidylate synthase inhibition after administration of fluorouracil with or without leucovorin in colon cancer patients: implications for treatment with fluorouracil. J Clin Oncol 1994; 12(10):2035–42.

58. van Laar JA, van der Wilt CL, Rustum YM, et al. Therapeutic efficacy of fluoropyrimidines depends on the duration of thymidylate synthase inhibition in the murine colon 26-B carcinoma tumor model. Clin Cancer Res 1996;2(8):1327–33.

59. Spears CP, Shani J, Shahinian AH, et al. Assay and time course of 5-fluorouracil incorporation into RNA of L1210/0 ascites cells in vivo. Mol Pharmacol 1985; 27(2):302–7.

60. Spiegelman S, Nayak R, Sawyer R, et al. Potentiation of the anti-tumor activity of 5FU by thymidine and its correlation with the formation of (5FU)RNA. Cancer 1980;45(5 Suppl):1129–34.

61. Machover D. A comprehensive review of 5-fluorouracil and leucovorin in patients with metastatic colorectal carcinoma. Cancer 1997;80(7):1179–87.

62. Drake JC, Voeller DM, Allegra CJ, et al. The effect of dose and interval between 5-fluorouracil and leucovorin on the formation of thymidylate synthase ternary complex in human cancer cells. Br J Cancer 1995;71(6):1145–50.

63. Modulation of fluorouracil by leucovorin in patients with advanced colorectal cancer: evidence in terms of response rate. Advanced Colorectal Cancer Meta-Analysis Project. J Clin Oncol 1992;10(6):896–903.

64. Alcindor T, Beauger N. Oxaliplatin: a review in the era of molecularly targeted therapy. Curr Oncol 2011;18(1):18–25.

65. Zwelling LA, Anderson T, Kohn KW. DNA-protein and DNA interstrand crosslinking by cis- and trans-platinum(II) diamminedichloride in L1210 mouse leukemia cells and relation to cytotoxicity. Cancer Res 1979;39(2 Pt 1):365–9.

66. Fischel JL, Formento P, Ciccolini J, et al. Impact of the oxaliplatin-5 fluorouracil-folinic acid combination on respective intracellular determinants of drug activity. Br J Cancer 2002;86(7):1162–8.

67. Arnould S, Hennebelle I, Canal P, et al. Cellular determinants of oxaliplatin sensitivity in colon cancer cell lines. Eur J Cancer 2003;39(1):112–9.

68. de Gramont A, Tournigand C, Louvet C, et al. Oxaliplatin, folinic acid and 5-fluorouracil (folfox) in pretreated patients with metastatic advanced cancer. The GERCOD. Rev Med Interne 1997;18(10):769–75.

69. Andre T, Boni C, Navarro M, et al. Improved overall survival with oxaliplatin, fluorouracil, and leucovorin as adjuvant treatment in stage II or III colon cancer in the MOSAIC trial. J Clin Oncol 2009;27(19):3109–16.

70. Weekes J, Lam AK, Sebesan S, et al. Irinotecan therapy and molecular targets in colorectal cancer: a systemic review. World J Gastroenterol 2009;15(29): 3597–602.

71. Cunningham D, Pyrhonen S, James RD, et al. Randomised trial of irinotecan plus supportive care versus supportive care alone after fluorouracil failure for patients with metastatic colorectal cancer. Lancet 1998;352(9138):1413–8.

72. Saltz LB, Cox JV, Blanke C, et al. Irinotecan plus fluorouracil and leucovorin for metastatic colorectal cancer. Irinotecan Study Group. N Engl J Med 2000; 343(13):905–14.

73. Shih T, Lindley C. Bevacizumab: an angiogenesis inhibitor for the treatment of solid malignancies. Clin Ther 2006;28(11):1779–802.

74. Keating GM. Bevacizumab: a review of its use in advanced cancer. Drugs 2014; 74(16):1891–925.

75. Van Cutsem E, Kohne CH, Hitre E, et al. Cetuximab and chemotherapy as initial treatment for metastatic colorectal cancer. N Engl J Med 2009;360(14):1408–17.

76. Yazdi MH, Faramarzi MA, Nikfar S, et al. A comprehensive review of clinical trials on EGFR Inhibitors such as cetuximab and panitumumab as monotherapy and in combination for treatment of metastatic colorectal cancer. Avicenna J Med Biotechnol 2015;7(4):134–44.

77. Bruera G, Cannita K, Tessitore A, et al. The prevalent KRAS exon 2 c.35 G>A mutation in metastatic colorectal cancer patients: a biomarker of worse prognosis and potential benefit of bevacizumab-containing intensive regimens? Crit Rev Oncol Hematol 2015;93(3):190–202.

78. Sanchez-Castanon M, Er TK, Bujanda L, et al. Immunotherapy in colorectal cancer: what have we learned so far? Clin Chim Acta 2016;460:78–87.

79. Fauquembergue E, Toutirais O, Tougeron D, et al. HLA-A*0201-restricted CEA-derived peptide CAP1 is not a suitable target for T-cell-based immunotherapy. J Immunother 2010;33(4):402–13.

80. Pardoll DM. The blockade of immune checkpoints in cancer immunotherapy. Nat Rev Cancer 2012;12(4):252–64.

81. Lee LH, Cavalcanti MS, Segal NH, et al. Patterns and prognostic relevance of PD-1 and PD-L1 expression in colorectal carcinoma. Mod Pathol 2016;29(11): 1433–42.

82. Schwartz RH. Costimulation of T lymphocytes: the role of CD28, CTLA-4, and B7/BB1 in interleukin-2 production and immunotherapy. Cell. 1992;71(7): 1065–8.

83. Linsley PS, Greene JL, Brady W, et al. Human B7-1 (CD80) and B7-2 (CD86) bind with similar avidities but distinct kinetics to CD28 and CTLA-4 receptors. Immunity 1994;1(9):793–801.

84. Riley JL, Mao M, Kobayashi S, et al. Modulation of TCR-induced transcriptional profiles by ligation of CD28, ICOS, and CTLA-4 receptors. Proc Natl Acad Sci U S A 2002;99(18):11790–5.

85. Schneider H, Downey J, Smith A, et al. Reversal of the TCR stop signal by CTLA-4. Science 2006;313(5795):1972–5.

86. Parry RV, Chemnitz JM, Frauwirth KA, et al. CTLA-4 and PD-1 receptors inhibit T-cell activation by distinct mechanisms. Mol Cell Biol. 2005;25(21):9543–53.

87. Schneider H, Mandelbrot DA, Greenwald RJ, et al. Cutting edge: CTLA-4 (CD152) differentially regulates mitogen-activated protein kinases (extracellular signal-regulated kinase and c-Jun N-terminal kinase) in CD4+ T cells from receptor/ligand-deficient mice. J Immunol 2002;169(7):3475–9.

88. Tivol EA, Borriello F, Schweitzer AN, et al. Loss of CTLA-4 leads to massive lymphoproliferation and fatal multiorgan tissue destruction, revealing a critical negative regulatory role of CTLA-4. Immunity 1995;3(5):541–7.

89. Waterhouse P, Penninger JM, Timms E, et al. Lymphoproliferative disorders with early lethality in mice deficient in Ctla-4. Science 1995;270(5238):985–8.

90. Ishida Y, Agata Y, Shibahara K, et al. Induced expression of PD-1, a novel member of the immunoglobulin gene superfamily, upon programmed cell death. EMBO J 1992;11(11):3887–95.

91. Freeman GJ, Long AJ, Iwai Y, et al. Engagement of the PD-1 immunoinhibitory receptor by a novel B7 family member leads to negative regulation of lymphocyte activation. J Exp Med 2000;192(7):1027–34.

92. Keir ME, Liang SC, Guleria I, et al. Tissue expression of PD-L1 mediates peripheral T cell tolerance. J Exp Med 2006;203(4):883–95.

93. Nishimura H, Nose M, Hiai H, et al. Development of lupus-like autoimmune diseases by disruption of the PD-1 gene encoding an ITIM motif-carrying immunoreceptor. Immunity 1999;11(2):141–51.

94. Nishimura H, Okazaki T, Tanaka Y, et al. Autoimmune dilated cardiomyopathy in PD-1 receptor-deficient mice. Science 2001;291(5502):319–22.

95. Okazaki T, Honjo T. PD-1 and PD-1 ligands: from discovery to clinical application. Int Immunol 2007;19(7):813–24.

96. Keir ME, Butte MJ, Freeman GJ, et al. PD-1 and its ligands in tolerance and immunity. Annu Rev Immunol 2008;26:677–704.

97. Terme M, Ullrich E, Aymeric L, et al. IL-18 induces PD-1-dependent immunosuppression in cancer. Cancer Res 2011;71(16):5393–9.

98. Fanoni D, Tavecchio S, Recalcati S, et al. New monoclonal antibodies against B-cell antigens: possible new strategies for diagnosis of primary cutaneous B-cell lymphomas. Immunol Lett 2011;134(2):157–60.

99. Barber DL, Wherry EJ, Masopust D, et al. Restoring function in exhausted CD8 T cells during chronic viral infection. Nature 2006;439(7077):682–7.

100. Sfanos KS, Bruno TC, Meeker AK, et al. Human prostate-infiltrating CD8+ T lymphocytes are oligoclonal and PD-1+. Prostate 2009;69(15):1694–703.

101. Ahmadzadeh M, Johnson LA, Heemskerk B, et al. Tumor antigen-specific CD8 T cells infiltrating the tumor express high levels of PD-1 and are functionally impaired. Blood 2009;114(8):1537–44.

102. Dong H, Strome SE, Salomao DR, et al. Tumor-associated B7-H1 promotes T-cell apoptosis: a potential mechanism of immune evasion. Nat Med 2002;8(8): 793–800.

103. Iwai Y, Ishida M, Tanaka Y, et al. Involvement of PD-L1 on tumor cells in the escape from host immune system and tumor immunotherapy by PD-L1 blockade. Proc Natl Acad Sci U S A 2002;99(19):12293–7.

104. Konishi J, Yamazaki K, Azuma M, et al. B7-H1 expression on non-small cell lung cancer cells and its relationship with tumor-infiltrating lymphocytes and their PD-1 expression. Clin Cancer Res 2004;10(15):5094–100.

105. Le DT, Uram JN, Wang H, et al. PD-1 blockade in tumors with mismatch-repair deficiency. N Engl J Med 2015;372(26):2509–20.

106. Phan GQ, Yang JC, Sherry RM, et al. Cancer regression and autoimmunity induced by cytotoxic T lymphocyte-associated antigen 4 blockade in patients with metastatic melanoma. Proc Natl Acad Sci U S A 2003;100(14):8372–7.

107. Ribas A, Camacho LH, Lopez-Berestein G, et al. Antitumor activity in melanoma and anti-self responses in a phase I trial with the anti-cytotoxic T lymphocyte-associated antigen 4 monoclonal antibody CP-675,206. J Clin Oncol 2005; 23(35):8968–77.

108. Beck KE, Blansfield JA, Tran KQ, et al. Enterocolitis in patients with cancer after antibody blockade of cytotoxic T-lymphocyte-associated antigen 4. J Clin Oncol 2006;24(15):2283–9.

109. Chung KY, Gore I, Fong L, et al. Phase II study of the anti-cytotoxic T-lympho-cyte-associated antigen 4 monoclonal antibody, tremelimumab, in patients with refractory metastatic colorectal cancer. J Clin Oncol 2010;28(21):3485–90.
110. Jocham D, Richter A, Hoffmann L, et al. Adjuvant autologous renal tumour cell vaccine and risk of tumour progression in patients with renal-cell carcinoma after radical nephrectomy: phase III, randomised controlled trial. Lancet 2004; 363(9409):594–9.
111. Berd D, Sato T, Maguire HC Jr, et al. Immunopharmacologic analysis of an autologous, hapten-modified human melanoma vaccine. J Clin Oncol 2004;22(3): 403–15.
112. Koido S, Hara E, Homma S, et al. Dendritic cells fused with allogeneic colorectal cancer cell line present multiple colorectal cancer-specific antigens and induce antitumor immunity against autologous tumor cells. Clin Cancer Res 2005; 11(21):7891–900.
113. Koido S, Hara E, Torii A, et al. Induction of antigen-specific CD4- and CD8-mediated T-cell responses by fusions of autologous dendritic cells and metastatic colorectal cancer cells. Int J Cancer 2005;117(4):587–95.
114. Gonzalez G, Crombet T, Catala M, et al. A novel cancer vaccine composed of human-recombinant epidermal growth factor linked to a carrier protein: report of a pilot clinical trial. Ann Oncol 1998;9(4):431–5.
115. Venook AP, Niedzwiecki D, Lopatin M, et al. Biologic determinants of tumor recurrence in stage II colon cancer: validation study of the 12-gene recurrence score in Cancer and Leukemia Group B (CALGB) 9581. J Clin Oncol 2013; 31(14):1775–81.
116. Yothers G, O'Connell MJ, Lee M, et al. Validation of the 12-gene colon cancer recurrence score in NSABP C-07 as a predictor of recurrence in patients with stage II and III colon cancer treated with fluorouracil and leucovorin (FU/LV) and FU/LV plus oxaliplatin. J Clin Oncol 2013;31(36):4512–9.

Index

Note: Page numbers of article titles are in **boldface** type.

Surg Clin N Am 97 (2017) 703–716
http://dx.doi.org/10.1016/S0039-6109(17)30061-0
0039-6109/17

surgical.theclinics.com

Moving?

Make sure your subscription moves with you!

To notify us of your new address, find your **Clinics Account Number** (located on your mailing label above your name), and contact customer service at:

Email: journalscustomerservice-usa@elsevier.com

800-654-2452 (subscribers in the U.S. & Canada)
314-447-8871 (subscribers outside of the U.S. & Canada)

Fax number: 314-447-8029

Elsevier Health Sciences Division
Subscription Customer Service
3251 Riverport Lane
Maryland Heights, MO 63043

*To ensure uninterrupted delivery of your subscription, please notify us at least 4 weeks in advance of move.

Printed and bound by CPI Group (UK) Ltd, Croydon, CR0 4YY

03/10/2024

01040395-0007